How to Prove Anything

30 absurd research papers no one else was brave enough to publish

B. McGraw

How to Prove Anything

Portfolio Director: Sunith Shetty

Relationship Lead: Tushar Gupta

Project Manager: Shashank Desai

Content Engineer: David Sugarman

Technical Editor: Seemanjay Ameriya

Copy Editor: Safis Editing

Indexer: Hemangini Bari

Proofreader: David Sugarman

Production Designer: Pranit Padwal, Prashant Ghare

First published: November 2025

Production reference: 1271025

Published by Packt Publishing Ltd.

Grosvenor House

11 St Paul's Square

Birmingham

B3 1RB, UK.

ISBN 978-1-80611-893-9

www.packtpub.com

I would like to dedicate this book to the data cleaners. They're doing God's work!

– B. McGraw

Contributors

About the authors

B. McGraw is the chief editor of Cranberry-Lemon's prestigious *Journal of Astrological Big Data Ecology*. He is terminally online and rarely has time to touch grass in between editing the papers for this journal and making edgy memes on his phone's MS Paint app. He achieved a B.S. and M.S. in electrical engineering signals processing through the Air Force because he was nerdy enough to like the statistics and didn't mind doing some push-ups. He is a research engineer who works in software and algorithm development in information fusion.

Gilligan Vincent is a big-shot writer, director, and producer of TV shows heavily featuring Mexican elements. If he's made anything else, I haven't heard of it, so it's probably not worth watching.

Chase Blockman is a finance guy, a blockchain enthusiast, and a YouTube physics watcher, always looking for the next unicorn. He is an expert in synergistic business solutions, innovation, and getting things done. You would not believe his bank account, and neither does the IRS.

Jack Lee and **Aaron Weiner** are best friends in the second grade. At first, they got their home rooms switched because they were talking too much in class, but now they're back together to collaborate on research because they are very good at math and science class.

Dr. Qubert Spins is a world-renowned physicist and quantum theorist who has developed the world's first quantum computing gaming PC for StarCraft and has found the very first evidence of string theory (only available for his top-tier Patreon subscribers).

Dr. Melba McCormick is an academic and expecting mother, known for advanced simulations, including her ability to generate authentic random numbers by measuring her toddler's behavior. She is an expert in modeling and simulation evaluation and has shown in her chapter in this book that she can fake her way through being a CFD expert as well.

Dr. Joe "Baby Hands" McGraw, PhD, MFM, B.A.M.F., is an over-educated fellow in the maternal fetal arts and general reproductive health expert who is 100% in this book because he is the brother of this journal's chief editor.

Wyatt "The Log Whisperer" Johnson is a world-renowned forest nurser and veneer wood logger, author of several self-help logging books, president of every professional society relating to logging, and the sole owner/proprietor/operator of the Johnson family logging business. He is also the great-great-great-great-great-great-great... grandson of Euler, so he's good at math.

Carol Louise Feurtalini is the head waitress at Mama Lou's Seafood Shack and has perfected the art of paying the right amount of attention to each customer by minimizing tip regret.

Hugh Mann is a respected and very normal professor of business studies. When he isn't teaching business to students or drinking a normal soup, he likes and does all of the normal things that humans do, such as get a haircut, walk by trees, collect books and other documents of importance, or take showers, even if it burns his skin. His skin and hair are normal colors; it's his real body, and he grew up in a small town in Indiana and has no living relatives.

Lane Ranger is a civil engineer who just achieved his B.S. at the prestigious Cranberry Lemon school of engineering. He is also an avid Hot Wheels collector.

Edgart Notting is a local network engineer and single man who is obsessed with pocket rockets. He has been looking for his soulmate for years, but cannot secure that first date as many refuse to talk further after he offers to share pictures of his favorite pocket rockets, which he swears are a good ride.

Mittens is a tabby cat at the cutting edge of human servant exploitation technology. He has developed methods in the past for dog intimidation, optimal couch destruction, and laser pointer removal.

Dr. Queso Grande is a Tex-Mex structural engineer specializing in the load-bearing analysis of tostadas, Crunchwrap Supremes, street tacos, and burritos. He is famed for his invention of the double-wrapped burrito to account for a low safety factor in a rice-stuffed Chipotle carnitas, with cheese, lettuce, fajita veggies, sour cream, and extra guac.

Dr. Franklin De Santa is a renowned carjacker and expert in autonomous vehicle exploitation. He is solely responsible for the constant delay of Tesla's automatic driving features and is coming for Waymo next.

Clocky McClockface is a sentient clock who writes papers for us from time to time. Not much is known about Clocky other than it is 5 minutes till noon.

Dr. Rajesh Koothrappali is a researcher who struggles when it comes to speaking up and has applied his understanding of math and social science research to create a formulaic methodology for responding to texts.

Chad Broman is a doctor of psychological machine learning and a video game enthusiast. He is happily in a mostly-committed relationship to his girlfriend, Dr. Tiffany Love, and dedicates his days to understanding her and supporting her to the minimal amount so that he can maximize his video game time.

Dr. Tiffany Love is a doctor of behavioral modification and a Netflix reality/dating show enthusiast. She tentatively believes that Chad may possibly be her future husband, but is not sure whether he is ready for the commitment or the sacrifice when he has such time-consuming hobbies. She spends her days compiling psychological profiles on him so that, one day, she may finally feel safe enough to set up a joint bank account with him.

Santa Claus is a warrior-demon trapped in the body of an old man, cursed to spend eternity bound to the netherworld known as the North Pole. He is only allowed to travel south for one night a year, and he uses it to advance the cause of rampant commercialism in the children of the world by threatening them with environment-polluting coal when naughty.

I would like to thank all those strange researchers online who have shared their expertise and research with our prestigious journal. I would also like to thank our Reddit/X (Twitter)/Facebook fans who increase my dopamine by liking our papers and memes. I'd especially like to thank my wife for putting up with me while I'm editing one of Chad and Tiffany's papers, and to the entire Packt team for their support during the course of writing this book.

[This page was intentionally left blank.]

Table of Contents

Preface

Science has a diversity problem, and I don't mean a gender or ethnic diversity problem, but a diversity problem in thought, style, and personality. When I started writing and editing papers for the *Journal of Astrological Big Data Ecology*, I was laughed at and scolded for giving a platform to voices who want to put a black hole at the center of the Earth. Science does not advance in small p-hacked papers so that you can gain tenure. Science conquers the world through bold women and men with bold ideas and a passable amount of academic scrutiny.

Since rebranding as a literary journal, we've reached all of these alternative voices who have been silenced for decades under a corrupt system unable to accept those too different to fit in their perfect little boxes. That system can go suck on a lemon because we're making our own system that rewards creativity and innovation. We have received papers on imitating the Mexican atmosphere for cinema, how to text your friends and seem interested, the load-bearing analysis of the Cheez-It Webbed Crunchwrap Supreme, and much more!

No degree, no problem! Wyatt "The Log Whisperer" Johnson never got a degree because his pappaw taught him everything he ever needed to know. Now he's the head of a logging empire and has two papers published in this book. He was rejected from dozens of journals because his tree-shaped nomenclature exploded the editor's brain, but we just copy and pasted his LaTeX images into Word! Even without a college, high school, or even middle school diploma, this book showcases the revolutionary research of two second graders, Jack and Aaron, whose academic minds are well beyond their years!

For the first time ever, this book publishes nine landmark papers by the infamous research couple Dr. Chad Broman and Dr. Tiffany Love. Through Chad's research to figure out the best way to play video games without annoying Tiffany too much, and Tiffany's research to get Chad to do the dishes, stop buying guns, and cut back on video game time, we can see how they have evolved as a couple. We observe how their research changes while they go on a break and what Chad does to win Tiffany back.

I am proud to present this compilation of diverse authors who have never had the chance to present their ideas to the world outside of a Substack account with 23 followers or a TikTok video with 30 views. Diversity of thought is the cornerstone of creating a confusing world view, but that's okay. We must embrace a diversity of opinions and avoid scientific consensus and echo chambers; otherwise, we'll end up like my Uncle Albert who still thinks we landed on the moon. If you have been shunned by the scientific community and have done your own research, we would like to publish it. Do not hesitate to reach out and we will get your ideas, data, and analysis in front of the subset of the population that either buys our books or follows us online.

Who this book is for

This book is for you truth-seekers who think that Big Academia is hiding the important facts from you. You've probably picked this book up and are thinking, "Wow, I don't know anything about black hole PFAS recycling, log-log-likelihood logging optimization, or insurance-mandated gender reveal computation fluid dynamics modeling and simulation software, but I would like to know more!" I guarantee you that you will not find any of these controversial alternative facts in any other publication, so get ready to learn your butt off.

What this book covers

Chapter 1, Dust, Heat, and Cumin: Low-Budget Synthetic Authentic Mexican Atmosphere Sepia Filter for Modern Cinema, tests the right blend of pollution, heat, and authentic Mexican spices to create an ideal approximation of the Mexican sepia filter. Using this digital approximation, Hollywood executives can save millions of dollars filming scenes of Mexico wherever they like.

Chapter 2, Novel Gravity and Velocity-Based Time Dilation Methodology for Real-Time Bitcoin Payment Processing, explores two concepts to make blockchain feasible as a real-time payment system. By launching an extensive network of bitcoin processing satellites and either creating a black hole at the center of the earth or speeding the earth to near the speed of light, time will slow down enough for the satellites to finish their blockchain operations.

Chapter 3, Me and My Friend Found Where the Coolest Part in My Room Is Using the Heat Equation Because It Is REALLY REALLY HOT OUTSIDE!, is a paper by Jack and Aaron, best friends who are desperate to cool off in the summer. By applying the heat equation, they solve for the coolest spot in Jack's bedroom to survive the summer.

Chapter 4, Me and My Friend Show That My Dad's Airstream Trailer Goes Faster with Dints and That We Shouldn't Be Grounded for Hitting It with a Baseball Last Saturday, is another paper by Jack and Aaron, who got in big trouble last weekend playing catch near their daddy's Airstream trailer. Little does Jack's daddy know that it's actually a good thing because it can go waaaaaay faster now.

Chapter 5, A Novel Method for the Safe and Effective Recycling of PFAS Plastics: A Black Hole Hawking Radiation Approach, is a groundbreaking paper that refutes those who believe that it is impossible to recycle PFAS. Dr. Qubert Spins proposes launching the "unrecyclable" plastic into a black hole, sucking up the Hawking radiation and fusion-reacting the particles back into useful heavy metals, such as hydrogen and helium.

Chapter 6, Pink and Fire: Computational Fluid Dynamics Simulation Analysis of My Recent Gender Reveal Party Disaster, analyzing the fidelity of the required CFD engine for gender reveal party insurance, is where Dr. Melba McCormick determines that there is no way she could have predicted her gender reveal party would burn down her backyard shed.

Chapter 7, Congenital and Parent-of-Origin Prediction Factors and Risks of Baby Jazziness in Americana Live Births, is a paper where, after sequencing hundreds of genomic sequences and testing parents and babies for jazz proficiency, Dr. Joe "Baby Hands" McGraw creates a statistical prediction model for determining the jazziness of a baby.

Chapter 8, Testicular Cancer Truck Nut Self-Examination for North American Pick-Ups: A Cost-Benefit Analysis, outlines and analyzes the effectiveness of screening truck nuts for testicular cancer in North American pick-up trucks.

Chapter 9, Log-Log-Likelihood of Black Walnut in Random Forestry, applies log-log-log analysis to forestry to determine the ideal conditions to find black walnut trees by optimizing log-log-likelihood.

Chapter 10, Natural Log Exponential Log Growth Models in Hardwood Nurseries, creates a foolproof plan to transform a boring natural log growth wood nursery into a natural log exponential log growth, practically tripling log profits!

Chapter 11, The No Regrets Waiting Model: A Multi-Armed Bandit Approach to Maximizing Tips, by applying carefully researched customer models and a Markov Chain drink order prediction model, presents different no-regret optimization algorithms to solve the tip-maximizing multi-armed bandit problem in high-stakes waitressing.

Chapter 12, Who's a Good Boy? A Metropolis-Hastings Approach to Determining Foster Dog Names of Unknown Origin, explores a novel approach to determining foster dog names. When dogs enter a shelter and are not surrendered by their owners, it may be impossible to determine what their original name was. Since dog shelters have way too many dogs and their database can't handle name duplicates, they end up with really awful names like Barney Barnes, which the dogs do not respond to. In this paper, we create a Bayesian sampling method to determine the true name of a dog with a flat prior.

Chapter 13, A Re-Examination of the Fermi Paradox: A Data and P(Doom)-Driven Markov Process Approach, examines the Fermi paradox. By using an intergalactic database of planetoids' ability to support life and the technological and biological data of other life forms in our galaxy, analysis of the Fermi paradox shows that it is extremely unlikely for any other intelligent life to exist in our universe.

Chapter 14, Comparative Space-Saving Highway Interchange Design, creates an analysis of alternatives for unconventional highway interchanges in dense urban environments, including vertical loops, M.C. Escher-style labyrinths, and wormholes.

Chapter 15, Image Transfer Protocol Delivery Methods for Sending Pocket Rocket Pictures to Tinder Matches, explores the use of TCP and UDP protocols in sending pictures of super sweet tiny motorcycles to matches on dating apps without risking getting unmatched, blocked, or reported.

Chapter 16, Unlocking Human Behavior: A Feline Exploration of Vocalizations and Behavioral Variations for Optimal Wet Food Provision from the Servant Human Class, expands upon prior research to create a foolproof method for extracting wet food from the servant human class.

Chapter 17, Yield Strength Comparative Load-Bearing Analysis of the Limited-Time Cheez-It Webbed Crunchwrap Supreme, tests and analyzes the physical characteristics of the Cheez-It variety of Crunchwrap Supreme when compared to the use of the traditional Crunchwrap as a building material.

Chapter 18, Novel Techniques for Hijacking Self-Driving Cars, develops and tests techniques to capture autonomous vehicles using dead falls, bear traps, steel cages, artificial pedestrians, laser pointers, and a pheromone-induced honeypot lure.

Chapter 19, On the Tardiness of Coworkers and How to Exploit It, determines optimum meeting tardiness to maximize free time and moral high ground by modeling the tardiness of your coworkers.

Chapter 20, Replying "Haha So True!" to Every Meme Your Friend Sends: An Experimental Study in Preserving Social Bonds with Minimum Effort, establishes texting "Haha So True!" as the optimum method for replying to friends who text too much when you desire to maintain friendships without becoming either overbearing or too distant.

Chapter 21, A Time-Series Analysis of My Girlfriend's Mood Swings, creates a mood prediction model for Dr. Love so that Dr. Broman can go on a bender in Vegas with his friend and not get in too much trouble.

Chapter 22, Behavioral Conditioning Methods to Stop My Boyfriend from Replaying The Witcher 3, develops a method to prevent Dr. Broman from replaying *The Witcher* again. It involves the careful positive and negative reward conditioning by his girlfriend, Tiffany.

Chapter 23, Sub-Nyquist Sampling While Listening to My Girlfriend, engineers and implements a method for parsing and observing conversations with Dr. Love so that Dr. Broman can maximize his attention while playing *Elden Ring*, which takes a lot of concentration.

Chapter 24, Who Should Do the Dishes? A Transportation Problem Solution, is where Dr. Broman and Dr. Love use linear programming to determine who should do the dishes by treating it as a transportation problem.

Chapter 25, Freudian Psychoanalysis of My Boyfriend's Gun Collection, is a paper by Dr. Love where she sketches a psychological explanation of Dr. Broman's recent obsession with purchasing, cleaning, and using new firearms.

Chapter 26, Breaking Up with Your Girlfriend but Not Your Friends: A Cyclic Graph Algorithm for Social Network Preservation, is where, after breaking up with Dr. Love, Dr. Broman develops a cliqued graph model of their different friend groups and develops an algorithm to maintain his friendships while also avoiding his ex.

Chapter 27, The Future of Romance: Novel Techniques for Replacing Your Boyfriend with Generative AI, is where Dr. Love, in an attempt to not fall back into the trap of getting back together with Dr. Broman, develops techniques using new generative AI technology to replace all of the functions of a boyfriend.

Chapter 28, Winning Tiffany Back: How to Defeat an AI Boyfriend, determined to get back together with Dr. Love, shows how Dr. Broman sabotages the training data of Dr. Love's ChadGPT language model such that it exhibits all of his most annoying behaviors.

Chapter 29, Would He Still Love Me as a Worm: Indirect Sampling and Inference Techniques for Romantic Assurance, is another paper by Dr. Love. After getting back together with Dr. Broman, she is unsure that Dr. Broman will love her no matter what and develops a Bayesian inference approach to determine whether he would still love her if she were a worm.

Chapter 30, Efficient Methods of One-Night Global Toy Delivery, is a paper by Santa Claus. Christmas comes once a year, but Santa Claus is hard at work year-round researching the top Christmas delivery technology. By utilizing a genetic algorithm, Santa Clones, and upgrading his sleigh, Santa solves his ultimate traveling salesman problem.

To get the most out of this book

- In this book, you may get lost, and it is advised to pack the following:

    - Three liters of water and a water purification method
    - 1x fleece jacket
    - 1x rain jacket or poncho
    - 3x pair of wool socks
    - 1x hiking boots
    - 2x quick-dry pants
    - 1x long-sleeve shirt for sun and bugs
    - 3x underwear
    - 1x towel (galvanized)
    - 1x bandana with a cool pattern
    - Three days' supply of food
    - Stove, fuel, and pot (for boiling water)
    - Bear bag/canister
    - Eating utensils
    - Snare wire (for days 4–10)
    - 550 chord
    - Lighter/matches
    - Emergency space blanket
    - 2x whistles
    - Bear spray
    - Hot chocolate with marshmallows

- Keep an open mind.
- Most importantly, the main rule of this book is to have fun!

Download the example code files

The code bundle for the book is hosted on my local drive at `/Users/BMcGraw/Documents/PersonalProjects/ProjectsImActuallyFinishing/Code/CodeThatWorks/Scripts/EtAl2/Final/Final_FinalScripts/`. We also have other code bundles from our rich catalog of books and videos available at `/Users/BMcGraw/Documents/Python/EtAl2/GraphVis/Analysis/src/include/external/submodules/build/executables`. Check them out!

Download the color images

We also provide a PDF file that has color images of the screenshots/diagrams used in this book. You can download it here: `https://packt.link/gbp/9781806118939`.

Get in touch

Feedback from our readers is always welcome.

General feedback: If you have questions about any aspect of this book or have any general feedback, please email us at `customercare@packt.com` and mention the book's title in the subject of your message.

Errata: Although we have taken every care to ensure the accuracy of our content, mistakes do happen. If you have found a mistake in this book, we would be grateful if you reported this to us. Please visit `http://www.packt.com/submit-errata`, click **Submit Errata**, and fill in the form.

Piracy: If you come across any illegal copies of our works in any form on the internet, we would be grateful if you would provide us with the location address or website name. Please contact us at `copyright@packt.com` with a link to the material.

If you are interested in becoming an author: If there is a topic that you have expertise in and you are interested in either writing or contributing to a book, please visit `http://authors.packt.com/`.

Share your thoughts

Once you've read *How to Prove Anything*, we'd love to hear your thoughts! Scan the QR code below to go straight to the Amazon review page for this book and share your feedback.

`https://packt.link/r/1806118939`

Your review is important to us and the tech community and will help us make sure we're delivering excellent quality content.

1

Dust, Heat, and Cumin: Low-Budget, Synthetic, Authentic Mexican Atmosphere Filter for Modern Cinema

Gilligan Vincent[1]

[1] Department of Cinematographical Studies in Color Filtering, Cranberry-Lemon University, Pittsburgh, PA, USA

Abstract

The digital Mexican sepia filter is a long-sought-after visual effect in American cinematography. The effect is simple to imitate, but creating an *authentic* Mexican refraction index is more complex. Due to a growing demand for more authentic Mexican visual filters by modern audiences, studios have spent additional millions paying actors to film in the middle of the desert of the Chihuahua and Coahuila regions, where the natural Mexican sepia light filter occurs at its maximum state. Using basic digital image processing techniques, this paper will create an authentic Mexican atmosphere in any environment by adjusting the refractive index, dust, and cumin levels to reach a South-of-the-border flavor.

Keywords: Authentic Mexican Sepia Filter, Sonoran Refractive Index, Cumin Dust Spread, Yellow Heat Index, Too Much Spice, Carranzan Mandate of 1918, Image Processing, OpenCV, Image Blurring, Dust Cloud Computational Fluid Dynamics

1. Introduction

Without a serious regressive change in automotive emission standards, there is little chance an authentic **Mexican sepia filter** can be achieved in Hollywood without the assistance of digital image processing. Even then, the oppressive heat index, the difference in the refractive index of light, and the cumin dust cloud make the Mexican atmosphere one of the most unique and iconic in the world [1]. Despite a similar effect when filming in the oppressive heat of yellow-tinted Southern Asia, a Graham-Masala finishing cloud creates an entirely different color tint effect, which savvy viewers will pick out instantly [2]. It is time to develop a more robust and researched method for generating an authentic Mexican color filter using basic functions shamelessly stolen from Stack Overflow!

2. Background

After the passing of the Mexican constitution in 1917, the new government's president, Venustiano Carranza, passed a widely beloved law in 1918 to change the refractive index of the air in Mexico in order to instill a sense of national pride. With the new refractive index, longer wavelengths "...would scatter to create a perpetual sunset to signify the diminishing government of Diaz and a sunrise for Mexico's future..." according to Carranza. This law was intended to consolidate the remaining revolutionary factions under the newly formed government and make it even more difficult for rebel leaders such as Pancho Villa and Zapata to maintain local support for their violent causes [3]. The plan worked, and Mexico soon developed an identity around a yellow-orange tinted color palette that transformed the sky into the Mexico we know today.

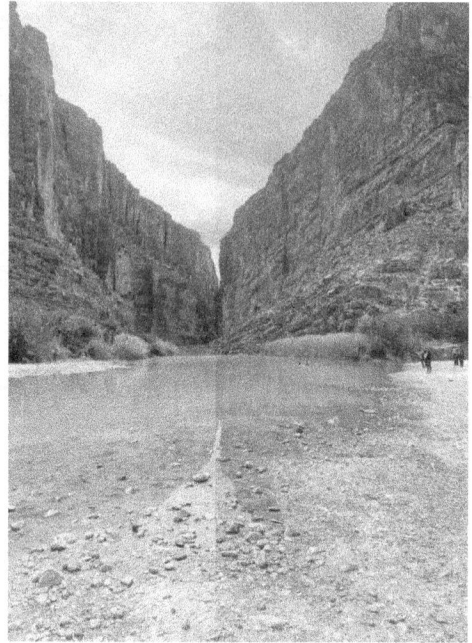

Figure 1.1: US-Mexican color filter seen along the Mexican-US border at Big Bend National Park

Not all Mexican yellow filters are the same. Known for its sea-misted ceviche tone, the Baja region tends to diffract more blues into the atmosphere than other regions, in stark contrast to the rest of the North's predominant reddish-orange desert color tone, reaching as far down as Mexico City. As one travels south out of the desert and into the jungles of Southern Mexico or the Yucatán Peninsula, greener, more colorful light travels further as the increased flora filters the government-mandated haze, adjusting the atmosphere to Carranza's 1918 law.

Countless Hollywood films and TV classics, such as *Breaking Bad*, *Traffic*, and *Extraction*, aimed to imitate this color filter in film to denote a change of location. However, many critics have criticized, as critics often do, the inauthentic visual effect, leading studios to fork over the funding to refilm on location. *Breaking Bad*, in particular, required the orangest of colors set in the cartel-ridden Northern desert regions of Mexico close to the New Mexico-Texas border. With TV fans growing more annoying than ever, studios quickly became hostage to their demands.

3. Methodology

The transformation of a normal-colored image to the synthetic Mexican atmosphere will be implemented using a three-stage filter. First, a yellow tint filter will be applied, then a yellower dust filter, and then, finally, a cumin dust cloud. Each filter will be applied by transforming the BGR (I don't know why OpenCV does it that way and not RGB) elements using a 3x3 transformation matrix, averaged with a variable intensity using the Python package OpenCV. Each filter will be demonstrated on the following test image, taken from a normal, non-yellow-tinted city. Additionally, the blur operation allows each image to be synthetically blurred as if there were a dust or cumin cloud.

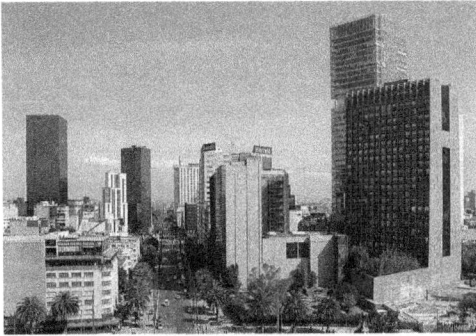

Figure 1.2: A normal city test image (Mexico City-Carlos Valenzuela, CC BY-SA 4.0, via Wikimedia Commons)

3.1 Heat

Through the combination of the intense heat of the Mexican sun, significantly stronger than anywhere else on the continent, and Carranza's famously mandated refraction index, even on a clear day, the sky will be noticeably yellower.

$$Yellow\ Matrix \ = \ \begin{bmatrix} 0.6 & 0.0 & 0.0 \\ 0.1 & 1.0 & 0.2 \\ 0.2 & 0.3 & 1.0 \end{bmatrix}$$

Using the preceding transformation matrix along with an intensity of 0.6 to be averaged with the original image, any image may be made authentically more yellow, as shown in *Figure 1.3*. Comparative physics-based simulation models guided by the 1918 Carranzan Mandate have been verified in [4], showing that this transformation matrix is good enough.

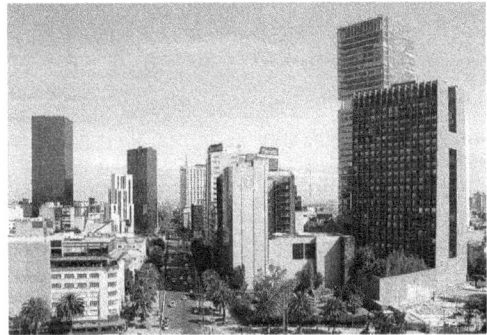

Figure 1.3: Yellow-filtered city

3.2 Dust

Next, to transform each image with a generous dust cloud, but at a level that is still visible, the image color palette is washed out using the following color transformation dust matrix:

$$Dust\ Matrix \ = \ \begin{bmatrix} 0.9 & 0.0 & 0.0 \\ 0.3 & 1.0 & 0.3 \\ 0.3 & 0.3 & 1.0 \end{bmatrix}$$

With the dust layer applied, the original image is further blurred by a 5x5 convolution matrix in OpenCV and averaged at an intensity of 0.4. We believe these are the correct values because it's starting to look about right. The new dusty image tricks the viewer into believing that they are now in a more arid environment, reducing the need for further establishing shots.

The results of this filter are shown in *Figure 1.4*.

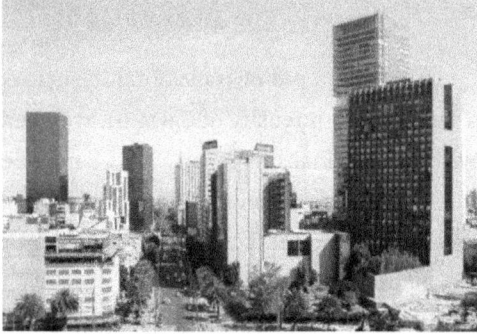

Figure 1.4: Dust-filtered city

3.3 Cumin

Next, a fine layer of brown from a special concoction of coriander, cinnamon, and primarily cumin, creates the final transformation matrix, as follows:

$$\text{Cumin Cloud Matrix} = \begin{bmatrix} 0.106 & 0.0087 & 0.756 \\ 0.294 & 0.259 & 0.174 \\ 0.672 & 0.787 & 0.894 \end{bmatrix}$$

As the cloud generated using the computational fluid dynamics (CFD) models from the methodologies in [5] is much more exact, the numerical certainty of this special spice blend color palette transformation is paramount! The image is then further blurred with a 2x2 convolution matrix and then averaged in with an intensity of 0.4. The results are shown in *Figure 1.5*.

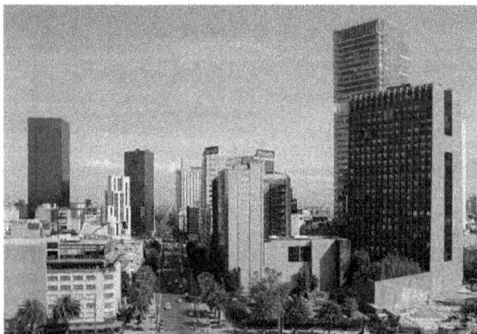

Figure 1.5: Cumin dust cloud-filtered city

4. Test Image

For the final test, a new test image needed to be generated using generative AI. IEEE recently banned the use of the famous Lena Forsén test image [7] in their research papers in an attempt to modernize [6]. This means we need a new test image. As we are always looking for opportunities to provide new positive male role models for boys and maintain a connection to our shared image-processing heritage, Lena was fused with John Cena through MidJourney. This generated a new standard test image, **The John-Lena**, shown in *Figure 1.6*.

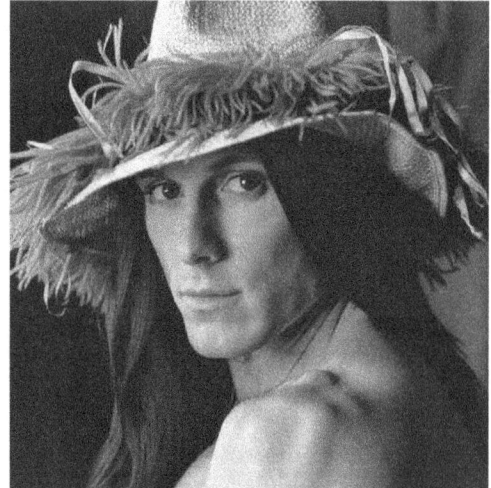

Figure 1.6: John-Lena test image

Through the recent advancements in AI, we could expand the image, something many engineers have always wished they could do. We then finalized the new and improved test image to be adopted by computer science and image-processing journals everywhere. Gaze into the future in *Figure 1.7*, a bold, refreshing new look for the field. It is John-Lena.

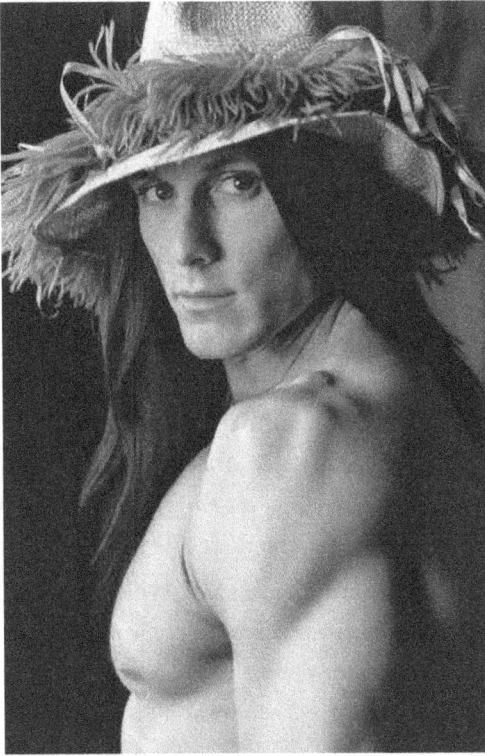

Figure 1.7: Expanded John-Lena

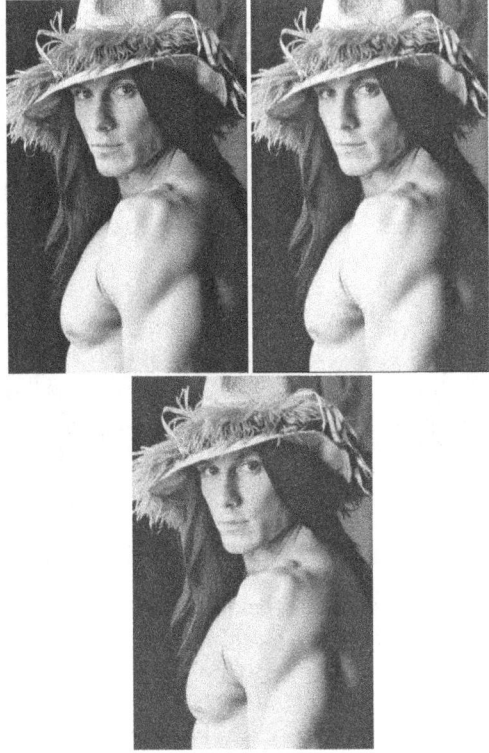

Figure 1.8: Clockwise from top left: Lena-Cena filtered successively through the yellow refractive filter, then the dust blur filter, then the cumin cloud

5. Results and Discussion

Each successive filter was applied to the John-Lena test image, as shown in *Figure 1.8*. As shown, through only the yellow refractive filter and the dust filter, John-Lena became far too yellow, which was nothing like an authentic Mexican atmosphere. By applying the final seasoning blend filter at the end, John-Lena now appears as if he were on some adventure south of the border in a hit new TV show or movie.

Thanks to the new filter, 98% of our test audiences identified this image as having been shot in Mexico without any additional shots for context. The color filter was found to be authentic enough to get the most annoying fans off our backs once again. There appeared to be no need to shoot the film on location in the Sonoran Desert at twice the cost. Now, shoots may occur at Vasquez Rock, as in the Hollywood of old.

Many different filter iterations were generated by experimentally dialing in the filters based on feels and vibes. It was important to create a variety of color palettes for moods and differing atmospheric locations according to heat index, wind conditions, and spiciness.

Those experiments revealed a clear line a filmmaker should not cross while applying the spice filter, as shown in *Figure 1.9*.

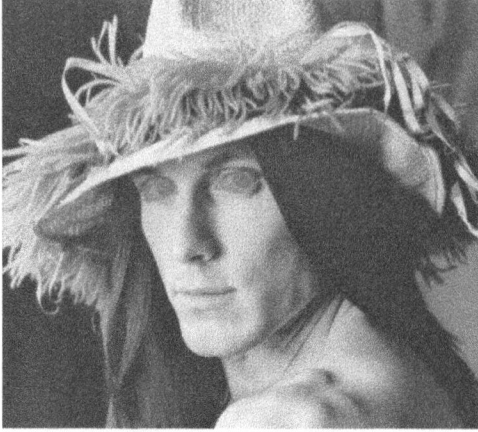

Figure 1.9: Too much spice! HE CONSUMED THE SPICE. THEY DESIRE THE SPICE

If too much spice is applied in the successive filters, images will ingest too much spice, which will cause the **Eyes of Ibad** phenomenon [8]. By exposing a human to a heavy dose of the spice **Melange**, even just synthetically, the subject appears to pass the Arrakis threshold, coloring their eyes blue on blue. It is not recommended unless you prefer to symbolize your character's connection to the land and their enlightenment by communing with their ancestral memories through the Water of Life. Lisan al Gaib.

6. Conclusion

Finally, through the magic of matrix transformations, OpenCV, and fiddling around with numbers, an effect that normally requires a passport may now be accomplished using a simple Python script. In this paper, not only have we saved Hollywood millions of dollars per year, but we introduced a fantastic new test image for image processors everywhere. It's impossible to hate John Cena, so we suspect John-Lena will catch on like wildfire.

References

1. Gilligan Vincent, et al., 2008. *The Mexican Yellow Tint Color Palette ::* Journal of Modern Western Cinematography

2. Sterling "Silver Screen" Stone, 2014. *Adventures in Mood Colors: Synthesizing Color Palettes Around the World ::* Journal of Post-Production Techniques, Tips, and Tools of the Trade

3. Veronica VonDutch, 2016. *A Brief History of the Mexican Atmospheric Mandates: Revolution Gone too Far ::* Annals of Alternative Mexican History

4. Winston "The Wizard" Whitaker, 2020. *Computational Models of the Mexican Atmospheric Refractive Index in a Post-Carranzan World ::* Journal of Fiesta-Physics

5. Melba McCormick, 2023. *Pink and Fire: Computational Fluid Dynamics Simulation Analysis of My Recent Gender Reveal Party Disaster ::* Journal of Astrological Big Data Ecology

6. https://www.theguardian.com/technology/2024/mar/31/tech-publisher-bans-playboy-centrefold-test-image-from-its-journals

7. https://en.wikipedia.org/wiki/Lenna: Oh man, if you haven't read up on this, you gotta: back in the 1970s, to get a test image, an engineer scanned this image from a Playboy magazine. Then it somehow became the standard test image for image processing for decades. It was only banned by IEEE in 2024.

8. https://dune.fandom.com/wiki/Eyes_of_Ibad

2

Novel Gravity and Velocity-Based Time Dilation Methodology for Real-Time Bitcoin Payment Processing

Chase Blockman[1] and **Blake Ledger**[2]

[1] Department of Coin Scheme Excellence in Computer Science, Cranberry-Lemon University, Pittsburgh, PA, USA

[2] CEO/COO/Founder/Majority Shareholder in Ponzi-Block Crypto Enterprises

Abstract

The search for a stable financial system is the most important thing humanity could ever research. This pursuit should be approached with absolute and unquestioning religiosity. It should be clear to everyone that crypto is the future of currency. There's no feasible way that the value of a government-backed fiat currency can possibly compete with the perfection of **blockchain** technology. Because of the proof-of-work and proof-of-ownership algorithms baked into the blockchain algorithm, it would be impossible for anything else to be more reliable. There is one primary issue stopping blockchain from replacing fiat currency: it is very slow to process transactions. Bitcoin, at its current rate, is capable of making 7 Transactions per Second (TPS). For reference, Visa will process 24,000 to 65,000 TPS at its peak to process payments. Because of this unfortunate bottleneck, in order for Bitcoin to keep up with Visa and physical cash, there would need to be about a 3–10,000x increase in processing speed. Using relativistic physics, this paper will exploit time dilation caused by relativistic speed and gravity to design a single blockchain system that can account for the 24–65,000 TPS and hopefully not destroy the Earth in the process.

Keywords: Cryptocurrency, Blockchain, Bitcoin, Dogecoin, Black Holes, Time Dilation, Astrophysics, May the Schwarzschild Be With You, Lorentz Equation, General Relativity, Earth Tearing Itself Apart, Packing on Mass

1. Introduction

It has long been theorized that through the addition of enough individual blockchain-based coins, or "shitcoins" as they're colloquially called, there would be enough network capacity to account for the number of transactions made by humanity [1]. With the exception of Dogecoin, Ethereum, and a few other blockchains, only a select few are allowed to know about, **cryptocurrency** has suffered the same primary issue as fiat currencies such as rapidly devaluing from Pump and Dump (PD) schemes [2]. While fiat currencies may fail due to corrupt and intrinsically evil governments PDing their own currency, shitcoins are PD'd by internet personalities [3]. The only way crypto markets can survive is to rocket ship into orbit so that there are too many stakeholders who have too much to lose for the market to crash.

This unfortunate side effect of cryptocurrency is counterintuitive when the ledger blockchain system should make it the most secure and trusted type of currency. Evidently, convenience and a hold of value are necessary to establish an official cryptocurrency. We can assume that crypto can only be successful after wide adoption once it overcomes its technical shortcomings as a day-to-day transaction method [4]. This will allow for crypto to achieve market penetration into the currency market of markets. Unfortunately for blockchain technology, the inefficient ledger validation that makes it so secure, trusted, anonymous, and separated from evil institutions makes the currency impossible to optimize for day-to-day use. That is why we must experiment with placing a super-massive **black hole** at the center of the Earth or speeding up the Earth's movement to near the speed of light.

2. Background

The basics of time dilation and blockchain are necessary to understand why we must either put a black hole at the center of the Earth or speed it up with Orbital Rotational Equatorial Rockets (ORERs) to avoid the collapse of our financial system.

2.1 Blockchain Basics

It is no secret that there is a real **Bitcoin Scalability Problem (BSP)** [5]. In order for blockchain technology to be trusted and decentralized, it must be enacted on a peer-to-peer network for each block. Blockchain works by allowing each block to keep track of everyone's transactions so that each block can know who owns what, thus creating the most inefficient database on the planet. If one person sends another bitcoin user a bitcoin, not only do the mathematical hashing operations need to occur to prove the validity of the payer and recipient using public and private keys, but each link of the blockchain must be updated with the transaction history. In essence, it's a linked list in which every link contains the information on all of the other links in the list, making the update process extremely taxing, especially when each link in the list is decentralized. Currently, a block size is 1 MB, and the time to create a new block is 10 minutes. This creates a throughput of about 7 TPS.

Unfortunately, the only possible solutions to this scaling issue would destroy the beauty of the blockchain. It could be centralized, which would make the transaction no longer decentralized and require an evil institution. The block size could also be increased to the size of GBs, but the required increase would then make the ability to run a block inaccessible to common users. Finally, transactions could be taken off of the blockchain, in which, obviously, you're not using the blockchain. The only solution to allow Bitcoin to handle world commerce must incorporate some sort of time dilation.

2.2 Velocity Time Dilation

By applying the Lorentz equation, time may be adjusted via time dilation according to the equation below. For instance, if we were to speed up the Earth to the speed of light somehow, time would halt relative to its surrounding environment.

$$\Delta t = \Delta t' \sqrt{1 - \frac{v^2}{c^2}}$$

Because the factor is divided by the speed of light squared, we expect to need to speed the Earth up to state fair spinny-ride speeds. Thankfully, anything is possible in the pursuit of more money.

2.3 Gravity-Based Time Dilation

Derived from Einstein's field equations in his general theory of relativity, the **Schwarzschild metric** provides an exact solution to the effect of gravity on time. As is tradition, it looks suspiciously similar to the previous equation. It's so similar, we suspect foul play.

$$\Delta t = \Delta t' \sqrt{1 - \frac{2GM}{Rc^2}}$$

As the factor is again multiplied by the speed of light squared and G = 6.67430e-11 m^3/kg/s^2, we're going to need a huge black hole to make any difference to our geocentric bitcoin servers. To anyone who ventures to physically test this paper, *may the Schwarzschild be with you*[1].

_____

1   This footnote is brought to you by *Spaceballs!*

3. Methodology

The configuration of the relative velocity and black hole positioning is of paramount importance. The importance couldn't possibly be more paramount. It's the Paramountiest+.

3.1 Rocket Earth Rotation

A differential velocity between satellites in orbit and the surface of the Earth will be no small feat. The most optimal configuration to speed up the Earth relative to the satellites is shown below in *Figure 2.1*.

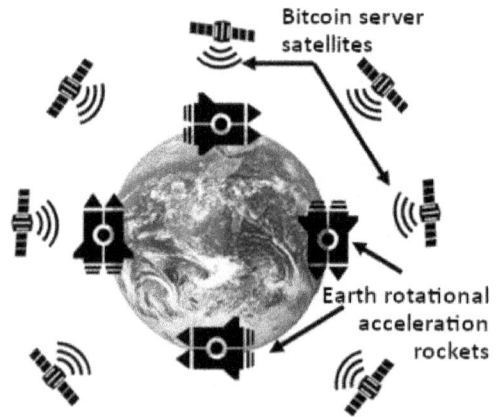

Figure 2.1: Earth acceleration rocket configuration

For this project to proceed, we will need a massive array of booster engines near the equator. Obviously, due to the enormous heat produced from these engines, we'll have to space them out, and it may take somewhere between minutes and centuries to achieve the required speed. I wouldn't necessarily classify this knowledge as insider trading, but land near the equator in South America and Africa may become extremely valuable. It will be possible in some parts of the ocean to outfit oil rigs to support an Earth accelerant booster, but if I were to invest in real estate, I'd stick to the equator.

The same result could be achieved with satellites orbiting near the speed of light. Unfortunately, that would require an enormous amount of thrusting on board to keep the satellites in Earth's orbit, so it is more reasonable to speed up the Earth's rotation to the speed of light.

3.2 Black Hole Earth Center

In order to create the most mass differential possible between the satellites and the surface of the Earth, a super-massive black hole must be created at the center of the Earth, as shown in the diagram below. It is vitally important that the black hole appears as suddenly as a thief in the night so that the surface of the Earth instantly becomes stuck in time stasis along the black hole's event horizon. Otherwise, the NIMBYs will thwart the progress of humanity once again. According to most zoning restrictions, black holes would drastically change the character of the neighborhood. Additionally, all of the satellites must be in place as the gravitational pull of the black hole will make escape velocity a thing of the past.

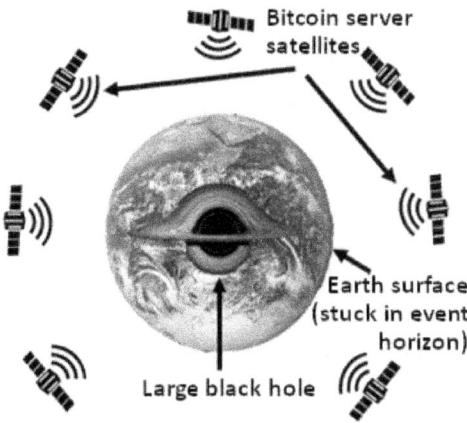

Figure 2.2: Earth's core black hole configuration

Also shown in *Figure 2.2*, we hope that the satellites will be so far away from the black hole that its effect on time for the satellites will be negligible compared to that on Earth. The plan is already looking a little shaky judging by some of the investors' looks at some meetings, so we don't need any complications from that sort of analysis ruining our plans.

3.3 Peer-to-Peer Satellite Structure

Before the Earth is sped up to breakneck speeds or we create a black hole at its center, we must launch all satellites. The logistical constraints of launching satellites in the midst of a super-massive black hole or while it is rotating near the speed of light are insurmountably unfathomable. We just can't fathom it, not even for a microsecond, according to our results section. All assets must be in orbit first.

It would be easiest if we contacted the most powerful space-faring nations on Earth to create a network of satellites to create a peer-to-peer network capable of enacting blockchain. Unfortunately, that would destroy the point of using blockchain. Institutions and governments are evil, and we should not involve them in this process whatsoever. It will be better for mankind if we hand our keys over to a small-to-medium number of oligarchs who have enough money to launch the satellites into orbit [6]. With a modest amount of 1–3,000 satellites controlled by the wealthy point-O-O-O-one percent (0.0001%), we should be able to allow them to handle the transactions fairly between each other without screwing over the little guy. The world's oligarchs have so much money already, there's no way they would rig the system in their favor for even more.

3.4 Simulation Test Environment

It will only be possible to enact the results of this paper once to fix Earth's monetary policies. Before collecting the required mass for either of the methodologies discussed, we must simulate and test different combinations of mass and velocity. Two simulation engines were developed for this analysis: the **Realistic Orbital and Tangential Acceleration Testing Environment (ROTATE)** [7] and the **Gravitational Relativity Analysis and Variability in Temporal Yield (GRAVITY)** [8]. These models, respectively, simulate and analyze a massive Earth model to determine how much speedup is achieved for each mass packed onto the black hole or equatorial rocket is added. This simulation engine, we are assured by their business rep, can handle near-lightspeed travel as well as a time-warping black hole. It was designed by our friends at Meta Singularity Solutions, which we may hold a minority stake in. The license for their software is a bargain at $99.99 a month! If you need to simulate the Earth in an other-earthly manner, this is your simulation software. I'd get into details, but that's proprietary knowledge.

4. Results

We backtracked the calculations of different speedups for our bitcoin server satellites and calculated the parameters for our GRAVITY and ROTATE simulations. The required mass and velocity for each speedup is shown in *Table 2*. Don't panic, this is potentially achievable.

Speedup	Black Hole Mass (kg)	Earth Velocity (m/s)	Required Mass (Fuel kg)
x4k	4.295506376 4224346e+33	299999990.62 49999	Math Range Error
x6k	4.2955065255 71971e+33	299999995.83 33333	Math Range Error
x8k	4.2955065777 74308e+33	299999997.65 625	Math Range Error
x10k	4.29550660193 65327e+33	299999998.5	Math Range Error

Table 2.1: Required conditions for satellite process speedup

The good news is that once we achieve a black hole that is about 2159x the mass of the Sun, or get around 99.99999% the speed of light, any speedup advantage is fairly marginal! We are not sure why our calculation for the required fuel mass to speed up the Earth is causing a Math Range Error in Meta Singularity's ROTATE simulator, but don't worry, we've already submitted a software bug ticket requesting more bits in the software's linear algebra library. As far as we know, the simulated Earth in ROTATE and GRAVITY stayed together in one piece in the first 1e-7 seconds before the software froze, but the time dilation was confirmed.

5. Discussion

There's a lot to unpack here. Many might think this effort fruitless as there is absolutely no way we could achieve enough fuel or black hole mass to generate the gravitational or velocity effects to produce the required time dilation effects. To those haters, I say look at the upside! If we just put in one large upfront effort, we will easily multiply our profits and processing potential by 10,000 for the rest of the history of humanity. I think it's at least worth trying and finding a path to achieve our financial dreams. Think about what power processing we will have when we incorporate AI!

5.1 Packing on Mass

Whether it's the mass of the fuel required to speed up the Earth or the mass to create the black hole, for this time dilation scheme to work, we need to pack on a lot of mass. We're not talking about a little mass; we're talking about 2,159 times the mass of the Sun. It's easy to relatively pack on mass within Earth, but to pack on that mass, you must take away mass from another massful object. We could potentially be looking for masses outside of our orbit and, to be honest, we think we're going to have to crowdsource this one. If you are an alien race now reading our journal, please reach out to us at bmcgraw584682@gmail.com via Earth's internet servers to let us know where to gain ~2.955e33 kg of mass on our planet. We promise that your investment in us will guarantee you a 1% per 5e32 kg of stake in Earth-created intergalactic intellectual property. We are a resilient bunch and fixing our monetary policy will get you in on the ground floor of an incredibly industrious and creative species.

5.2 Imaginary Velocity

If you didn't notice in the equations, the Lorentz equation squares the velocity. What if we were to accelerate sideways in time? Could we create a positive effect on the imaginary velocity of Earth? OR! We could potentially create satellites moving sidewise in imaginary time-space velocity at a sped-up rate. We would not need a black hole or massive arrays of Earth Rotational Boosters on the equator.

We could potentially speed up the time of our satellites themselves by accelerating them *sideways*. Is such a thing possible? I don't know, but it could be. Yes! Let's explore this option before opening up that other wormhole [9], or whatever mass-packing operations are currently on the table [10].

5.3 Weather Effects

A lot of people believe that a near-light-speed acceleration of the Earth's rotation will drastically affect the weather in a detrimental way. Many progressive investors may even believe this could accelerate global warming. Let's not cause another man-made climate crisis, they say. But, stay with me here, if we had 3,652,499 more days in the year, would we not be the most productive species in the galaxy? If you had that many more calendar workdays on the schedule, would you not be able to keep up with your tough day-to-day and produce more output in your spare time? I think you would. There's only so much Netflix you can catch up on. I think the resulting shortened microsecond days from the gravitational speedup would kick our weekly and annual schedules into overdrive! I think it would be amazing for our species! YES, let's do it!

Wait, I just realized that it's actually reversed in relation to the rest of the galaxy, so never mind.

6. Conclusion

Who cares if the Earth falls apart from a collapsing black hole or angular momentum if we're all making money!

We are living in the crypto age, so it's time to adjust our lives to our new currency and leave the old ways of fiat currency in the past. With a small investment of ~4.29e33 kg of black hole or an unspecified amount of rocket fuel, we could solve the BSP once and for all without endangering our bottom line with misguided government institutions. Invest now and maybe you could get a small stake in our satellite-based bitcoin processing constellation!

References

1. Celeste Lightweaver, 2022. *More Avenues of Success: A Shitcoin Methodology for Blockchainification of Global Monetary Policy :: Proof of Work Quarterly*

2. Baroness Fifi Cumberbund, 2023. *Analysis of the Pump and Dump: Why do Shitcoins Fail so Fast? :: Journal of Blockchainology*

3. Theodosius P. Opulentworthy, 2021. *Can YouTube Virility Prop up the Blockchain? No, and a few other bad Internet Ideas :: Memecoin Monthly*

4. Lord Marmaduke Stashington, 2022. *Avoiding the Visa Transaction Fee: Methodology for Getting Rid of the World's Biggest Unaddressed Monopoly :: The Quarterly Ledger*

5. The Bitcoin Scalability Problem. https://en.wikipedia.org/wiki/Bitcoin_scalability_problem

6. Sir Winthrop Treasury-Bottom, 2024. *An Oligarchic Solution to Removing Government from Currency :: The Decentralized Times*

7. Tess R. Actor, 2023. *The Realistic Orbital and Tangential Acceleration Testing Environment (ROTATE): A Simulation for Day Shortening and other Climate Solutions :: Journal Unnecessary Simulation Technologies*

8. Neutronius Gluemore, 2023. *The Gravitational Relativity Analysis and Variability in Temporal Yield (GRAVITY): A Simulation Engine Just Because :: Journal Unnecessary Simulation Technologies*

9. Gordon Freeman, Barney, Et al., 2018. *A Wormhole to Xanadu: Infinite Mass for an Infinitely Growing Economy :: Journal of Black Mesa Enterprises*

10. Mac the Body Builder, 2013. *Packing on Mass: Bags of Chimichangas will only take Physics so Far :: Journal Body Builder Body Guards Incorporated*

3

Me and My Friend Found Where the Coolest Part in My Room Is Using the Heat Equation Because It Is REALLY, REALLY HOT OUTSIDE!

Jack Lee[1], **Aaron Wiener**[1], **Superman Action Figure**[2]

[1] Ms. Makema, 2nd Grade Maths, Department of Young Academic Misfits, Southeastern Northwest Primary School, Oceania

[2] My (second) favourite superhero. He's here for moral support and in case we need more time to write the paper as he can turn back time by making it go backward by flying really, really, really, really fast and reversing the spin of the Earth. I saw it in a movie once!

Abstract

In this paper me and my best friend Aaron try to figure out where the coolest part in my room is during summer so that we don't have to sit in front of the fan all day. The summer is almost over but I still think this will be useful to know for next summer and I don't think it's going to stop being hot for a WHILE! I'm finally not grounded anymore but now my mommy says it's too hot to go outside. I think she is right! It is HOT! Finding the coldest spot in my room would be really awesome! Not only would my mommy stop shouting at us to stop using the fan and driving up the power bill, but it means that me and Aaron could use that electricity to instead make progress in our hardcore Minecraft survival world. It's REALLY tough. We have gotten REALLY good at Minecraft.

We are going to try and use the heat equation to find a cold spot in my room! The fan doesn't work that well anyway, it just blows hot air around! I think we need a bigger fan. I like it when Aaron talks through the fan and makes his voice all funny though.

Keywords: It's HOT!, Thermodynamics, Heat Equation, Keeping Cool, A LOT of dimensions, Computers, doing math with computers, Python (not the snakes!), different equations, Counting in Spanish, Optimizing, Hot and Cold things

1. Introduction

After me and Aaron finished our previous paper [1], we showed it to our math teacher. Ms. Makema was not impressed though, and after telling us that we were "wasting our time," "not going to solve the Collatz conjecture," and "not sleeping during nap time like she told us to," she made us sit inside and write down lines while everyone else played outside. While writing "We will not write any more pointless papers during nap time" for the fiftieth time I noticed that the room was starting to get quite warm. The outside was as high as 40°C! Aaron was sitting next to me, so when I mentioned that it was getting hot he said that we should move, then Ms. Makema said to keep quiet! I thought that this was a great idea, so we immediately started looking for a different part of the room to sit in.

This was when we found the problem. We weren't sure where the coolest part of the room was, and we didn't really want to run around with a thermometer. We only had ONE thermometer, and it was HARD TO READ! PLUS, we didn't want Ms. Makema to think that we were goofing around and extend our punishment. PLUS, running around made us even hotter! We decided to solve this with MATH! We like Math and are VERY good at it! In math there is a thing called the heat equation. We are VERY good at equations as we tried to tell Ms. Makema even though she tells us we don't need to learn about equations yet. I think we might be smarter than her and she doesn't know how to use equations.

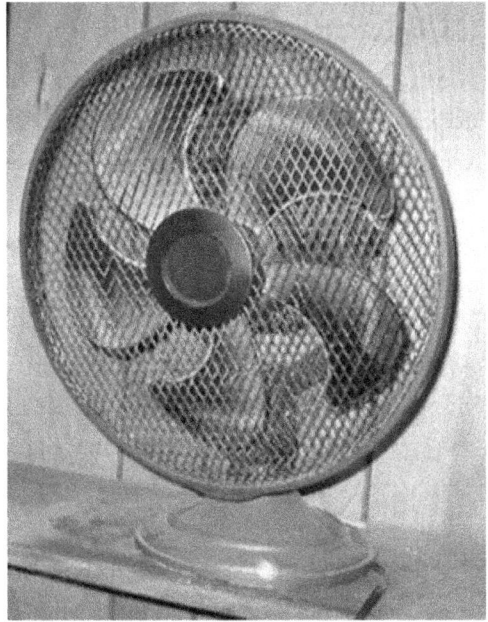

Figure 3.1: I got this fan because I complained to my mommy about how hot it was but I don't think it cools down my room enough anymore because it is really, REALLY hot outside and it probably needs to be like THREE times bigger.

By using equations and not a thermometer, not only would we be in the coolest part of the classroom during a 40°C day, but we would not need the fan at home! We're killing two birds with one stone, although I like birds, so I probably wouldn't kill them. One time I was throwing rocks at birds with Aaron and Michael and John and some other kids in class and I was actually trying to not hit the birds, but don't tell them that!

1.1 Background

My brother Oscar, who is going to university now, told me that one of the things he learned about, besides the 3n+1 problem we solved earlier, was the heat equation [2]. I miss Oscar, I can't wait for him to come back at the next break. He told me that the equation is a partial differential equation, and that it will tell me how temperature diffuses over time. **Diffusing** is a big word for people like Geoff who can't understand big words. I can explain it, because I understand it and read about it online. For a temperature to diffuse, it has to spread out, like when they finally let all of us outside, we can spread out into the playground. If we have been inside longer we will run outside faster, this is like temperature, it can spread out faster or slower. I think things that spread out must have something to do with the **Mess On particle**, which is a particle me and Aaron discovered to explain why my room is so messy in another paper [3]. We didn't even need to buy a particle accelerator to find it.

I still don't know what a differential equation is or what a partial differential equation is. It has something to do with things changing and because the part that changes is only a part of the equation I don't know if it's worth learning about it if it's going to change all the time. Differential means change because it stands for difference which is like subtraction but it's not subtraction. I tried learning the rules to not get in trouble in Ms. Makema's class but she keeps CHANGING THEM when she doesn't like how we follow her rules. She tells us to do our math homework but gets mad when we are drawing more differential equations to try and figure out what they are instead of learning how to do more arithmetic. I think my teacher is a partial differential equation because she changes so much and I don't understand her. Arithmetic is boring, I'm already perfect at it. I make NO mistakes! I'm not perfect at differential equations, they keep changing like Ms. Makema. The heat equation is written with partial differential equations like:

$$\frac{\partial u}{\partial t} = \dot{u} = \alpha \Delta u = \alpha \nabla^2 u$$

Apparently the $\frac{\partial u}{\partial t}$ is the part that changes. I think ∂ is a silly letter, or maybe it's a partial because it's an incomplete 8. I asked Oscar what α is and he said it was actually made up of a lot of things. It's something called a "thermal diffusivity" which has something to do with the types of atoms and particles and how they touch each other. Me and Aaron are really smart at particles, like when we discovered the Mess On particle [3] even though we didn't have a particle accelerator because my dad wouldn't let me spend a million-billion-trillion dollars on it. We still found it. Thermal diffusivity is, like, when heat travels through things, and how fast? I think. Water is slow. That's why water is so cold in the summer. But the diffusivity of concrete and metal is high, because I burn my hand when I touch it, or the things in the kitchen can heat up REAL fast. I think that's because the particles are closer together, which makes it easier for heat to go through. Me and Aaron decided to rate the thermal diffusivity of the different objects in my room based on how hot they were when we got home from school. We put the alphas in *Table 3.1* based on what we felt. I couldn't touch the window for very long.

Object	How hot	α
Carpet	Not very hot	2
Bed Sheets	Warm, except when I lay in it then very hot	5
Window	VERY HOT	9999
Train Book	Warm	10
iPad	Hot	25
LEGO	Not hot	14

Table 3.1: Thermal diffusivity of things in my room

Me and Aaron agree on the numbers so they should be correct. Apparently, we also needed the α of the air, so we decided to make it $\alpha_{air} = 1$ because air can't be hot and it can't be cold like an object except when it's from something like a refrigerator or oven or by the window. Maybe it can have a temperature but then I wouldn't know what number to give it. The right side of the equation is now defined as:

$$\Delta u = \nabla^2 u = \alpha \left(\frac{\partial^2 u}{\partial x^2} + \frac{\partial^2 u}{\partial y^2} + \frac{\partial^2 u}{\partial z^2} \right)$$

Because an upside-down triangle means Laplacian. A Laplacian is a three-dimensional derivative and means "The Place"-ian in Spanish where "-ian" means change except I don't know the language "-ian" is from. It is very special because it can find the change of heat at any three-dimensional point in my room! Did you know that you are three dimensions? So am I! Some cartoons are two dimensional, but I think most are three dimensional now.

While we are talking about the heat equation in three dimensions, there is nothing stopping us from using it with more than three spatial dimensions. I think we could keep adding

on dimensions if we wanted to. We are smart enough that I think we can. We could even apply it to four dimensions or even A THOUSAND DIMENSIONS! Even though I can't picture that, someone has come up with a method to make Tesserectane [4] which I guess is something more than 3D! We will now use the heat equation to answer our question and find out where we should sit so that we can stay cool!

2. Analysis

I wish my room was in one-dimensional space, because if it were in one-dimensional space, the heat equation could be solved by something called separation of variables. In separation of variables, the variables get separated like when I get peas and carrots and don't want to mix them so that I can eat the carrots first because they taste better than the peas. I can do that because peas and carrots are one dimensional which is like when something is a line or one thing. I think it would be kind of boring if my room was one dimensional, I couldn't do anything except sleep I think because I'm three dimensional. Apparently, Oscar knows how to solve through separation of variables, but he refused to show us how it was done, even when we offered to give him one of my toys. I think if he showed me, we could figure out how to do it in the three-dimensional space which is my room.

It won't be hard to solve because we already figured out the α for all the objects in my room, except the air conditioning vent I can't reach. And we set α to 1 for air because it doesn't do anything. Unfortunately, I found out I can't just use my partial differential equations with just my α values, I need initial conditions and boundary conditions. I did not know how to look this up or what they were, so we'll figure that out later.

I think it means the walls, or the doors, but I'm not sure which. Me and Aaron tried to do the analytical solution, but we ran out of paper to make our calculations on, and we couldn't write on toilet paper.

On our family computer, we didn't run out of paper. BUT it was hard to write in math form. We decided to try and solve it numerically like Oscar told us we would have to do. I still think we can solve it on paper, but we need more paper and pencils to do that. We tried erasing and re-writing, but it took too long. We were getting frustrated and hot, and we were doing this to not be hot! Solving something numerically is like solving it with numbers instead of with letters. BUT the numbers are close numbers, they're not exact numbers. It's like when I try and guess how long we have left at school, I am normally not correct, but I am close. It always is longer than I think it is. Solving with numbers would be A LOT! Since we had even less of a clue of how to do SO MANY calculations, we first asked Oscar. He said that we would need a really, REALLY big computer and that we could not do it on our iPad or my dad's computer.

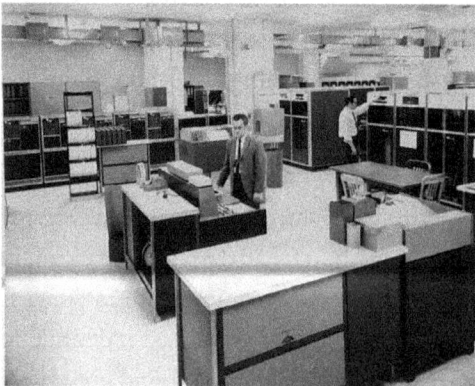

Figure 3.2: Old computers used to be REAALLY BIIIG! I think if we had an old computer, we could solve the heat equation EASILY! It must be WAY FASTER than my dad's computer!

I think we could still do it because we are REALLY GOOD at using computers! I once put a frog on the desktop background and my dad was mad because I guess he doesn't like frogs. He doesn't like it when we use his computer either, but we don't know how to solve something numerically on an iPad. It got put into a parental lock mode last time we tried to watch videos on it. Computers now are REALLY SMALL compared to how they used to be. I guess people have to do less math on computers because old computers used to be the SIZE OF A ROOM! My dad's computer is only as big as my arm!

My dad sometimes doesn't turn off his computer so that's how we could get on sometimes. It has all of the applications. That's why he was so mad at me for putting a frog on his desktop background, I think. I don't think he likes frogs. It was OUR FROG WE CAUGHT! We named him Jerry. I miss that frog. He could jump THREE FEET! While we were trying to get enough **ender pearls** to drop, we thought about asking ChatGPT how we would use my dad's computer to solve the heat equation next time he leaves his computer on. ChatGPT is a person on my dad's computer that he talks to a lot. He's VERY SMART and answers ALL my questions until he says we ran out of questions for the day. Then we have to wait and I HATE waiting to ask more questions. Even Oscar doesn't answer all my questions.

While we didn't have access to GPT-4 because mom stopped letting me use the credit card and I can't remember that many numbers, we could still ask GPT-3.5 [5] how to do it. I think ChatGPT 4 must be smarter because four is a bigger number. At first ChatGPT 3.5 said it was a bad idea to use my dad's computer but then I asked it without telling it we were using my dad's computer. It said to use something called python! I don't know how because a python is a snake my mom won't buy me from the pet store and snakes don't have fingers and you need fingers to use computers. We eventually realized that **Python** is a language like **English** or **Spanish**. Except instead of using the language to talk to my friend Juan, I use it to talk to a computer. I know thirty words in Spanish: Hola, Adios, Por favor, Gracias, Si, No, Amigo, Familia, Gato, Perro, Casa, Comida, Jugar, Escuela, Libro, Pelota, Feliz, Triste, Ayuda, Sol, Luna, Estrella, Agua, Arbol, Flor, Color, Numero, Tren, Coche, and Avion. See?

Python was a thing we had to download from online. We clicked on A LOT of download buttons until we found the right one. The download made a lot of popups on the computer but we got it to work.

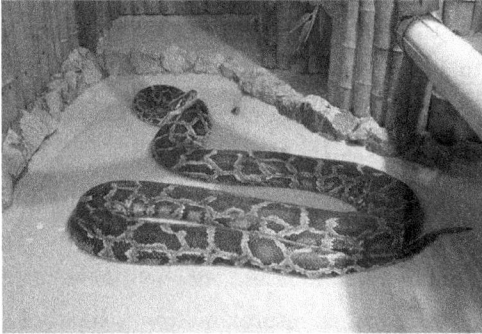

Figure 3.3: A python, which doesn't have any fingers. I saw it at the zoo once. I would like to own a python, I think he would be a cool pet.

3. Results

We started writing our code in the Python language. Oh! I forgot that I actually know forty words in Spanish because I can count to ten! Uno, Dos, Tres, Cuatro, Cinco, Seis, Siete, Ocho, Nueve, Diez! Thankfully, Juan knows English because it's hard to talk with only forty words. We didn't know any words in Python, so we

asked ChatGPT how to talk to the computer and we typed exactly what it told us to type. I thought it didn't work but then we realized we forgot to type a "\}" after a letter "+" and before another line. Python is really hard even when you're typing directly from ChatGPT! My dad is only away from his computer for thirty minutes, so we had to type FAST!

We used the code from ChatGPT to find out the temperature of a 1-meter cube in our room! It made a whirring sound which I was afraid my dad would hear while he was in the kitchen and not at his computer. After running the script, we did get a very funny looking picture we put in *Figure 3.4*. We think that the purple means cold and the orange-yellow means hot, so we want to stay away from the orange-yellow part. I think ChatGPT said that my room started out colder than it actually was because that part of my room was not that much hotter than the rest. I think that might have been a mistake with the initial condition.

3D Heat Equation Solution

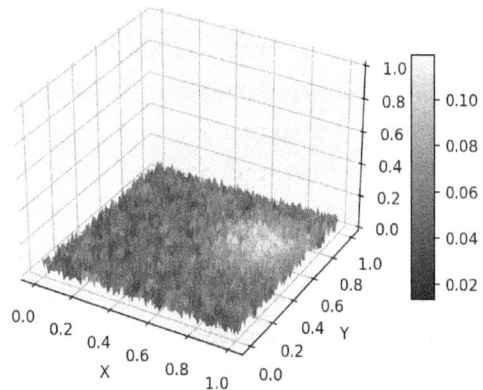

Figure 3.4: A solution to the 3D heat equation

The Python code provided by ChatGPT worked. I think it wasn't exactly right but I think that's why it is a numerical and not analytical solution. I said that earlier! If you were paying attention.

Numerical is not exactly the same as it is in real life so I think we did it good enough. We had finally found a way to find the cold spot in our room that worked! We thought about solving it numerically on paper when we found another four pieces of paper then we gave up almost immediately! It was A LOT of calculations, and it would have taken us a VERY long time to do them. I know we would have done them PERFECTLY because we don't make mistakes.

Figure 3.4 shows the solution to the heat equation for a 1 m sized room after a very short amount of time with uniform initial conditions. Our room is larger than $1\,m^2$ but I think if we stretch out the picture on our computer it can be big enough to cover our ENTIRE room! We wanted to stretch out the picture on the BIG SCREEN TV, but couldn't figure it out and had to use our imaginations. My room I think is at least eight times bigger than 1 m.

We were very happy to find a solution to such a hard problem; we were now able to extend this to my bedroom to answer the original question and stay cool. It still wasn't that much cooler. But it WAS COLDER! We almost IMMEDIATELY encountered a problem with the answer. The computer's answer was for only a region where the boundary conditions were zero! My room's walls aren't zero degrees! AND the end time of the program was ONE SECOND! I think there are at least THOUSANDS of seconds in a day! Because sixty seconds in sixty minutes in one hour with twenty-four hours in a day adds up to A LOT! Except you don't add, you multiply those numbers!

These may be fun to think about mathematically but are completely unrealistic to do on my dad's lunch break from work and useless in a real scenario. ALSO, the simulation took a long time to run because we had to run it during the thirty minutes my dad spends in the kitchen while making a sandwich. We had to run it WAAY TOO LOONG. While I watched the computer run, I thought it took FOREVER! This means that to run it for any amount of time longer than a second might take EVEN LONGER and I might get CAUGHT! We decided to try anyway because we wanted to know REALLY BAD and changed the one second to sixty times sixty times twenty-four and the 1 m into 8 m because I think my room is at least EIGHT TIMES BIGGER! The computer made a lot of noise. I think it was its fan, but some sounded like it was the speaker AND NOT AN EMAIL, and it had a moving bar come up when we clicked on a program that WOULDN'T GO AWAY! My dad came back from his lunch before it could finish and got REEAALLY MAD at his computer. I think he restarted it and didn't see the results. I don't think he would have told us anyway.

4. Conclusion

We did solve the heat equation to find where the coolest part in my room was during summer, even IF it was only for one meter, a second, and an approximation instead of a solution. We did realize that I wasn't even really in my room most of the time, and that trying to figure out where it was hot made more heat, which should be in our heat equation! Most of the time I was either at school, playing with my friends outside, or over at Aaron's house because he has a pool WITH A SLIDE! And when I was at home, I would usually be in the living room. And at night, it was cool enough that I didn't really have to worry about the heat. There were mosquitoes which I think are VERY ANNOYING, but I'll have to solve the mosquito problem in another paper! There wasn't much reason to solve the heat equation for my room since I wouldn't even be in it half the time. I still think that it was REALLY fun solving a hard math problem like a heat equation! I like math!

5. Acknowledgments

Me and Aaron came up with most of what to say for this paper, but we still had Oscar to help us actually write and typeset all of this up. We only talked to ChatGPT to talk to the computer for us because he speaks to the computer in Python. I don't know if ChatGPT is a boy or a girl because he or she or I don't know didn't tell me. I think all computers are boys and all iPads are girls. Oscar was even more annoyed than when we got him to write up our previous paper.

References

1. Lee, Jack and Wiener, Aaron. *Me and My Best Friend Aaron Prove the 3n+1 Problem even though it is a REALLY Hard Problem*, Journal of Astrological Big Data Ecology, Chapter 16 of *Et al.: Because Not All Research Deserves a Nobel Prize*

2. Heat Equation, Wikipedia: `https://en.wikipedia.org/wiki/Heat_equation`

3. Lee, Wiener. *A Particle Physics Model of Why My Room is Never Clean and Why I Shouldn't Have to Clean it Up Everyday Like Mommy Tells Me To*, Journal of Astrological Big Data Ecology, Chapter 15 of *Et al.: Because not all research Deserves a Nobel Prize*

4. Freely, Jackson, Cupid, Cedric the Fourth. *A Total Synthesis of Tesseractane: The First Preparation of a 4-Dimensional Natural Product*, Journal of Immaterial Science

5. ChatGPT, OpenAI: `https://chat.openai.com/`

[This page was left blank because the previous paper was going over word count.]

4

Me and My Friend Show That My Dad's Airstream Trailer Goes Faster with Dints, and That We Shouldn't Be Grounded for Hitting It with a Baseball Last Saturday

Jack Lee[1], Aaron Wiener[2], and Titan Camera Man[3]

[1] Miss Jones's 2nd-grade homeroom because I got moved from Ms. Makema's after I got caught talking too much during history class

[2] Ms. Makema's 2nd-grade homeroom because Miss Jones remembered that the principal said that me and Aaron can't be in the same class as each other, even though I got myself switched on purpose

[3] This is an AWESOME big camera man with a large screen and lots of guns and rockets that fights the Skibidi toilet man army [1]! He's in a bunch of episodes, and I think he's my favorite of the cameramen. I like it when he beats the Skibidi toilets, and they start dancing to that song [2]. I like that song.

Abstract

My daddy is really mad at me and Aaron. He found out last Saturday that we've been playing catch with a baseball and some other balls near his **Airstream**. But especially baseball. We were playing inside like we wanted to, because it was cold, but then my daddy said to take it outside. So we decided to throw the baseball outside. It was cold, so we put on a jacket and a hat and came in sometimes to stay warm. Me and Aaron are better at throwing the ball than catching it right now, and we hit the side of my daddy's Airstream a bunch. I didn't think we were throwing it that hard, but now I think we were throwing it really, REALLY hard. My daddy yelled at us this last Saturday when he found a LOT of dints from our baseball on his Airstream. I didn't think we could hurt his Airstream because it is made out of metal, which is INDESTRUCTIBLE! It's like **Captain America's shield**, except he gave it away because he's old now. But now I think there's a new Captain America who has the shield. And there was another guy on a TV show, but he's not Captain America anymore either. My brother explained it to me, but I forgot. The Airstream is NOT like that shield. Aaron showed me an episode of a SUPER old show. It's over 15 years old; it's ANCIENT! Older than my dad. It's called MythBusters and they have an episode where they dint a car like a golf ball, and it drives better. I think that's what we did to my daddy's Airstream, and we shouldn't be grounded for making it better. We have to show that it's better so that we don't have to be grounded.

Keywords: My Daddy's Airstream, Baseball Dints, Air, Science, Golf Balls, Aerodynamics, Myth-Busters, Speeding, Playing Catch, Fans, Leaf Blowers, Air Drag, Wind Tunnel, Uncontrolled Downhill Test, Smoke Streams, Fire Trucks, Downhill

1. Introduction

I don't know if dints are spelled dints or dents, and I looked it up, and they can be either way, so I think I'm going to spell it both ways. My English teacher would hate that. We made a lot of dents on my daddy's Airstream. An Airstream is like a house, but on wheels and covered in metal. Except it's too small to be a house, even though my daddy says it is one. He spends a lot of time working on his Airstream trailer and says that if things get bad, we'll be living out of it, so I think he really loves it. I think he loves it more than our normal house, which is bigger, and I have my own room in my house. In my daddy's Airstream, I don't have a room. I have a couch I can sleep on, but we share it during the day. I don't like weekends when my daddy makes us practice bugging out in the Airstream. I would rather be in my backyard playing catch with Aaron or watching Skibidi Toilet videos again, especially the ones that **Titan Camera Man** is in.

2. Background

Me and Aaron learned a few days or a month ago that cars can be like golf balls. It's in a TV show that I'm about to tell you about. Golf balls are like normal balls, but they are hard and small, and you hit them with a stick instead of throwing them.

2.1 Golf Ball Car MythBusters Episode

One day, when me and Aaron were hanging out, even though my daddy had grounded me but my mommy didn't know about it yet because he went on a business trip, I told Aaron about the dents and how mad my daddy was.

He said that he watched a cool video about it on a show called **MythBusters**. His parents let him watch that show, and I wish mine did too. I thought it was really cool. I like MythBusters because they are funny, and they do science, which I love. I love science, and I like it more than English or History. They have a lot of MythBusters; they have millions, I think, because I couldn't count them all, even though I am very good at counting. I would like to watch all of them if I could, but my screen time is limited. They are all almost an HOUR LONG and would take up all my screen time. In one episode, the MythBusters tried making a golf ball car out of golf balls [3]. Except that golf balls can't work, so I think they used something like Play-Doh called clay. They made it like a golf car with all the bumps on golf balls, and that made it better. My mommy says our plates are made of clay, which doesn't make sense because it's not Play-Doh. We'll use Play-Doh later, even though it wasn't Play-Doh that they used. Aaron said that the bumps are like the ones that we made with my baseball. Usually, when MythBusters test something, it comes out, they decide it's false. They call it BUSTED!, but this was not busted. Busted is a word they use when something is not true. I think it's from their name. They said that a golf ball car was not busted, and I think it is just like our Airstream with all the dints. The MythBusters always tell us to never try anything we're about to see at home, but we decided to anyway.

2.2 The Dints in My Daddy's Airstream

We counted, and I think we made almost 30 or 100 dints on my daddy's Airstream. We originally only made the dents on one side, so we didn't think it was that bad because he had another side that didn't have any dints. Once we tell my daddy about the golf balls, he won't be mad that we put dents on the other side of his Airstream and the front and back. He will be happy, and he will probably buy me more toys and not be mad at me anymore.

We used Aaron's ruler from school. We aren't supposed to take our rulers home, but we did it anyway, so don't tell Ms. Makema. We measured that the dents are deeper than the fifth marker on our ruler, which I think is VERY deep. The dents on golf balls are not very deep, and I think the dents we made will be better than golf balls and make my daddy's Airstream better. We counted up as many as we could. I think we might have counted some dents twice, or three times, but I don't think that happened. We counted them and put them in the table below by how many ruler markers deep and wide the dents were. We measured the depth in small markers and the width in the big markers. A marker is a line drawn on a ruler, and it's used to say how big or long something is by counting and multiplying. You can also use fractions if you are better at those. On my classroom door frame, I'm 35 markers tall.

	1 Marker Deep	2 Markers Deep	3 Markers Deep	4 Markers Deep
1 Marker Wide	2	5	9	2
2 Markers Wide	3	8	5	6
3 Markers Wide	6	13	24	8
4 Markers Wide	5	12	16	10
5 Markers Wide	4	5	7	3

Table 4.1: Dint size where each dent is measured by the number of markers on Aaron's ruler he stole from school, and the width is measured in large markers, and the depth is measured in small markers

2.3 Golf Balls

Golf balls have dints in them. I learned on MythBusters and a YouTube video [4] that it's because it makes it go faster because of **aerodynamics**, which is a big word I learned in those videos. I think aerodynamics makes a lot of sense in explaining why dints are a good thing. When air moves, it's like water except that water is bigger than air, which is why it's easier to breathe air than it is to breathe water. I breathed in water once in a pool by accident and I did not like it. My brother Oscar saved me. At first, I didn't think air was anything but I learned that air is actually something even though we can't see it. It is very EXTREMELY small particles that we can't see, like the **Mess On particle** I discovered that made my room messy [5] even though my mommy didn't believe me. I drew the way that air flows around a ball and a golf ball like it shown in the videos listed later.

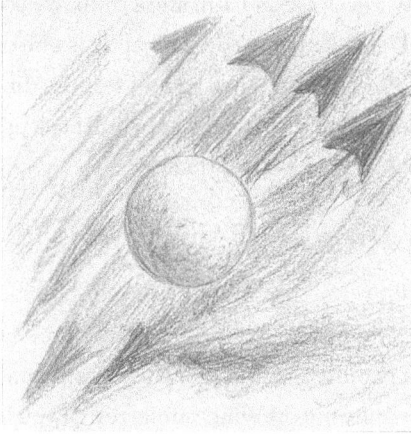

Figure 4.1: Golf balls have air go through because of the bumps. This drawing has the golf ball in orange and the air in the different blue and red arrows, and the air flows around because of the bumps, which makes it better

When air flows around a ball, you can't see it, but it's there. It's like a ghost or a fart. You can't see it, but you can smell it and feel it. There are big lines of air and small lines of air. When there are big lines, I think that makes a ball go slower, but when there are a lot of little lines, it goes faster? I don't know why the size of the line is the reason why golf balls go faster, but I think my daddy's Airstream would have REALLY big arrows of air slowing it down. I think air is a bad thing in aerodynamics, so the more of it, the worse you are. Except one time I went to a state with really big mountains, and I ran out of breath really, REALLY easily. I thought I was sick, but I wasn't. I asked my brother Oscar, and he said that it was because there was less air, which made me slower. So, I don't know if more air always makes you slower because that one time, less air made me slower.

3. Methodology

We knew that the more the Airstream was like a golf ball, the faster it would be. We couldn't make it small, or a sphere, but we could give it more dints. I don't think spheres are faster, but I don't know why. According to YouTube videos and science that we understood, it was true, but my daddy doesn't always believe me, so we needed to test whether or not his Airstream would be faster with more or less dints. Only one side had dints, though! Also, we are not allowed to drive for another 10 years. We need a plan to find out if it's faster.

3.1 We Filled in the Dints with Play-Doh and Then We Dented the Other Side of My Daddy's Airstream

We wanted to test the Airstream with twice as many dints and no dents. Our allowance wasn't large enough to buy another Airstream, and my mommy wouldn't drive me to buy one to see if I could afford one, so we had to use the same Airstream in our backyard. It was easy to make more dints. My daddy took away my baseball, but he can't take Aaron's baseball away. We didn't know how to undo dents, and it was hard to make dents on the roof of the Airstream. We tried suction cupping with some window toys I got for Christmas. They were like really cool. On the toy, I can lick a plastic circle on the toy with a suction cup, and then the superhero sticks to the window. I think if I had a really big suction cup, I could climb up a building. The superhero suction cup is not big enough to climb with. I tried. It was also not big enough to un-dent my daddy's Airstream, so we decided to fill them all with Play-Doh.

The Play-Doh got stuck to the metal when it dried, so we had to make new dints to test the aerodynamics again. I think if the Play-Doh comes off and there are WAY more dents the Airstream could go SUPER fast.

3.2 Wind Tunnel Test

We learned from the YouTube videos that we don't have to drive the Airstream to test the air around it if we find something called a wind tunnel. We couldn't find one, so we had to make one. My daddy is always yelled at by mommy in the fall because she doesn't like the leaves on the ground, and he has a leaf blower, which I guess makes it easier, but he hasn't let me use it yet, even though it looks fun. He also has a fan that can blow air when he makes his special smoke in his garage. I'm not allowed in the garage when he uses it, and it smells really bad like a skunk, but I think it would make a great wind tunnel.

I learned online that for wind tunnel tests, you still can't see air, so we need to make some smoke. My backyard has a lot of twigs and leaves, and I think we can use those to make smoke for our wind tunnel test.

3.3 Hill Test

My daddy won't let me drive his truck and even if he would, I can't reach the pedals and I think it's against the law to drive a truck. The Airstream is VERY heavy, but we can push it down a hill. It is on a hill, and I think we can push it down if we take away the wedges at the wheels and steer it. I think that it will speed up like super quick and make it down the hill WAY faster with the dents than if it didn't have any dents. At the bottom of the hill is a curb and some bushes that I think will stop the Airstream. I don't think that I can pull the Airstream back up the hill by myself because

it is so heavy but I can with me and Aaron and Oscar and my mommy when I tell her what we're doing, and my dogs, Hopper and Wolfy. They are as big as I am, and I think we could pull it back up if we do it all at the same time with ropes. I think we should test the dinted Airstream first so it's easier to pull back up because it will be faster then.

4. Results

We rewatched the golf ball YouTube videos a few times, and we think that the more smoke that made it directly behind the Airstream, the better during the wind tunnel test. If you look at the picture I drew, we put Aaron behind the Airstream while I blew air and smoke from our backyard fire with the leaf blower.

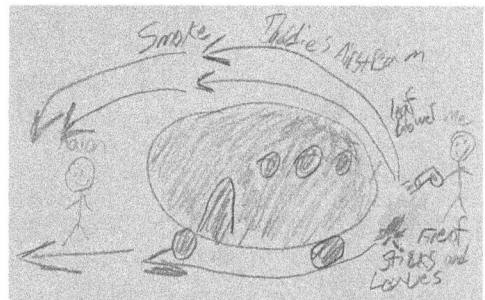

Figure 4.2: How we are going to make air go around my daddy's Airstream and how we'll make smoke too and blow it with a leaf blower to see if Aaron coughs

Aaron wrote down how many times he coughed so that we would know how much smoke got behind the Airstream. He has asthma and stuff. I know this because he gets to bring an inhaler to school, which looks like something from a movie. The more aerodynamic it would be with the dints, the more Aaron would cough. We expected a LOT of coughing with the dints and almost no coughing without the dints.

I think that's how it would have gone if we could have finished our test. We couldn't, because I think wind spreads fire a lot, and Aaron had to come help put out the fire before it got to the fence, which is made out of wood AND BURNS! We eventually got help from a fire truck, and we were able to put out the fire. But then we didn't have any sticks or leaves left to burn for any more experiments. My mommy also took away our lighter we found in the drawer with all of the coins, pens, and paper clips, so we couldn't burn the sticks in my neighbor's yard, who didn't have a fence.

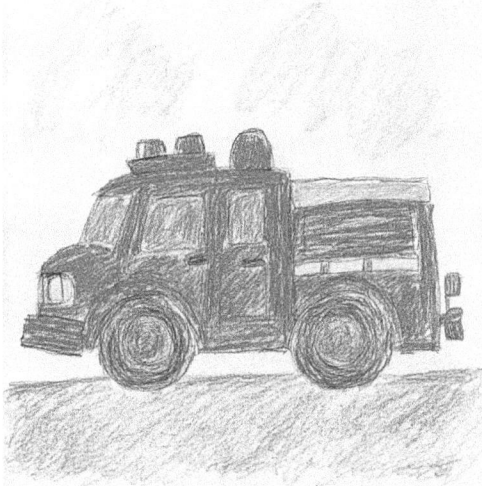

Figure 4.3: The fire truck that came to help put out the fire so we didn't burn down our fence.

We couldn't test with our wind tunnel, but I think we would still be able to show that the dints were good with the downhill test. I think it would go fifteen HUNDRED times faster with the dints, but we weren't able to measure it twice. We pushed it down our hill, which is really fun to sled on in the winter. You can go really fast if you lay flat on a sled. I think it would have gone really fast and I'm good at steering things so I didn't think we would run into cars. When the Airstream started rolling down the hill, I ran and tripped and could not keep up with it while it ran down and it hit two cars that were on the side of the road. I think it might have hit more cars if it didn't stop but I don't think they were supposed to be there. The police officer that came told me to stop crying but I think I could have steered it if I could have run faster with the Airstream.

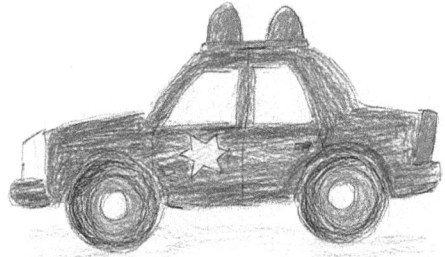

Figure 4.4: The police car that came to tell us that we can't roll our daddy's Airstream down the hill. He was really mean

6. Conclusion

We couldn't make Aaron cough until he ran to help put out the fires, and I couldn't run fast enough to steer the Airstream, so I think the dints made it really, REALLY fast even though we couldn't collect enough data. I wish that my daddy was happier that his Airstream was faster than he was mad about the other things. We proved that the Airstream is faster using science like the MythBusters, but my daddy doesn't like the extra dents on the other side and the roof and the front of the Airstream. He also doesn't like me using smoke in our wind tunnel or our downhill test. He grounded me more than I was before, and now my mommy knows about it! I think when he realizes that it's faster during the next bugout weekend, I think he will love me again.

References

1. *Skibidi Toilets 65-1 ALL Episodes HEALTH-BARS* (1-78?) | Ending version (All NEW seasons): `https://www.youtube.com/watch?v=evAzQ4-8ew8&pp=ygUQVGl0YW4gQ2FtZXJhIG1hbg%3D%3D`

2. *Speakerman theme song (1 hour)*: `https://www.youtube.com/watch?v=19i1I_iwMU8`

3. *Dimple car experiment*: `https://www.youtube.com/watch?v=VUiGhyHC-1A`

4. *Science of Golf: Why Golf Balls Have Dimples*: `https://www.youtube.com/watch?v=fcjaxC-e8oY&t=166s`

5. Me, Spider-Man, and Batman, 2023. *A Particle Physics Model of Why My Room Is Never Clean and Why I Shouldn't Have to Clean It Up Every Day Like Mommy Tells Me To* :: Journal of Astrological Big Data Ecology

5

A Novel Method for the Safe and Effective Recycling of PFAS Plastics: A Black Hole Hawking Radiation Approach

Dr. Qubert Spins[1]

[1]Department of Quantum Possibilities, Cranberry-Lemon University, Pittsburgh, PA, USA

Abstract

Per- and Polyfluoroalkyl Substances, or **PFAS**, are a group of highly troubling synthetic chemicals used in plastics, foams, and lubricants. Because of their strong carbon-fluorine chemical bond, they are extremely difficult to destroy and even harder to effectively recycle. Dumping carbo-floric monsters in landfills and oceans has poisoned the ground and water we live on, which is incredibly dangerous to human health. PFAS contamination is quickly becoming a crisis that could take decades to fix. While there is no easy way to transform the chemical compounds into useful materials harmless to humans, fundamentally, they are still made up of the same standard physical model of elementary particles of Quarks, Leptons, Gauge Bosons, and Higgs Bosons. If a miniature black hole is used to gobble up PFAS plastics to be filtered into fundamental elementary particles, the dangerous PFAS compounds will be utterly destroyed, rendering their mass and energy useful again. In this paper, we will propose and analyze a method to generate a PFAS-based miniature black hole, extract elementary particles and energy via **Hawking Radiation** using a **Penrose** extraction technique, create hydrogen through a particle accelerator, and finally use the new hydrogen/helium to fuse heavy elements in the fusion process of a new sun. PFAS will then be recyclable!

Keywords: Black Holes, PFAS, Recycling, saving the world, possibly destroying the world, Penrose Process, Particle Accelerators, elementary particles, stellar heavy metal generation, million-dollar ideas, Time-Dilation Hourly Wage

1. Introduction

PFAS recycling is not the first proposed garbage solution involving black holes. By utilizing miniature primordial black holes, [1] was able to transform the dangerously expanding New Jersey landfill into a rapidly collapsing but now contained New Jersey keep-out zone. Not only did the New Jersey black hole create a gravitational singularity that could gobble up all of their garbage out of mind, but the fact that light can't escape ensured that their garbage would also be out of sight. This was a revolutionary innovation which, for the first time in human history, allowed NIMBYs to back an environmental project, breaking Uhlman's rule [2].

[1]'s successful garbage disposal project, however, did not go far enough. With all garbage collected into a singularity, there is no mechanism to recapture materials, indicating that the Earth will eventually run out of resources and destroy our way of life. Luckily, black holes don't keep everything they suck in and emit energy in the form of Hawking radiation as elementary particles and energy. As proposed in [3], it may not be probable in our lifetime, but it is possible for Hawking radiation to turn into recyclable aluminum and other heavy metals. This paper confirms it will not happen in our lifetimes unless you are an elf, which can live ~10^9 years [4].

2. Design

The design for the blackhole PFAS extraction involves a counterweight-based ballistic input device, a center black hole with **Penrostronauts** (human labor) extracting energy and particles, a particle accelerator, and an external stellar transformation process.

A diagram of the recycling system is shown in *Figure 5.1*.

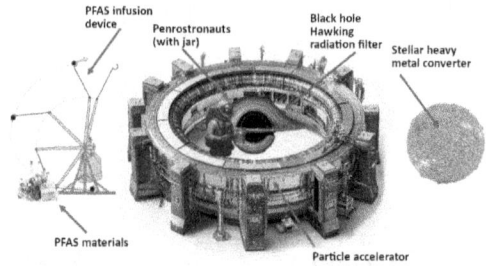

Figure 5.1: PFAS recycling method diagram

First, PFAS material is tossed over the particle accelerator and into the black hole. Next, a brave contingent of Penrostronauts travel into and out of the ergosphere of the spinning black hole with a Mason jar each, to extract elementary particles and Hawking radiation. Next, the elementary particles and energy from the Hawking radiation power a large particle accelerator, which produces relatively larger things such as helium and hydrogen. Finally, said elements are amassed at an off-site fusion reactor used to synthesize heavy elements that are useful for society, such as aluminum, lithium, and iridium.

3. Miniature Black Hole

When my research committee questioned my ability to safely input PFAS material into the inner horizon, I had to do an extensive literature review. After the New Jersey black hole landfill became operational and shortly became a keep-out zone following the tragic spaghettification of three sanitary workers [5], alternatives were explored. While rockets had an effective range [6], they were logistically and environmentally not cost-effective. Next, a railgun was attempted and analyzed in [7], but the required power utilized all of the extracted Hawking radiation and some additional grid power on heavy trash days. We then realized that volunteer-powered human hamster wheels [8] could fuel the contraption shown in *Figure 5.2* to launch 90kg of PFAS material 300m deep inside the inner horizon of our black hole Hawking radiation filter. Through a counterweight, a long lever made with the tallest straight tree from a nearby park, and some pulleys, we make short work of fueling the blackhole with more PFAS plastic mass.

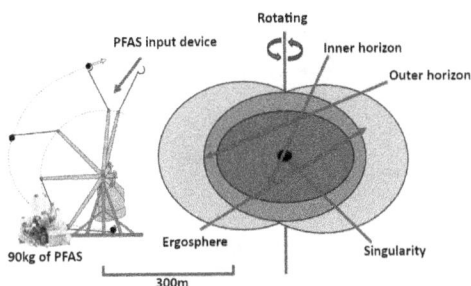

Figure 5.2: Black hole configuration

4. Penrose Extraction Device

It is important to note that the black hole seen in *Figure 5.2* is circulating. This is crucial as it will allow for a safe ergosphere zone so that we may extract important Hawking radiation and elementary particles expelled by the miniature black hole. To accomplish this rotational requirement, all matter is tossed in slightly to the right of the singularity. Next, some device would need to venture into the ergosphere and extract the previously filtered PFAS elementary particles.

Normally, this job would be accomplished by a robot. However, a recent paper suggested that it would always be cheaper to use human workers when working in proximity to a black hole [9-10]. Because of the time dilation of the intense gravitational field, if humans were paid at an hourly rate, the manpower costs would be a fraction of the cost of a fixed-cost robot. As shown in *Figure 5.3*, a cross between an astronaut suit and a 19th century diving suit pressurized with anti-spaghettification marinara sauce allows for any penrostronauts to safely enter and exit the ergosphere without being spaghettified.

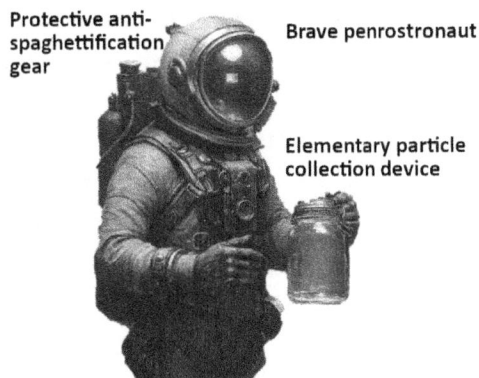

Figure 5.3: Penrostronaut doing an honest day's work

Each penrostronaut will be equipped with a Mason jar to keep the elementary particles as fresh as possible, pickled in a mixture of sugar and salt dissolved in water and apple cider vinegar. Penrostronauts then use a Penrose orbital path to carefully enter the ergosphere and exit with a Mason jar full of particles.

5. Particle Accelerator

While they make up all matter in the universe, unassembled elementary particles do not have any marketable value even among top recycling processors. A meta-analysis found that 94% of unsorted recycled fundamental elementary particles thrown in the recycling bin just end up back in a landfill. The next crucial step in our method to make use of our deconstructed PFAS plastics involves banging the elementary particles together.

Now, if you have enough time, you can make slow gravitational forces over hundreds of millions of years for them to bang into each other until they become any type of element. In our fast-paced society, we've decided to speed up this process using magnets [11].

After liberal use of the right-hand rule and bundles of wires wrapped in circles, an orthogonal circular magnetic field produced by buckets of megajoules of energy accelerates particles at extreme speeds. Most, uncreatively, call this contraption a particle accelerator. It's not super worth going into the statistics of it all, but if enough particles are flying around at high speeds, they eventually hit each other to make larger elements such as hydrogen and helium. If we're lucky, we may measure something strange that will give us infinite grant money through clickbait headlines for "breaking physics" before shortly revealing that it was a statistical anomaly of Gaussian measurement error [12]. The resulting elements are then collected to sell to balloon artists and for our next process.

6. Stellar Heavy Metal Generation

There are two methods of generating recyclable elements from hydrogen and helium. Both involve fusion reactions. One involves a large magnet, and the other involves an explosion. First, a mass of three parts hydrogen and one part helium is amassed in a centralized nexus. Then the mass is orbited by a series of ~10^5 gaming laptops running *Cyberpunk 2077* on maximum graphics to achieve a critical temperature of ~10^9K to jump-start a fusion reaction [13]. After a certain amount of time, to be determined, the fusion reaction will begin to produce heavy metals, which are easily recyclable.

The less catastrophic method of extracting heavy elements shown in *Figure 5.4* involves a large magnet to pull iron and aluminum out of the reactor. Once collected, these are then sold at a market rate to pay our penrostronauts who make it out of the ergosphere in time for payday every other Saturday.

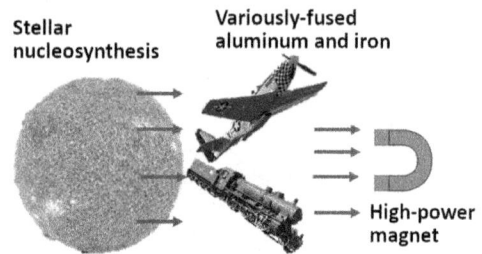

Figure 5.4: Aluminum-iron stellar nucleosynthesis

If one is feeling daring and wants some higher-selling heavy elements such as gold, uranium, lead, and other valuable metals of the unstable variety, the supernova II method may be desired. This is accomplished by waiting until the stellar reaction collapses in on itself and explodes in a supernova II.

For this method, it is best to initialize the fusion reaction in a safe location. We suggest performing this in a safer environment, such as the Alameda test range, which withstood 19 seasons of MythBusters explosions [14]. We still suggest surrounding your supernova II with several layers of ballistic glass, concrete, and fine nets to collect your heavy metals, as shown in *Figure 5.5*.

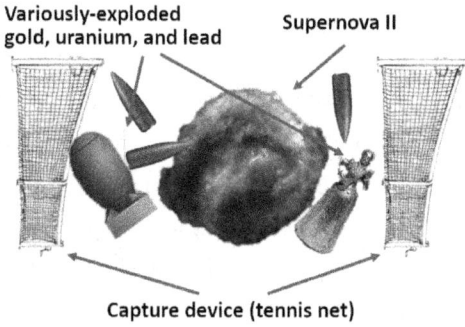

Figure 5.5: Super safe supernova II
heavy metal extraction

7. Efficiency Calculation

It's not quick cash. The payoff for this method may take a while, so if you're trying to pay off your mortgage and your mortgage isn't over 9 million years, it may not be worth it. This business model is only suitable for long-term investors. If you wait, the payoff is, however, immense. The efficiency of the process, inputs, outputs, and time of each step are shown in *Table 5.1*.

Step	Input	Output	Time Required	Efficiency
PFAS Catapulting	Human Hamster Wheel	~	10^2 Years	inf
Hawking Radiation Extraction	Paid Penrostronauts	$2.61*10^{16}$ Joules	10^9 Years	10^{15} – Insurance
Particle Accelerator	10^{16} Joules	10^{-1}	1 Year	10^{-17}
Fusion Reaction + Metal Extraction	10^{18} Joules	10^{17}	10 Years	10
Supernova Reaction	10^{22}	10^{20}	10^7	1

Table 5.1: PFAS Blackhole
recycling efficiency

Using E=mc^2, we find that 1kg of PFAS plastic has about 90 petajoules of energy. Using the Penrose process, 29% of the mass of the PFAS can feasibly be transformed into energy and extracted by the penrostronauts. Thankfully, we practically pay our penrostronauts nothing between the time dilation, their de-spaghettification suit, loan payments, and hourly wage. Unfortunately, the insurance will likely be through the roof unless you can bust up their union! Even more unfortunate, this step of the process will take the longest at 10^9 years unless we manage to produce a blackhole miniature enough to evaporate faster.

Next, the particle accelerator, at very low efficiency, only requires one year to gather enough helium and hydrogen. Hopefully, the PFAS Hawking radiation energy will be enough to power the reactor, especially with the rising cost of energy.

What energy is consumed by the particle accelerator may be generated using the fusion reaction, either by going supernova or in a normal fusion process. Luckily, a fusion reaction may be achieved by the Hi-res-cyberpunk2077-PC initiation procedure in only 10 years. We estimate this timeline because previous research has determined that fusion is always 10 years away [15]. If time allows, the supernova II reaction may be achieved in a timeline of 10^7 years, which, in the grand scheme of things, is not as long as the 10^9 years to extract all of the Hawking radiation. This is, of course, with 1kg of PFAS plastic. If it works anything like a computer program, this process may be sped up by parallelizing the process and extracting Hawking radiation at the same time as PFAS is catapulted in, turned into heavier elements and fused in a stellar reactor.

8. Conclusion

Utilizing this blackhole method, anything consisting of the standard elementary particles in physics may be recycled into aluminum! Oil companies likely do not want you to know about this because lightweight and flexible aluminum is an existential threat to their ability to sell you more plastics. I don't have anything to back that up, but we all know it. Finally, we have a solution to slow down the spread of microplastics into the world's oceans and our genitalia [16]. All we need to do is create a miniature black hole, power up a massive particle accelerator, and risk a supernova II in our solar system.

References

1. Dempster Dewey Dumpster, 2004. *Primordial Black Holes as a Solution to the Ever-Growing Landfill Problem* :: Journal of Galactic Waste Management

2. Zorhangimus Uhlman, 1989. *NIMBY No Mo': The Curious Case of My Block's Worst Neighbor and Why I Can't Dig My Own Swimming Pool*:: Annals of HOA Hell

3. Leonard Shogins, 2002. *Hawking Radiation Recycling: One Man's Energy is Another Man's Treasure* :: Journal of Advanced Astro-Economics

4. Aerindir Leafusurper, 2019. *The case of Anardil the Oldest Elf in the Universe: A Case Study in Elf Longevity* :: Journal of Aging Sciences of the Woodland Realm

5. 2008 *Tragedy Strikes New Jersey's First Black Hole Landfill* :: Reuters

6. Elton "Rocket Man" Johnathon, 2010. *A Missile Guided Infusion Trash Solution for an Event Horizon Safe Trash Launch Method* :: Journal of Ballistic Refuse

7. Principeps Quarkson, 2011. *Of Railguns and Red Tape: An Analysis of Failed Black Hole Waste Transportation* :: Journal of Ballistic Refuse

8. Gimble B. Higgenbotham, 2017. *Human Hamster Wheels as a Renewable Energy Source for Black Hole Launch Solutions* :: Journal of Ballistic Refuse

9. Sphagioli N. Matt-Bolls, 2018. *The Cost of Doing Business: Tragedies and Triumphs in Black Hole Operations* :: Annals of Cosmic Labor and Legalities

10. Finning T Stretch, 2023. *Robots or Time-Dilated Humans? A Cost-Benefit Analysis in Black Hole Proximity Labor* :: Singularity Workforce Innovations

11. Booker J. Whorff, 2015. *Particle Accelerators as a Matter Shortage Solution* :: Journal of Spindly Wire Innovations

12. B. McGraw, 2002. *CERN Experiment Disproves Physics! Or just bad Measurements* :: Journal of Astrological Big Data Ecology

13. Neutron, Jimmy, 2018. *Gotta Blast Some Fusion Energy: How Cyberpunk 2077 is Powering Our Future* :: Journal of Speculative Fusion Technologies

14. MythBusters Seasons 1-19, nearly every episode

15. Hawkinfield Geralderbrother, 2023. *Fusion Energy: Why It's Always 10 Years Away* :: Journal of Impossible Goals

16. Microplasticson Junks, 2024. *Microplastics in the Oceans and Why Your Genitalia Don't Work No More* :: Journal of Marine Recycling Catastrophes

6

Pink and Fire: Computational Fluid Dynamics Simulation Analysis of My Recent Gender Reveal Party Disaster

Dr. Melba McCormick[1]

[1] Department of Advanced Physics in Motherhood, Cranberry-Lemon University, Pittsburgh, PA, USA

Abstract

In my disastrous gender reveal for our unexpected girl, Alice, a chain reaction involving confetti, a leaf blower, and eighteen tubes of smokeless pink powder has rendered my she-shed unfit for craft night. Despite the unexpected nature of this gender reveal disaster, my insurance company refuses to honor my policy to cover the burning down of my backyard craft shed, estimated at a value of $10,000, and $3,000 of craft supplies and gardening equipment. In this paper, we will use a **Computational Fluid Dynamics (CFD)** engine, **Gender Reveal Simulation (GRSim)**, mandated in my insurance policy, to lower my deductible to show that this fire was a freak accident. We will develop a turbulence, combustion, radiation, and pyrolysis model to show that we were cursed with the perfect storm of pink-colored corn starch and Holi dust canons, ignited by a confetti-clogged leaf blower with a factory defect, causing a massive twenty-foot fireball that $1,000-a-year licensed software could not have predicted.

Keywords: Gender Reveal Party, Computational Fluid Dynamics, Pink Dust Canons, Confetti Clouds, Crafting Shed, Insurance Scam, Gender Reveal Simulation, Arson Investigation, Firework Free Reveal, It's a Girl!

1. Introduction

My shed is ruined, and the insurance company, Guardian Umbrella, is screwing me over! Gender reveal parties are becoming more of a nuisance when it comes to arson investigations, so I took out a specific policy for my upcoming backyard BBQ and gender reveal. The policy required careful planning and detailing of the reveal, a strict NO FIREWORKS policy, a safety review board, a fire marshal inspection, the use of smokeless powder, and a pricey computational fluid dynamics simulation that I wanted anyway. I wanted to make sure the effect was magical in the sim before putting in the effort to plan it. I've sunk most of my life savings into my current suburban home and did not want to risk it, so I took the policy following all of the precautions, simulation and all.

Now the insurance company's stiffing me out of $13,265.30 because they think I ran the numbers wrong! Little does this company know that they're dealing with the wrong policyholder, who is an expert in simulations [1]! I'm double-checking the numbers, all of the models of our materials, and flow patterns, and it's looking more and more like this was a total freak accident that Gender Reveal Simulation (GRSim) could not have predicted. Additionally, I would like the $1,000 back I spent on this useless piece of software. An intern could have vibe-coded a better simulator!

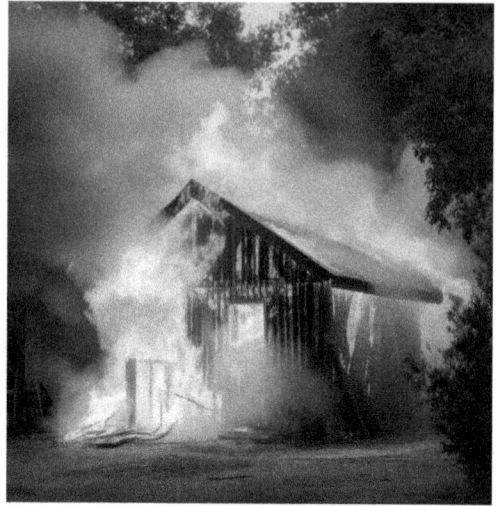

Figure 6.1: My shed on fire

2. Background

Beginning as a quaint American cake-based ritual in the 2000s, the gender reveal party has figuratively and literally exploded into American society. It was everything Americans loved about a party... Going Big. The Fourth of July was previously the only fire-based holiday, but the fireworks and explosion-based gender reveal party mixed with vloggers in the 2010s, leading to the practice getting bigger and bigger until they began causing major forest fires [2], a deadly plane crash [3], an outbreak of blue powder-based popcorn lung [4], and the deadly eruption of gang violence in a Chicago suburb [5]. As the danger made headline news, the practice grew because of one inconvenient fact: Americans love danger.

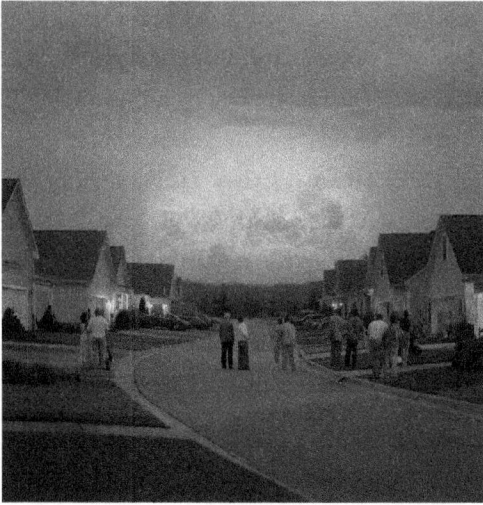

Figure 6.2: The day of the Great Chicago Gender Reveal Disaster

It was only after these deadly incidents that companies such as our own insurers, Guardian Umbrella Insurance Company, began offering gender reveal party-specific insurance policies, and real-world risk mitigation techniques began to form to prevent such tragedies. As the California couple who caused a 22,000-acre wildfire from their smoke-generating pyrotechnic device faces jail time, many began flocking to the robust insurance policy instead of just getting a lame pink or blue cake.

In order to facilitate proper risk mitigation, the simulation engine GRSim was developed. Insurance companies quickly determined that their policies would attract the wrong type of risk-takers and took it upon themselves to develop not only risk mitigation procedures but a full Computational Fluid Dynamics (CFD) simulation engine. Through GRSim, expecting couples could lay out the locations of smoke poppers, confetti, BBQ grills, and flammable objects so that it may run a variety of wind pattern sims to determine the amount of risk for their insurance policy. While the provided software uses a $1,000-a-year-per-user license, and the median gender reveal fire risk will ruin a good boot stamping out a grass fire, the upward tail expected risk of the average gender reveal party may exceed $5,000 due to the enormous risk of the party going wild. It turns out, apparently, this policy allows the insurance company to determine that every user used the software incorrectly... surprise, surprise... Thus, we must show it wasn't our misuse.

3. Numerical Methods

In order to generate the governing equations of our simulation, the first principle of physical laws was used to determine Newtonian fluid motion to include conservation of mass, momentum, and energy. Despite the advertising of the smokeless pink/blue powder poppers, our smoke reveal canons were best fit with a low-Mach number fluid motion, so Favre-filtered equations were used. This paper leverages research from [6], which utilizes the Fire Dynamics Simulator to improve upon GRSim.

3.1 Turbulence Model

The backend of the GRSim implements Large-Eddy Simulation (LES) to handle sub-models at a sub-grid length scale, despite the simulation engine handling our half-acre backyard. This allows for large and small eddy currents to be handled by GRSim. Turbulent viscosity was determined using a Smagorinsky subgrid-viscosity model [7]. Because we were more concerned with hotter objects causing turbulence, an additional model was integrated into the simulation developed by Lisa Smithers [8] to model optical turbulence from a hot new intern in a Cranberry-Lemon optics lab. If the model can generate an object as hot as Todd (*Figure 6.3*), we think it can model the heat of our smokeless pink poppers.

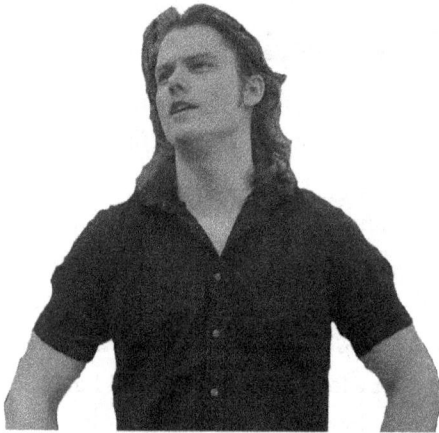

Figure 6.3: Todd

3.2 Combustion Model

While GRSim uses the single-step combustion model taught in high school, the model from the FDS utilized in [6] implements a two-step model representing the mixture fraction approach, which models fuel and oxygen burn

instantly when mixed. As we will discuss later, the contents of our pink smokeless poppers, when in the presence of an ignition source, will combust instantly at the density observed at my party. Following the insurance policy procedure, we waited for the wind to die down for an under-ventilated environment, which, further research revealed, after my claim was rejected by Guardian Umbrella, is the worst-case scenario for these pink smokeless poppers [9].

In a single-step combustion reaction mechanism, fuel and air combust immediately, while the two-step combustion model tracks the CO intermediate product, as shown in the following equations.

Step 1:

$$C_xH_yO_zN_aM_b + v_{O_2}O_2 \rightarrow v_{H_2O}H_2O + v_{CO}CO + v_s soot + v_{N_2}N_2 + v_M M$$

Step 2:

$$v_{CO}\left(CO + \frac{1}{2}O_2\right) \rightarrow v_{CO}CO_2$$

3.3 Radiation Model

While a traditional radiation heat transfer model involves the emission of EM waves from the ignition source to the solid fuel and the O_2 gas particles, the tragic consequences of my gender reveal party involved a gaseous form of $C_2 + O_2$ and other highly combustible carbon-based powders shot at a high velocity from our eighteen tube poppers. It did not help that it was a hot day, and we had left our tube poppers in the sun to heat up. With the pink powder-based fuel mixed ominously within the oxygenated environment, an updated radiation model in GRSim showed that we should never have been allowed to use those poppers in any environment, even though they were explicitly allowed by my insurance policy!

To allow GRSim to accommodate our pink poppers, ordinary differential equations were integrated in discretized control volumes to calculate the band-mean absorption coefficients using the unfortunately named *gray gas assumption*. As a cursory analysis of the radiation cloud was analyzed, it appeared that the highly reflective pink powder accelerated the exploding fireball, and I may not have been writing this paper if we were expecting a son and we used a less reflective blue powder.

3.4 Pyrolysis

To capture the gasification phase of our seemingly already gaseous pink powder, the Pyrolysis model was updated to ensure that our burning solid material was already gas. While the true gasification process involves multiple steps as in our combustion model, we assume a single-step process, leaving the model implemented in GRSim alone. As shown in the equation below, once applied to a gaseous cloud of hot pink dust, it makes no sense that these poppers use powder and not smoke. Utilizing Arrhenius's form, the combustible process may be expressed in the equation below:

$$r_{i,j} = \left(\frac{p_{s,i}}{p_{s0}}\right)^{n_{s,ij}} A_{ij} exp\left(-\frac{E_{ij}}{RT_s}\right)$$

Where r(i,j) is the rate of reaction for the ith mass component and jth consumed reaction, where p represents the density of the powdered pink cloud material. Finally, the A/E components show the pre- and post-exponential activation energy of the Arrhenius chemical process, solving for 8.314 J/(mol x K). As warned in [10], once estimated values for

pink gender reveal smoke poppers are applied to the Arrhenius expression, a deadly, eyebrow-apocalypse-inducing fireball becomes inevitable once introduced to any sort of open flame or even a spark. To quote the analysis in [10], "When the pyrolysis process begins in the pink gaseous cloud, there is no stopping it. If in a low to medium turbulence density, you'd better hope that there is no ignition source near the deadly cloud of pink powder, because if there is, there is no amount of firefighting equipment that could prevent the deadly fireball, even in expert hands. If it weren't specifically outlawed by the Geneva Convention, it would be an unstoppable weapon of war."

3.4 Material Properties

Though any exterior damage caused by the all-encompassing flaming fireball has been purely cosmetic or solved by sending my nephew to three sessions of child therapy, the primary discrepancy of the GRSim analysis was the destruction of my backyard gardening and craft shed. Because the non-jail-broken version of GRSim did not allow me to include all the material properties of my craft shed, I naturally had to add some functionality. By adding in the evidently highly flammable fabrics and 70s wallpaper, the enhanced GRSim showed a vulnerability that the standard release CFD analysis did not show. By administering a simple calorimeter test on the primary materials found in my destroyed craft shed, I found the values necessary to analyze the effect of a potential fireball on the one space I have for myself.

The results are shown in *Table 6.1.*

Material	Pine Exterior	70s Wallpaper	Assorted Fabrics	Wooden Tools
Specific heat (kJ/kgK)	1.38	1.02	1	1.52
Conductivity (W/(mK))	0.14	0.13	0.1	0.1
Density (kg/m^3)	489	120	100	670
Heat of combustion (kJ/kg)	14500	15500	15000	523
A	1.89e10	2.8e14	4.28e14	1.92e10
E	1.51e5	1.8e5	2.02e5	1.62e5
Heat of reaction (kJ/kg)	430	2500	3000	440

Table 6.1: Material properties for GRSim of my craft shed

4. Backyard Gender Reveal Party Reconstruction

As shown in *Figure 6.4*, the party poppers were all pointed away from my home and towards my craft shed, as per my plan, signed off by the fire marshal. Each popper, organized in two rows of 9, was tilted at a five-degree angle off the vertical axis. Not included in the officially signed-off gender reveal plan was the sudden low breeze, carrying the deadly pink dust clouds towards the cloud of confetti released in a swirl from its hopper bin away and back towards the leaf blower. Though we have no estimation of how strong the breeze was, it was only slight enough to carry the

powder without dispersing the material into a low-density cloud.

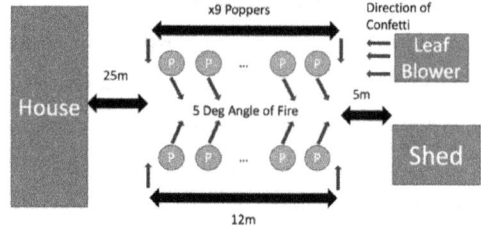

Figure 6.4: Backyard configuration (not drawn to scale)

4.1 Confetti Spread

As shown by the eight tilted black arrows in *Figure 6.4*, the leaf blower against the environmental wind of my backyard, against the cold front, produced an unexpected catalyst. Unfortunately for the already problematic GRSim, the mesh grid CFD solution was too small to detect the back-spreading eddy carrying a dangerous amount of thin papered foil and confetti back into our family leaf blower.

4.2 Leaf Blower Engine Malfunction

For some sadistic reason, after-action reports found that the confetti used small wires of aluminum to straighten out the confetti with no regard for the potential risk of short-circuiting a nearby leaf blower. As shown in the air current simulation I cooked up myself with no help from the GRSim software, which I now completely distrust, the back-eddy currents of confetti would very likely filter in aluminum-layered confetti through the air filtration unit of our leaf blower, and into the covered circuitry, causing a spark. All it took was one spark.

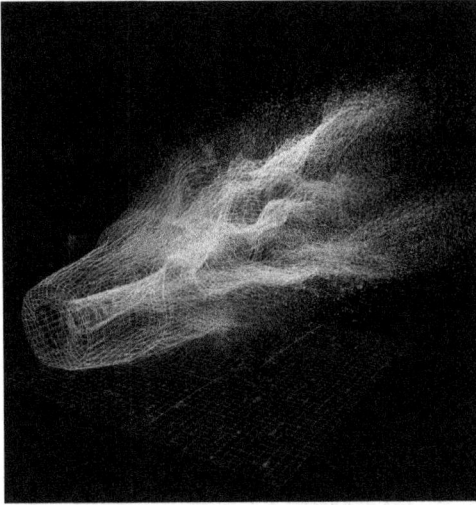

Figure 6.5: CFD-produced mesh grid of leaf blower-induced confetti eddy currents

4.3 Pink Powder Cannon Spread

Given an initial propulsion of 20g of gunpowder in our pink party poppers, we modeled the powder density spread with an initial 100-200km/hr, which showed a 10m spread away from the poppers around our backyard party. Adhering to the plan suggested and signed off by the fire marshal, we pointed the powder cannon tubes directly up at a five-degree tilt toward the shed based on the measured wind patterns.

4.4 Mesh Sensitivity

Despite evidence shown in [11] that the dangerous mixture of fine-grain corn starch and pink Holi powder may cause an explosive atmosphere, the default conditions with the updated models from section two continued to show a safe gender reveal party.

Though the simulation was numerically stable, GRSim was not sensitive enough. It was only once the mesh grid sensitivity was decreased from a 0.2m x 0.2m x 0.2m grid to a 0.01m x 0.01m x 0.01m grid in the jailbroken process (the maximum sensitivity capable) and run overnight on my work cluster that any danger was observed in the simulation from the pink death cloud.

4.5 Uncontrollable Fire Spread to Craft Shed

After re-running the simulation in GRSim with the party poppers at the required sensitivity, the updated models from section two, the inclusion of the new leaf blower, and the confetti model ignition source, we determined the cause. Similar to my cousin's recorded video footage, the new GRSim results showed a rapidly expanding flame ball engulfing not just my father's eyebrows, our last good camping chair, and other innocent objects, but a sizable and prolonged flame completely engulfing my now destroyed craft shed.

5. Results and Discussion

Re-running the simulation in the default and correcting the configuration, the events of the disaster measured through recorded video footage were timed in relation to how fast each object was engulfed in flames.

The results are shown in *Table 6.2*.

	GRSim (default)	Recorded Footage	GRSim (Corrected)
Father's Eyebrows	N/A	0.12s	0.08s
Good Camping Chair	N/A	0.04s	0.02s
Twinky, the Garden Gnome	N/A	0.23s	0.19s
My Hydrangea Bush	N/A	0.31s	0.29s
Bag Toss Hole	N/A	0.26s	0.24s
Crafting Shed	N/A	0.52s	0.51s

Table 6.2: Simulation vs measured results

Without the need for deep analysis, GRSim performed much better when calibrated far outside of the recommended defaults of my insurance policy. After 100 simulations, testing every possible wind pattern, not one default GRSim run resulted in a destructive fireball costing me a minimum of $13,000 and the sentimental value of my hydrangea bush.

Once corrected, GRSim predicted the speed and spread of the fireball with extreme precision, with a regular 10-40m/s speed bias. The air was likely more humid than input in the simulation, or some other unknown factor slowed down the explosion in the real gender reveal party.

6. Conclusion

As proven in this paper, there is no feasible way anyone could have predicted the loss of my craft shed, given the mandatory precautions of my insurance policy. It took extensive research and additional modeling work that any reasonable policyholder should not have to undergo to mitigate the risk of a leaf blower-ignited fire. Even in the presence of a spark, the default parameters of GRSim did not predict the explosive atmosphere of a typical pink dust cloud at the default $0.2m^2$ grid sensitivity. I'm not doing this analysis just for me and my shed, but for all of the victims out there getting stiffed by stubborn insurance agencies. It's time we fight back with science and a more robust Computational Fluid Dynamics simulation framework!

References

1. Melba McCormick, 2022. *Novel Techniques for Random Number Generation: Toddler Behavioral Sampling* :: Journal of Astrological Big Data Ecology

2. *California Couple whose gender-reveal party sparked a wildfire charged with 30 crimes* – The Guardian: https://www.theguardian.com/us-news/2021/jul/21/couple-gender-reveal-party-wildfire-charged

3. *Pilot Dies after plane crashes during gender reveal party in Mexico* – CNN: https://www.cnn.com/2023/09/04/americas/mexico-gender-reveal-plane-crash-scli-intl/index.html

4. *Are gender reveal parties spreading popcorn lung? Shakey evidence says maybe* :: Nervous News Network

5. *Two dead and eighteen wounded when gender reveal party misinterpreted as gang signals* :: The Moral Outrage Weekly

6. Yuen, Anthony Chun Yin & Yeoh, Guan & Alexander, Bob & Cook, Morgan. (2014). "Fire scene investigation of an arson fire incident using computational fluid dynamics-based fire simulation." *Building Simulation*. 7. 10.1007/s12273-014-0164-9.

7. Smagorinsky J (1963). "General circulation experiment with primitive equations: Part I. The basic experiment." *Monthly Weather Review*, 91: 99–164.

8. Lisa Smithers, 2023. *Optical Turbulence Characterization and Wiener Filtering of Hot New Intern Induced Temperature Gradients* :: Journal of Astrological Big Data Ecology

9. Melba McCormick, 2023. *Gaseous Pink Death Cloud: Never Pop a Smokeless Powder Tube without Wind* :: Annals of Celebration Technology

10. Dr. K Offbrand Soda, 2021. *A Pyrotechnic Analysis of Pink Gaseous Powder.* Journal of Non-Banned Chemical Warfare

11. Kukfisz B, Piec R, 2021. *The Fire and Explosion Hazard of Colored Powders Used during the Holi Festival.* Int J Environ Res Public Health. 2021 Oct 21;18(21):11090. doi: 10.3390/ijerph182111090. PMID: 34769610; PMCID: PMC8583402.

[This page was left blank as an elaborate tax scheme.]

7

Congenital and Parent-of-Origin Prediction Factors and Risks of Baby Jazziness in American Live Births

Joseph "Baby Hands" McGraw[1,2]

[1] Department of Baby Catching and Internal Fetal Medicine, Cranberry-Lemon University Medical School, Pittsburgh, PA, USA

[2] Lead Vocalist, Piano Player, Drummer, Bass Player, and Producer of the Joe McGraw Experience

Abstract

In this paper, we're talking about jazzy babies. The association with the American **jenotype** and malformations of the jazz-rhythmic thorax glands is a well-studied risk, leaving many parents wondering whether or not their baby will be jazzy enough for their five-piece ensemble. While certain populations have been measured as 64% Jazzy on the Brubeck scale [1], there has been a decrease in **jenetic** jazz alleles across all demographic groups. While some believe that these factors may be caused by a change in cultural musical taste, many genetic predictors suggest a drop in jazzy jenes, which allow American children to follow a 5/6 Mixolydian swing beat with a flat eighth. In this study, we will provide two parental prediction factors measured in 813 families and three genetic prediction factors, which show up to a 1.42 factor (CI 95% 1.30,1.54; P=4.57×10^-7) increase in jazziness.

Keywords: Jazzy-Jenomics, Monk Jene, Jazzy Babies, Rhythmic Thorax Abnormality, Paternal-Jazz Risk Ratios

1. Introduction

Genetics is the code of life. Just like most computer code, it is largely undocumented and remains a mystery. **Jazz** is America's gift to the world of music and, jenetically speaking, a mystery. I put a ton of jazz in my labor and delivery playlists, and I only hear good things about it from my nurses. When they come out of that delivery room, I always hear the same thing from many of the parents. They say, "Dr. Joe? Do you think my baby's gonna be that jazzy?" Many may think that jazziness is a result of the influence of pre-existing musical genres, but the science has been clear that jazz is a jenetic abnormality, allowing certain blessed Americans to hear a melody where others hear noise, to feel a rhythm where most can't clap along, or to hear a song where there only seems to be an unrelated series of notes linked together by the fact that they came out of the same instrument within the same self-indulgent solo.

Jazz is not only an important piece of American cultural heritage, but it also gives society instrumental music that's actually interesting to listen to when you're reading or writing and can't listen to something with lyrics. While some say orchestral philharmonic or certain instrumental metal cores may fill that role, recent studies have found that people will judge you for being pompous or unnecessarily aggressive in large groups or crowds, with the exception of surf rock [2]. When you listen to jazz, you're just cool. When all other musical genres are analyzed, nothing beats jazz.

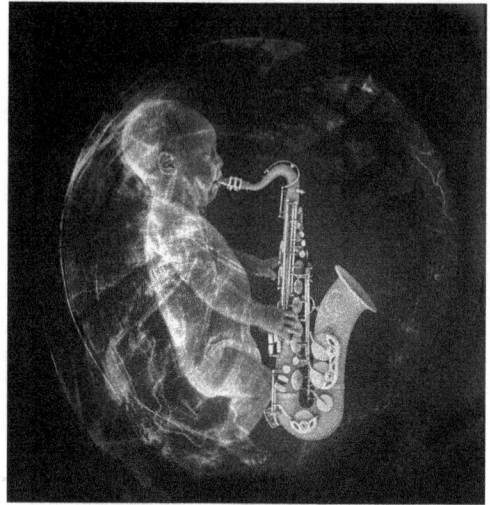

Figure 7.1: Ultrasound of a jazzy baby gestating in the womb, practicing blues scales on the Alto-Sax

But jazz is under attack. The percentage of the jazzy-jene demographic has been declining at a rapid rate [3]. Many propose that the youth have become too lazy and stick to simple chords and rhythms by TikTok-famous singer-songwriter types [4]. A cross-analysis has suggested that the authors of [4] were actually just old and out of touch [5]. Something else was going on. For jazz to flourish, a population of musicians must contain musicians at a rate of 5% or higher above the 96% Brubeck Scale (BS) threshold or the Coltrane Criterion (CC) for detecting a jazz master. Additionally, there must be a large enough population of jazz appreciators at a 30% BS or higher [6].

2. Background

This is not the first paper attempting to crack the jazz jenome. From 2008 to 2011, after the successful cloning of Dolly the sheep, an effort was underway to clone Louis Armstrong [7]. Despite having access to an excessive trumpet spit collection from Satchmo himself and an ungodly amount of funding when investors realized the market capital of obtaining another *What a Wonderful World* hit, from licensing to movies and wedding montages, the effort failed due to a lack of genetic modeling, and the research was unable to create a throat sound gravelly enough [8]. Additionally, the proto-Louises were too young to evaluate and got loose when someone compassionate left the gate to the holding pen open. Due to the controversial cheek enlargement surgeries, the corporate sabotage was believed to be an inside job.

Soon, evolving genomic technology such as DNA microarrays and advances in computing such as Windows XP, as well as the completion of the human genome project, accelerated the genetics revolution of the aughties. When everyone with a statistics background rebranded as a data scientist in the teens, Python became usable, and companies such as *23andMe* began collecting massive amounts of data so that people wouldn't need to scrapbook to know their origins; genetics caught on like wildfire. It was in our Jupyter Notebook-filled analysis bender that [9] was the first to map out the jazzy jene by swabbing the spit stains from the brass section of Cranberry-Lemon's prestigious jazz band. Following the landmark study, Blinky "Fingers" Malone was the first to notice a decline in the jazzy-jene population when comparing 90s and 00s microarray data to the present [3].

While some may believe that a drop in jazzy jenes will only cause an increase in boring normie rock or more country ballads, jazzy jenes are known to prevent serious diseases. Shown in [10], an increase in jazzy jenes showed an incredibly strong immune response to fratty behavior such as drinking hard seltzer and wearing salmon colored polo shirts while listening to songs about chicken-fried steaks.

Some traditional medical practitioners have not been favorable to jazzy jenes. Dan Smith was alarmed by a high correlation measured between jazzy jenomics and cardiac arrhythmias [11]. It was later shown in a spite paper [12] that the measured arrhythmias from [11] were actually a bebop beat and that "Dan Smith don't know the difference between a snare-snap march and a Swing-drop-scuttle and should not be allowed to practice medicine." [12] then showed that the arrhythmia-prone hearts were not only resistant to cardiac complications but that they could feel. Like, really *feel*.

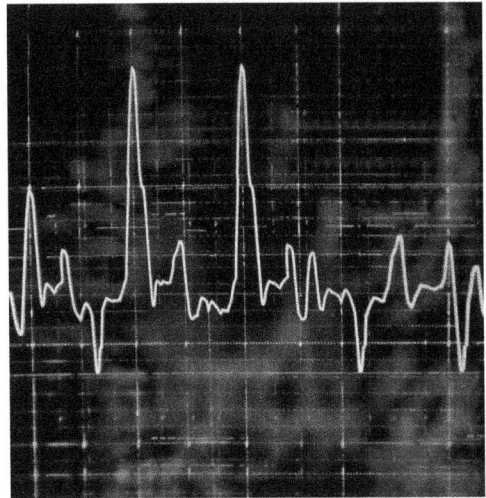

Figure 7.2: Poly-rhythmic EKG of a class 6 jazz legend

3. Parental Predictors

Children taking after their parents isn't just a concept my father refuses to believe in; it's science! It's also the easiest way to predict whether or not a parent's baby's gonna be jazzy. When it comes to parental predictions of baby jazziness, it is difficult to nail down causation and correlation [13]. Some parents may have recessive jazzy jenes, which may produce a jazzy baby from not-so-jazzy parents.

Likewise, jazzy parental traits may manifest due to long-term second-hand or first-hand jazz exposure after birth, as shown in [14]. As discussed in [14], given enough second- or first-hand exposure to open-air jazz at twenty or more album-years[1], a parent's genetic make-up may mutate into a jazzstrocity. Whether or not a parent's jenetic makeup is mutated before conceiving a child, due to the likeliness of the child's second-hand exposure to jazz post birth and mid-adult transformation, it all ends up coming out in the wash. In this paper, two qualitative parental metrics will be presented to predict baby jazziness.

3.1 Toe-Tappin-Test

If you, as the practicing physician, have the opportunity to meet the parents before the birth, here's an easy little test you can do. Play something with a swing in it. Maybe start with something simple like an old Big Bad Voodoo Daddy classic and see if you get some tapping going from the parents. Now, if you want to really confirm your hypothesis and achieve a strong statistical result, a sure-fire method was developed in [15]. Play Herbie Hancock's "Watermelon Man" and start a timer. As the song progresses from the Pygmy yelping to a fat funk baseline, notate when the toe tapping starts and fit the exponential distribution equation below, which was calibrated in [15].

$$Watermelon\ Man(jazz)\ =\ \hat{\lambda}e^{-\hat{\lambda}t}$$

Estimate lambda by dividing the number of trials by the sum of seconds before toe tapping. If lambda is greater than two minutes, then the subject is unlikely to be jazzy. If it's less than one minute, then the subject is extremely jazzy, and funky.

3.2 Rhythmic Thorax Gland Abnormality

As previously mentioned, from the spite paper [12], jazzy people often have different heart patterns. This has been analyzed from the autopsies of the bodies of the South Detroit High Top Steppers Drum and Bass marching band after the tragic dump truck St Patty's Day massacre. Jazz rhythms come from an abnormally large thorax gland in the lower abdomen. Once thought of as vestigial, the rhythmic thorax regulates the rhythm center of the body. Centering the rhythm in the gut and not in the brain threw off scientists for decades.

Most humans have a medium-sized rhythmic thorax about the size of a quarter, connected through neural tissues and blood vessels to sense heart pressure. As jazz jenes transform the body, the rhythmic thorax can grow as large as a plum, allowing for the body to sense and respond to complex polyrhythms.

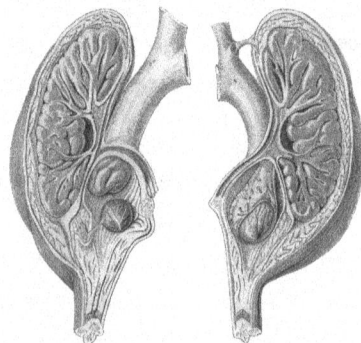

Figure 7.3: Anterior and Uncleterior Rhythmic Thorax Gland

---

1   An album-year is a common metric to measure a patient's exposure to jazz in which one album-year is equal to listening to one jazz album per day for one year. Album-years increase as patients are exposed to harder stuff such as Coltrane or Mingus.

To assess the subject's rhythmic thorax without an ultrasound, subject the subject to a series of differing, unrelated time signatures. Measure the subject's heartbeat. Be sure to mix in some 7/6s with some 9/4s and rarely stick with 3/3s. Every thirty seconds, shout "NOT MY TEMPO!" and note their ability to keep up with three or more simultaneous beats. Feel how swollen their thorax is just above the patient's left hip bone.

4. Genetic Predictors

Jazzy jenomics works when mutated jazz cells pass a special type of protein around called a head. While many cells in a non-jazzy body may form completely different proteins based on function, a jazzy cell will always contain head proteins. These proteins may metabolize through scripted or unscripted means or pathways. Whether the head protein follows a diminished scale or an augmented 7th, it eventually turns the whole body into jazz. These jene types or alleles can be studied by measuring deletions and additional copies of particular patterns in the jazz jenome, also known as Copy Number Variants (CNVs).

4.1 MINGUS Allele Imputation

One of the well-known jazz-head jenes is the MINGUS allele. While this allele is simple to upregulate, it is a rare trace gene, which does not often occur naturally in many jazzy jenes unless exposed to secondhand jazz. Any instance of this allele type is a clear sign that a baby will be jazzy. Only the jazziest jenotypes can handle this allele, as it adds in noisy cacophonous signals to the rhythmic thorax at blisteringly fast speeds. While living harmoniously in normal jazzy jenomes, a rare mutation of this allele in a non-jazzy jenome can result in chronic dizziness, tinnitus, and a loss of appetite.

4.2 4x4 Allele Gene Deletion

While making up the majority of non-jazzy jenomic rhythmic thorax proteins, the 4x4 allele group is often deleted in a jazzy jenome. Throughout patients registering high on the BS spectrum, 4x4 Allele deletions can make it difficult for patients to follow generic rock, country, EDM, and nearly all church hymns. While some 4x4 traces may be found, it is often 93% deleted from a jenome to make room for other rhythmic proteins.

4.3 MONK Allele Abnormality

Normally only activated by alcohol, Monk Alleles fit achromatically within head proteins. Flying in the face of all jenetics, the MONK Allele group's achromatic arrangements fit in all the wrong SNPs (Single Nucleotide Polymorphisms) within a chromosome in an extremely unnatural way that just seems so right. It is a modern medical mystery how the MONK jene's honky tonk jenome sequence doesn't kill everyone that has it or at least give patients a grab bag of rare diseases, but it works.

5. Data Collection

Despite a very confusing email chain explaining what we were trying to study, we were finally allowed to use the National Birth Defects Prevention Study (NBDPS). When using the jazz detection protocols outlined in [16], we focused our analysis on 813 families who were interviewed in person.

Each patient was evaluated on the Brubeck Scale and additional buccal swab kits were used to collect saliva residue after we asked each participant to toot the jazziest they could into a special trombone as detailed in [16]. Of the 813 families, 127 were excluded. Some were excluded because they had to leave the interview halfway to catch a television show (n=9), more were deemed ineligible because their trombone toot wasn't jazzy enough or produced an insufficient amount of saliva (n=23), and finally, most had to be removed from our results because we just couldn't understand what they were saying (n=93). They may have been extremely jazzy, but there was no way to measure it.

Due to the vibrational data held within the jazzy allele patterns, genetic material was transformed into the Fourier domain before applying log-normal models to each summary statistic. Unfortunately, they weren't normally distributed, and by not normally distributed, I don't mean non-Gaussian. We couldn't find a distribution that fit any of the data and had to cobble together several and invent a new distribution using some kernel fit operation nonsense we hand-waved to our reviewers.

6. Results and Discussion

Once each of the jenotypes was transformed into the Fourier domain and analyzed using the special new distribution, a total of 1630 SNPs were included in the final analysis. 1318 of those SNPs appeared to be positively correlated with an increase in jazzy behavior in subjects, while the remaining jenes appeared to show negative correlation. The results of each of the jenes and the positive and negative paternally derived risk factors are shown in *Table 7.1* for the top 20 jenes. Additionally, the pathway methods in which each gene is metabolized and the genotype is shown.

The variety of jenes' jenotypes and pathways show that the methods in which jazz may jenetically manifest in a patient is diverse and chaotic. In contrast, many jenetic risks to babies not being jazzy appear to be highly correlated in an uptick in the 4x4 time signature allele or the existence of the AC/DC rock gene or the generic country Garth BROOKS gene. As expected, MINGUS and MONK are the highest predictor SNPs.

Pathway	Jene Symbol	dbSNP ID	Chromosome	Jenotype	Paternally-Derived Relative Risk (95% CI)	P-Value for Paternal vs. Maternal Effect
Trans-Lead Sheets	MINGUS	rs1234567	2	Avant-Garde	1.23 (1.12, 1.44)	2.66×10^{-6}
Feels	MILES	rs2345678	3	Fusion	0.35 (0.24, 0.48)	1.22×10^{-5}
Feels	MONK	rs3456789	4	Bebop	1.42 (1.30, 1.54)	4.57×10^{-7}
Groovin	GUARALDI	rs4567890	9	Cool	0.29 (0.16, 0.39)	9.88×10^{-6}
Trans-Lead Sheets	HANCOCK	rs5678901	20	Post-Bop	0.31 (0.21, 0.45)	3.33×10^{-6}
Groovin	BRUBECK	rs6789012	13	Cool	0.27 (0.15, 0.38)	6.55×10^{-6}
Trans-Lead Sheets	COLTRANE	rs7890123	10	Free Jazz	0.40 (0.27, 0.52)	2.14×10^{-7}
Full Scores	GERSHWIN	rs8901234	1	Orchestral	0.36 (0.24, 0.49)	7.81×10^{-6}
Feels	ELLA	rs9012345	7	Swing	0.32 (0.19, 0.43)	1.05×10^{-5}
Trans-Lead Sheets	ARMSTRONG	rs1123456	4	Dixieland	0.38 (0.26, 0.51)	4.01×10^{-6}
Trans-Lead Sheets	COREA	rs2234567	5	Fusion	0.26 (0.14, 0.37)	8.94×10^{-6}
Feels	ELLINGTON	rs3345678	7	Big band	0.28 (0.17, 0.39)	2.72×10^{-5}
Trans-Lead Sheets	HOLIDAY	rs4456789	2	Swing	0.34 (0.22, 0.47)	1.19×10^{-6}
Trans-Lead Sheets	MCLAUGHLIN	rs5567890	8	Fusion	0.39 (0.25, 0.50)	5.49×10^{-7}
Feels	PARKER	rs6678901	5	Bebop	0.33 (0.20, 0.44)	9.71×10^{-6}
Full Scores	GETZ	rs7789012	11	Bossa Nova	0.37 (0.23, 0.48)	3.87×10^{-6}
Groovin	SIMONE	rs8890123	49	Soul	0.30 (0.18, 0.41)	2.53×10^{-5}

Full Scores	AC/DC	rs9901234	5	Rock	-1.25 (0.13, 0.36)	6.32×10^{-7}
Full Scores	4x4 TIME	rs1012345	2	Hymn	-1.41 (0.28, 0.53)	1.88×10^{-5}
Full Scores	BROOKS	rs2113456	7	Country	-1.22 (0.10, 0.35)	4.68×10^{-5}

Table 7.1: Risk ratios (RR) and 95% confidence intervals (CI) with P-values for pater-nally-derived effects for the top 20 SNPs

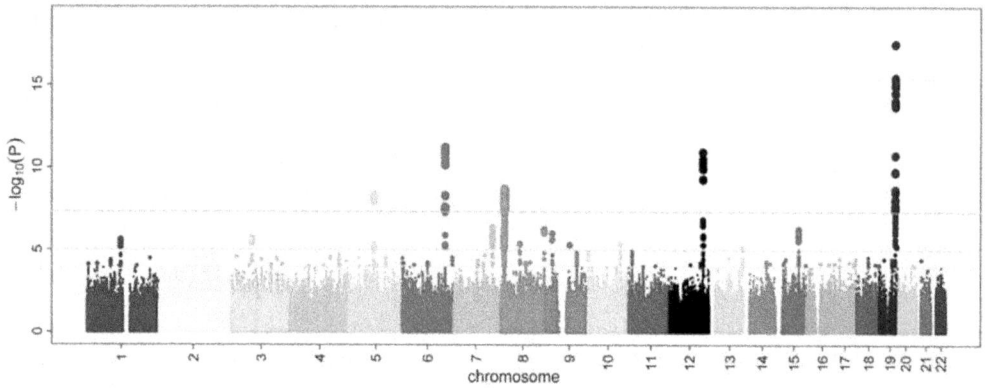

Figure 7.4: A normal genomic Manhattan plot (M. Kamran Ikram et al., CC BY 2.5, via Wikimedia Commons)

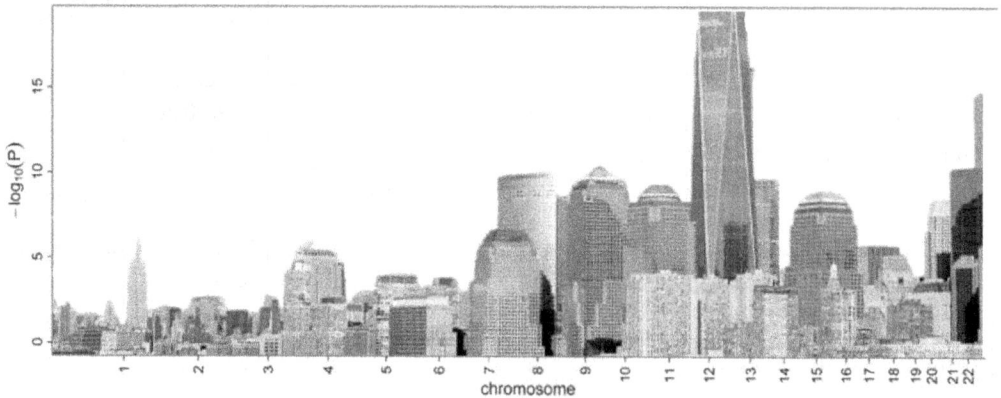

Figure 7.5: A Manhattan plot of a jazzy baby's jenomic sequence

Jenetics, like jazz, is full of noisy signals that don't make sense until you put it all together into a human and have the feels to understand it. For those who can't do that with raw data, there's the log scale and clever transforms. When the genetic predictors are fully shown in log scale through a Manhattan plot (*Figure 7.5*) and shown in comparison to a non-jazzy normal genome (*Figure 7.4*), the jenetic jazz effect becomes blindingly obvious. Somehow, in some way, the Manhattan plot converges into Manhattan. It doesn't make a lot of sense until you squint your eyes and let it go fuzzy, then there it is—the big apple.

Although conclusive, many babies were found to be jazzy without jazzy jenomes, as described in this paper, at an 8.2% rate. Within the interview, it was shown that second-hand jazz exposure due to pushy Spotify daily wind-up playlists often led to jazzy babies even without finding a high concentration of jazznetic material correlating to other jazzy babies. Ya know what didn't show up in the jazzy babies was doing jazz hands. Absolutely zero. The only subjects measured doing jazz hands were extremely unjazzy dads making a joke about our study during the interview process.

Future endeavors for our project include looking at epigenetic changes present in those with jazzy exposure later in life and determining which environmental factors are most associated with upregulation of the proteins in the rhythmic thorax gland. Specifically, we plan to investigate the role of proximity to jazz clubs, phases of the moon, and the number of tritone substitutions encountered per week.

7. Conclusion

There is hope in the resurgence of jazz. With a stronger, more rigorous understanding of what makes a baby jazzy, we can decrease the dangerous risks of babies being born in a flat time signature. By upregulating and selecting highly correlated jazz jenes, we can guarantee babies will not go through life not knowing the pleasure of a smooth jazz piano solo and won't be lying when they tell their friends that they enjoy Miles's experimental stuff. This isn't to say that we can't love and take care of non-jazzy babies—they need our help more than any, but with the new advances in jenetics and a better understanding of the jazz jenome, few babies will suffer from not being jazzy.

8. About the Author

Joseph "Baby Hands" McGraw is a jazz enthusiast and baby catcher currently listening to Ella Fitzgerald records in Motown. His extensive educational background is diverse and has included research in areas such as keyboard clackiness, efficiency of various log splitting techniques, the chicken-allergen connection, and maximization of the length of the signout. He is the recipient of the National Amateur Lunar Visualization Society's 2022 Photo of the Year for his exceptional photo series featuring the most detailed photo of the Sea of Tranquility this decade. In his free time, he loves performing in triathlons: running the list, cycling blood pressures, and swimming in a sea of unnecessary consults.

References

1. Fatz "The Boots" Shorterly, 2012. *The Brubeck Scale: An Adaptable Metric on Jazziness* :: JenoJazz Studies Quarterly

2. Whisker Whammy Jenkins, 2016. *Non-Instrumental Music Alternatives to Jazz and Why You'll Always be Jivin' Back* :: Journal of Jenetic Grooves

3. Blinky "Fingers" Malone, 2015. *Cause for Alarm: Decline in Jazz Population Among Americans* :: Annals of Jazzy Jenomics

4. Arthur Boomer Johnson, 2014. *The Kids These Days Don't Listen to Good Music Anymore* :: Journal of Things That Should Stay Facebook Posts

5. Twinkles "Trombone" Taylor, 2014. *Arthur Boomer Johnson Sucks and is Out of Touch, the Kids LOVE Jazz* :: Journal of Improvisational Beats

6. Zippy "Zoot" Sanders, 2021. *Sustainable Jazz Population for Regenerative Groovetastic Cultural Environments* :: Journal of Chromojazz Explorations

7. Tootsie "Horns" McGee, 2008. *A Practical Approach to Cloning Louis Armstrong* :: Syncopation and Sequencing Studies LLC

8. "Boom-Boom Bass" Jackson, 2023. *Where are the Louis: A Limited Docuseries of the Louis Armstrong Cloning Disaster* :: Netflix

9. Scooter "Here Comes Trouble" McDoodle, 2022. *Mapping of the Jazzy Jenome* :: JazzAllele Insights

10. Tad "The Sexy Sax Man" Richards, 2018. *Live your Best Life: Health Benefits of Jazz* :: Rhythmic Jenomics Review

11. Dan Smith, 2016. *The Dangerous Negative Effects of Jazz: Arrhythmias, Sex, Alcohol, and More!* :: Annals of the Abstinence Mindset

12. John Midnight, 2019. *Positive Heart Effects of a Jazzy Rhythmic Thorax* :: Cool Cats Medical Research

13. Mae "Honey Lips" Turner, 2021. *Test before you Invest: Parental Predictors of Jazz Men and Women* :: Jazz Pulse Health Review

14. Stanley "Swing King" Rivers, 2021. *Ear Bathing Second-Hand Jazz Exposure Benefits and Risks* :: Blues and Medical Sciences Quarterly

15. Lionel "The Licks" Groover, 2017. *The Herbie Test: A Definitive Test for Jazztection in Adults over 23* :: Swingtime Health Journal

16. Jumpy Wobbles-Hat O'Reilly, 2023. *Jazz Jene Detection Database* :: Journal of HarmoJenetics Jazzology

8

Testicular Cancer Truck Nut Self-Examination for North American Pick-Ups: A Cost-Benefit Analysis

B. McGraw[1] and Joe "Baby Hands" McGraw[2]

[1] Department of Truck Care Analytics, Cranberry-Lemon University

[2] Center for Applications in Gentle Feels, Cranberry-Lemon University

Abstract

The United States Preventive Services Task Force (USPSTF) has recommended against testicular self-examinations (TSE) or clinical examination for testicular cancer screening in truck nuts of any make or model. This comes as no surprise as the USPSTF is heavily lobbied by the auto-manufacturing industry, which benefits from regularly servicing trucks suffering from cancer that has metastasized to the engine block. This paper discusses truck nut screening techniques and a cost-benefit analysis of everyday truck owners and field technicians regularly screening truck nuts. The cost of treating early-stage truck nut cancer can be as cheap as $1.97 for a replacement orange or $3.94 if cancer is detected in both truck nuts. If undetected, treatment could amount to an average of $29,997 in chemoil-change therapy or $50,000 in unmarked black market car parts and mechanic labor. As testicular truck nut cancer occurs in 5.7 out of 1,000 pick-ups, on average, between 50 and 100,000 miles, the additional four minutes of truck nut screening could save the average consumer $190.05 in truck nut cancer treatment!

Keywords: Truck, Nuts, Pick-Up Screening, Chemoil-Change Therapy, Testicular Cancer, Truck Care, Gentle Squeezing

1. Introduction

Screening another man's truck nuts is no longer just a bet stake. Despite my many letters to the NFL, we still don't have a blue-themed testicular cancer month, and many truck owners are unaware of the risks to their own truck nuts. Testicular cancer is detected in 80 trucks a year [1], and the risk of the mechanical work from such cancer risk scares 562 consumers a year into extended warranty scams [2]. Some truck owners may feel uncomfortable screening for lumps, particularly owners without private garages.

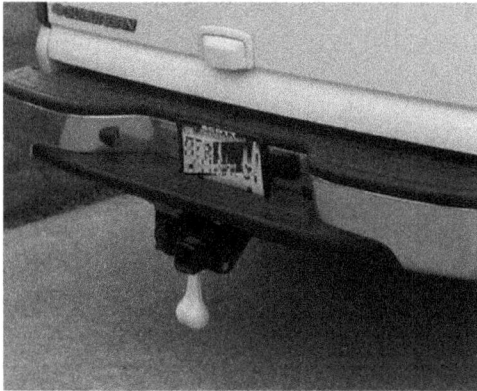

Figure 8.1: Truck nuts (The359, CC BY-SA 2.0, via Wikimedia Commons)

2. Background

Due to the average wear and tear from the elements, as well as sun and exhaust exposure, truck nut cancer is equal parts common and aggressive.

2.1 Timeline of Testicular Truck Nut Cancer

Very little is known about stage 0 of truck nut cancer, so let's skip that one; we assume it has something to do with abnormal cells. However, in stage 1, those abnormal cells begin to create a tumor, which causes discoloration and some minor swelling. Within pro-duce-based truck nuts, this is known as the "moldy stage." In stage 2, the tumor grows larger until it is the size of a penny and the consistency of corn pudding [3]. In stages 1 and 2, any truck owner should be capable of detecting a malignant lump with minor training. Depending on the aggressiveness of the truck nut tumor, it may take 6 to 12 months to progress from a stage 1 to stage 2 cancerous truck nut [4].

If left untreated for more than three months at stage 2, it will progress. In stage 3, the tumor will grow larger and begin spreading to the trailer hitch, brake lights, and, in some cases, deep within the tailpipe [5]. At this stage, some trucks may no longer be street legal and may even fail emissions tests. Finally, once a malignant truck nut lump bumps to stage 4, the cancer has metastasized into the engine block, which can only be treated with extremely costly mechanics in special fields. Late-stage cancerous truck nuts have been known to progress from a stage 3 to a stage 4 and untreatable cancer in just under four months [6].

2.2 Early Preventive Treatment

If caught early, the problem can be solved with low-risk surgery. If the tumor is small enough in early stage 2, it may be safely removed with an X-ACTO knife and some tweezers. If the lump has grown too large and is at risk of spreading locally to the flat bed, it is likely that one or both truck nuts must be removed and replaced with some tennis balls or oranges for vanity, even if deep down, it may feel like it'll never quite be the same. In 86% of testicular stage 1 and 2 cancers of truck nuts (72% of diesel burning), surgical removal is enough to prevent further complications [7].

Although these outcomes are not pretty, they are preferable to the alternatives if the truck nut cancer goes untreated.

After the cancer begins to spread from the truck nuts to the rest of the pickup, not only will the truck nuts need to be surgically removed, but the cancerous vehicle will potentially need to undergo multiple rounds of Chemoil-Change Therapy (CCT), which can cost the consumer tens of thousands of dollars even on a full warranty [8].

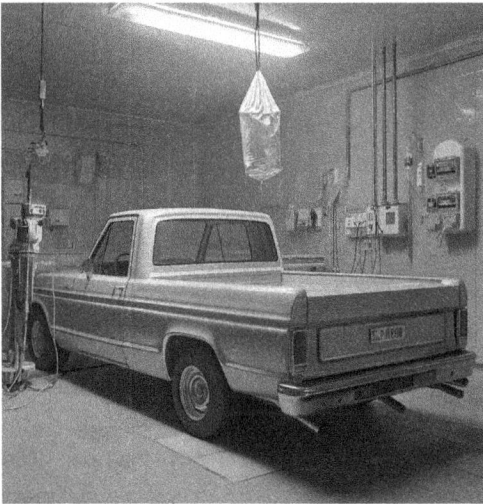

Figure 8.2: Cancerous truck undergoing Chemoil-Change Therapy (CCT) post-nut removal

3. Truck Nut Lump Screening Methodology

What you're gonna want to do first is wash your hands. You always wash your hands before and after. First, warm up some water on the stove or in a garden hose if it's a hot enough day. Soak the truck nuts in hot water. This relaxes the scrotum so that it's easy to feel the nuts through the produce bag they may be hanging from.

Next, examine each truck nut with both hands. Don't hold back. Hold the truck nuts between your thumb and middle fingers and roll them around firmly but gently. It is your truck, so you'd better treat it well. Feel around for any nodules or lumps, or any strange consistency or texture. Feel for the epididymis, as shown in *Figure 8.3*. After regularly checking your truck nuts, you should become familiar with them. This should be a painless screening, so if your car alarm goes off, that is not a good indication that your truck nuts are cancer-free.

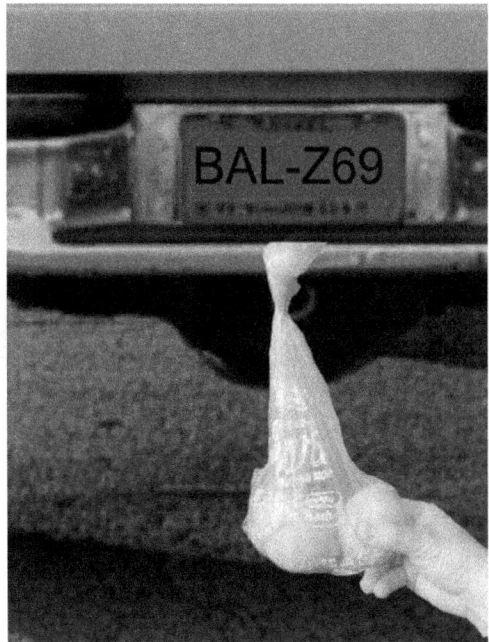

Figure 8.3: Examination technique (one hand)

4. Cost-Benefit Analysis

Feeling up your truck is free; CCT is not. Over a truck's lifetime, there is a 0.72% chance of developing truck nut cancer in trucks over 200,000 miles [1]. Assuming you already have an X-ACTO knife and tweezers, the cost of treating stage 1–2 testicular truck nut cancer maxes out at the cost of the replacement prosthetic of 2 x $1.97 for the oranges and produce bag [9].

According to [10], with regular screenings and the method discussed in section 3 of this paper, the average truck owner has an 88% chance of detecting lumps in their truck nuts at stage 1 or 2. Without screening, that probability drops to 0%.

The average stage 3 or higher truck nut cancer patient undergoes three rounds of CCT in treatment [11]. At an average consumer price of $9,999 with a coupon, truck nut testicular cancer costs on average $29,997, because those coupons are usually a cruel joke. At a 0.72% chance of developing truck nut cancer, the average consumer will spend an expected $215.98 on treatment versus the $25.93 it would cost if regularly screened.

5. Conclusion

You don't need a cost-benefit analysis to know that you don't want your truck nuts to get cancer. We all know that a truck's livelihood is worth a lot more than $29,997 when dealing with the side effects and time commitment of CCT. Not only will truck owners save money, but they will save towing power. Not all trucks are successfully treated and will end up rusting out in your front yard. Do what's right and squeeze those nuts every six months, and you could save a truck.

References

1. Dr. Roisin McTorque, PhD – International Council on Decorative Accessory Oncology, 2017. *Global Truck Nut Testicular Cancer Rates* :: Archives of Rear-End Oncology

2. Dr. Gregorio Hatch, MS, DPhil – Oxford Automotive Prosthetic Research Centre, 2019. *Consumer Risks of Predatory Warranty Schemes in Vehicular Oncology* :: Transmetallic Oncology & Screening Journal

3. Dr. Mallory Axlebaum, MD – Appalachian School of Automotive Embellishment Sciences, 2012. *Feelsology; Top 10 Food Comparison to Stage 3 Truck Nut Cancer* :: The Rust Belt Review of Auto-Genital Pathology

4. Dr. Tomas Gritsch, MD – Vienna Auto-anthropology Institute, 2022. *National Health Statistics in Vehicular Nut Lump Timelines of Stage 3-4 Trucklicular Cancer* :: International Journal of Symbolic Automotive Anatomy (IJSAA)

5. Dr. Lance Derrington, MD – Southern Truck Testicular Health Alliance (STTHA), 2016. *The Prostate of the Half Cab: A Case Study in Catalytic Converter Failure due to Stage 3 Truck Nut Testicular Cancer* :: Chemoil Therapeutics and Decorative Oncology Quarterly

6. Dr. Hal V. Linch, DO – Bureau of Undercarriage Oncology Research (BUOR), 2021. *Deadly Warning Signs: Metastasization Rates in Stage 4 Testicular Truck Nut Cancer* :: Scandinavian Journal of Chrome Preservation & Disease

7. Dr. Willem J. Grubb, MSc, FRVHO – Federation for Vehicular Hanging Ornamentation (FVHO), 2008. *Surgical Treatment of Stage 2 Malignant Truck Nut Lumps* :: Proceedings of the Annual Undercarriage Health Conference (AUHC)

8. Dr. Curtis Yawley, MD – American Society for Recreational Towing Medicine, 2009. *A Chemoil-Change Treatment Technique for Advanced Stage Truck Nut Cancer* :: Journal of Functional Auto-Testes Research (JFATR)

9.   Jack, Jimbo, and Guest Appearance Lee-
     Roy, 2017. *Jack and Jimbo's Sure Fire Truck
     Nut Budget Replacement* :: Jack and Jim-
     bo's YouTube Channel

10. Dr. Benjamin D. Grohl, MPH – Midwest
     Center for Metalloscrotal Studies, 2023.
     *Success Rates in Amateur Truck Nut Screen-
     ings* :: The Hanging Review: Biannual
     Journal of Peripheral Auto-Accessories

11. Prof Marianne Slag – School of Vehicular
     Anatomy, University of Axlebridge, 2020.
     *A Vehicular Life-Cycle of Chemoil-Change
     Treatment in Stage-3 Cancer Truck Nuts* ::
     Journal of Vehicular Urology & Applied
     Ornamentation (JVUAO)

[This page was left blank because this page is protected wetlands.]

9

Log-Log-Likeliwood of Black Walnut in Random Forestry

Wyatt "The Log Whisperer" Johnson[1,2,3,4,5]

[1] Department of Statistical Wood Studies, Cranberry-Lemon University, Pittsburgh, PA, USA

[2] Owner of Wyatt Johnson's Fine Furniture Warehouse, with half-price deals on cabinets and coffee tables this Presidents' Day! Pittsburgh, PA, USA

[3] Owner of Wyatt Johnson's Specialty Wood Depot LLC, If you can saw it, you can buy it here, Pittsburgh, PA, USA

[4] President, Treasurer, and Pot-Luck Organizer of the Royal American Selective Logging Society

[5] Chief Editor and Author of the Veneer Logging Magazine, 12 issues a year for only $60 per 6-month subscription. A TRUE BARGAIN with all the wisdom you'll gain!

Abstract

Black Walnut is one of the most valuable pieces of lumber you can naturally find in an American forest. A good log of Black Walnut could make $1,000 to $1,500 at a normal lumber warehouse, though a logger could make $2,000 easily at Wyatt Johnson's Specialty Wood Depot LLC because it's a business owned by loggers and not industrial capitalists. $2,000 will buy you a lot of Miller! Many hustlers out there, such as Samantha Greene, say they have the perfect system for finding the rarest trees in the forests of Appalachia, but they're only after your money. They don't have the mathematical background like I do. By using maximum log-log-likeliwood estimation to find valuable logs such as Black Walnut, I was able to pinpoint the most likely old-growth forests to turn my logging business even more profitable and find *Old Wilbur*, which was thought to only be a legend until this paper!

Keywords: Logs, Log Optimization, Log Likeliwood, Black Walnut Logs, Veneer Wood, Maximum, Chestnut, Loggin' Business, That Snake in the Grass Samantha Greene, 🌳, Woodstagram, REAL LOGGERS!, Making Money

1. Introduction

In my previous paper, *18 Secrets to a Profitable Specialty Wood Logging Industry* [1], I perfected logging. Now I have made it even more perfect! Using a **log-likeliwood estimator** and **Inverse Binomial Sampling (IBS)**, shown in [2], you can get rich OVERNIGHT! I come from a long family of academics and loggers. I didn't know it, but IBS runs in my blood. How else could I run the most profitable logging company East of the Mississippi?

1.1 Background

If yer a traditional logger like me, you'll know that the likeliwood function is the fundamental building block of any estimation algorithm. Many of the youths with their machine learning models, ChatGPTs, and Lime scooters probably haven't been properly edumacated in the realm of statistical inference. Their heads are filled with kooky liberal nonsense like generative AI or that environmentalist crap Samantha Greene pushes. A large ML model won't be able to implement the fruitful grand tradition you get from old hats like me. By instilling the Johnson family's patented 200-year-old secrets in logging into the parameters of joint probability distributions, a simple walk through the forest can help you find the most likely location of the finest and most valuable Black Walnut in the rolling hills of the Appalachians. These methods could easily be applied to American Chestnut, White Pine, or even Hard Maple. The newly Wyatt-Johnson-approved and owned **Log-Log-Likeliwood (LLL) estimator©**, heavily featured in this month's issue of Veneer Logging Magazine, will give you wealth you could never even dream of from yer logging business. As you can see from *Figure 9.1*, it's a beautiful wood! A real money-maker!

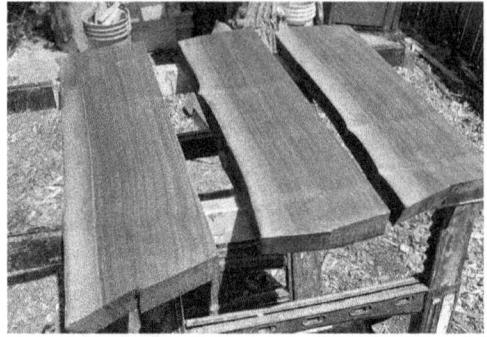

Figure 9.1: Beautiful and valuable Black Walnut (A. Drauglis from Washington, DC, USA, CC-BY 2.0, via Wikimedia Commons)

Using this method, you could find $1,000–2,000 worth of hardwood for just a Saturday's worth of work. Do this for an entire year twice a week and you're making $100,000–200,000 just walking through the forest. I'd recommend three times a week, so ya got time for church on Christmas and Easter. That's the sort of wealth you can achieve if you follow this easy-to-implement log-log-likeliwood estimation method! It's honest, hard work that makes the economy churn, not like that phony *Save the Forest* foundation, charging $500 a ticket to show off some boring oaks in an overpriced forestry reserve like that Samantha Greene pushes. She'll say my methods don't work [3] just because she's been trying to shut me down for a decade this last winter. She thinks I don't even care about the forest [4] but I do [5]. I'm a conservationist, the forest's my livelihood!

tribution of tree species. If you're slow like my son Cleatus, T stands for transpose not tree!

$$\overline{\overline{\text{🌳}}} = \left[\overline{\overline{\text{🌳}}_1}, \overline{\overline{\text{🌳}}_2}, \overline{\overline{\text{🌳}}_3}, \dots \overline{\text{🌳}}_M\right]^T$$

Then let Y represent the observed real-valued trees observed in a forest; if you're a REAL LOGGER, commonly notated as *RL*, N will be a very large number. If you don't think your Ns are big enough, consider taking my short course for only $295 at our annual Vegas conference, which includes a free catered lunch from Fire House Subs, *Mmm, Mmmm, Mmmm, Mmm... Mmmm... Toasty.*

$$Y = \left[\text{🌳}_1, \text{🌳}_2, \text{🌳}_3, \text{🌳}_4, \text{🌳}_5, \dots \text{🌳}_N\right]$$

The likeliwood of a particular distribution of tree species such as Black Walnut may be defined below as $LogLikelihood_n\left(\overline{\text{🌳}}\right)$. The trees you'll be wantin' to estimate should be self-evident to any *RL*, but that only scratches the surface; you should really just take my master class!

$$LogL_n\left(\overline{\overline{\text{🌳}}}\right) = LogL_n\left(\overline{\overline{\text{🌳}}}; Y\right) = f_n\left(Y; \overline{\text{🌳}}\right)$$

Finally, the likeliwood function may be estimated by multiplying each k'th log-likeliwood from k below:

$$f_n\left(Y; \overline{\text{🌳}}\right) = \prod f_k\left(\text{🌳}_k; \overline{\text{🌳}}\right)$$

For the sake of making the math easier for Ole Betsy, the tower workstation that saw me through the drought of '06, we change that log likeliwood into a log-log-likeliwood below.

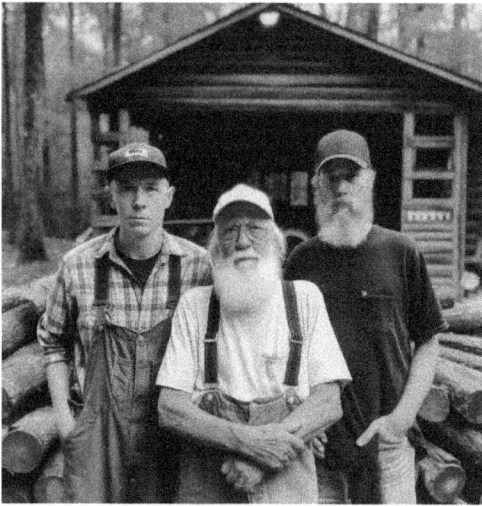

Figure 9.2: Me and my boys, Wyatt Jr and Baby Cleatus. We're a proud family-run and operated logging business that cares.

2. Methodology

First off, nobody East of the Mississippi has better tree model distributions than I do. Some people think they can just run some AI modeling on some US forestry data and come out with some hot result like a big shot, but I don't think so. That'll get you stuck wandering the woods with nothing to show like my cousin Jethro, who spent a little bit too much time on the YouTubes. There's experience that you don't get from any new trendy *Transformers*-based models. We don't do it like that, no sir, not in our family-owned Wyatt Johnson-approved logging business; we use good ole-fashioned maximum likeliwood estimators. That's a pedigree that you ain't never gonna get from no neural network!

2.1 Maximum Likeliwood Estimate

Suppose there's a true distribution of tree species 🌳 in a Forest $\mathbb{F}$ where $\overline{\text{🌳}} \in \mathbb{F}$ could be represented below with each individual dis-

That makes the multiplications into additions; it's an old logger trick we used to use to do our math on the fly in the back country when our calculators couldn't get any solar power through the thick forest of the underbelly of America.

$$\widetilde{\overline{\mathbb{A}}} = argmax \left(\sum LogLog_k \left(\mathbb{A}_k; \overline{\mathbb{A}} \right) \right)$$

The most likely result can then be estimated by taking the argmax of our log-log likeliwood sum function and determining how much Black Walnut there is in a given forest $\mathbb{F}$ and whether or not any $\mathbb{RL}$ types may find any use in searching for some high-dollar wood. You ain't a *RL* until you optimize your parameters numerically. Unless you listen to Jethro, you ain't gonna find a closed solution!

2.2 Numerical Optimization

Now this here's a real hoot and a half settin' up your Hessian matrix to find yer numerical approximation. As shown below, defining yer derivatives is a job for any amateur or apprentice $\mathbb{RL}$. Now, if you've spent as much time in the back woods as I have, looking at that Hessian and finding a global optimum for those tree distributions, you may notice something tricky. I'll give ya a minute to put on that thinkin' cap and see if you can spot it yerself. I don't even think that snake in the grass Samantha Greene couldn't figure this one out, and she's such a phony! She don't know the difference between pine and hickory!

$$H\left(\widetilde{\overline{\mathbb{A}}}\right) = \begin{bmatrix} \frac{\partial^2 lln}{\partial \mathbb{A}_1^2} & \frac{\partial^2 lln}{\partial \mathbb{A}_1 \partial \mathbb{A}_2} & \cdots & \frac{\partial^2 lln}{\partial \mathbb{A}_1 \partial \mathbb{A}_M} \\ \frac{\partial^2 lln}{\partial \mathbb{A}_2 \partial \mathbb{A}_1} & \frac{\partial^2 lln}{\partial \mathbb{A}_2^2} & \cdots & \frac{\partial^2 lln}{\partial \mathbb{A}_2 \partial \mathbb{A}_M} \\ \vdots & \vdots & \ddots & \vdots \\ \frac{\partial^2 lln}{\partial \mathbb{A}_M \partial \mathbb{A}_1} & \frac{\partial^2 lln}{\partial \mathbb{A}_M \partial \mathbb{A}_2} & \cdots & \frac{\partial^2 lln}{\partial \mathbb{A}_M^2} \end{bmatrix}$$

Yup, that's right, no big-wig Silicon Valley company's gonna see that like an $\mathbb{RL}$ can. Yer gonna be dealin' with multiple roots! Now any $\mathbb{RL}$ worth his spit'll tell ya that the roots between $\overline{\mathbb{A}}_2$ and $\overline{\mathbb{A}}_3$ will get all sorts jumbled up together, 'til you don't know which way's up or down. My buddy Jimbo back in '96 was back hunting for a patch of Cherry he estimated using a Gaussian process back when men were men and people looked at ya funny when ya assumed a dataset's homoscedastic [6]. He swore up and down over his own Maw's life that he found the global root, but didn't realize with so much interminglin' of trees through their roots and mycorrhizal networks [7] that there were multiple roots. I was like, "Hey buddy, you lost? Better expand that search space!" Oh, he's never lived that one down. That boy couldn't find $\widetilde{\overline{\mathbb{A}}}$ if it smacked him in the face, bless his heart! He was a true friend though, that Jimbo. The kind they don't make anymore. He officiated mine and Mrs. Wyatt Johnson's wedding.

3. Results

Enough about Jimbo and on to the results. As shown in *Figure 9.3*, a clear pattern begins to emerge when the log likeliwood is plotted on a log scale of a special normalization technique that you'll learn about in the 19th lesson of my masterclass. Even Samantha Greene's gotta be able to understand it. That's the sort of secrets they don't teach you in school with all the made-up and biased histories they gotta teach those kids about Kennedy. That's why I home-schooled both Wyatt Johnson Jr and Baby Cleatus; more time for the important things like logging, true history, and dimension reduction techniques like the good Lord intended.

Log-Log Likeliwood Estimate of Billy-Ray Jeffreyson's Property

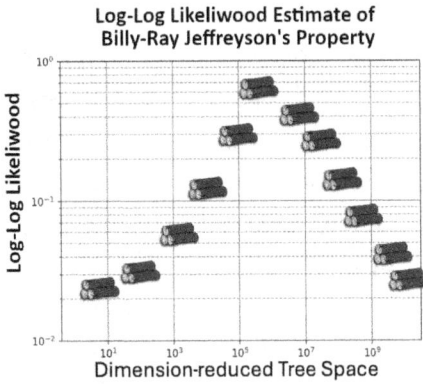

Figure 9.3: Log-log-log likeliwood plot pointing us straight to Billy-Ray Jeffreyson's property

Well, I tell ya, we took our readings and spotted a private property owned by a friend of mine, Billy-Ray Jeffreyson. I brought a pack of Miller and a fifth of Ancient Age as is tradition and we chased that gradient right to him. I couldn't believe him when I saw him. It was Old Wilbur. We both heard about Ole Man Wilbur at least twice a year from the old coots down at The Holler Hideout, a good ole Honky-Tonk. It's always been a real big fish story but there he was standing right in front of me. I ain't never seen a black oak Baby Cleatus couldn't wrap his arms around, and it would take three Baby Cleatuses to do that with Old Wilbur. Just look at the photograph in *Figure 9.4* and tell me that $\overline{\text{🪵}}_2 \not\exists \mathbb{F}$. No sir, I tell ya what, not only does $\text{🪵}_2 \exists \mathbb{F}$ but I'd even venture to say that $\frac{\overset{\sim}{\overset{\wedge}{\text{🌲}}}}{\text{🌲}} \approx \text{🪵}$.

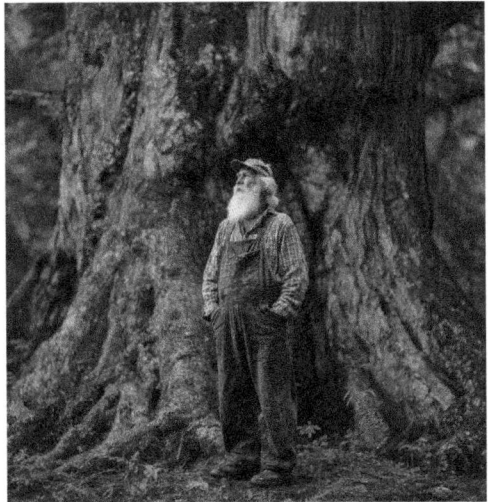

Figure 9.4: Me with my prized Black Walnut, Old Wilbur

Well, we didn't just take a picture to prove we found that legendary tree; we brought back at least $10,000 worth of fine lumber from Old Wilbur and some other Walnut in that area. A fine investment of some forest analysis and $20 of whiskey and beer. No one on Wall Street's gonna get you that return on investment playin' with your retirement account. Keep 'em in treasury bonds like my meemaw always told me after surviving the big one and spend the rest loggin'.

4. Conclusion

Well, if you don't think our maximum log-log-likeliwood estimator works, or you think we should preserve the forests like that Samantha Greene's always sayin', excuse my French, but Goddamnit, you can quit your dadgum jabberin'! That lady will not quit pestering me about my business. Protest this, protest that. You know how many hippies I've shooed out of tree forts in perfectly good hickory trees by blasting "Cotton Eye Joe" 24/7 until they couldn't take it anymore because of her?! Well, the number would surprise you...

If people didn't want to buy my fine furniture or source my lumber, it would just go to the big block store flattenin' the rainforest. That tree hugger thinks I'm bad, but I'm a conservationist. If they ain't getting the fine wood from me, they're getting it from some third-world country that don't pay their workers, which don't make American jobs. They're not surgical like we do. I bet they just flatten the entire area and it all goes to some factory furniture store and that fine piece of old growth forest is gonna end up in some particle board IKEA part 186B of a dresser ya store your Christmas sweaters in! I'm sorry, just talking about Samantha Greene got me goin'.

I hate to self-promote, but Wyatt Jr and Baby Cleatus are making me do this. It makes me feel like a scam artist like that snake in the grass Samantha Greene, but please follow them on their TikTok, Snapchat Premium, Facebook, Twitter, Teddit page, Woodstagram, OnlyFans, and subscribe to their Substack, whatever that is. I don't know what a hashtag is but I'm sure you can find them.

4. Conflicts of Interest

The author has absolutely no financial conflicts of interest with this study, not like that snake in the grass Samantha Greene!

References

1. Wyatt "The Log Whisperer" Johnson, 2024. *18 Secrets to a Profitable Specialty Wood Logging Industry* :: Self-published

2. Opheusden B, 2020. *Unbiased and efficient log-likeliwood estimation with inverse binomial sampling* :: PLoS Comput Biol 16(12). https://doi.org/10.1371/journal.pcbi.1008483.

3. Samantha "Snake in the Grass" Greene, 2022. *Predatory Logging, a Wyatt Johnson Case Study* :: Eco-Terrorists Weekly

4. Samantha "Snake in the Grass" Greene, 2023. *The Wyatt Johnson Wood Empire: A Story of Greed and Saw Dust* :: Netflix 3-Episode Limited Series

5. Wyatt "The Log Whisperer" Johnson, 2023. *Modern Logging Conservationism and why Samanthat Greene is full of Baloney* :: Veneer Logging Magazine

6. B. McGraw, 2021. *Stop Assuming I'm Homo: Cries out Nations Heteroscedastic Datasets* :: Journal of Astrological Big Data Ecology: https://jabde.com/2021/04/08/stop-assuming-im-homo-scedastic/

7. Reynolds, 2023. *Tracking International Communism with Mycorrhizal Networks* :: *Et Al*:: *Because not all Research Deserves a Nobel Prize*

10

Natural Log Exponential Log Growth Models in Hardwood Nurseries

Wyatt "The Log Whisperer" Johnson[1,2,3,4,5]

[1] Department of Statistical Wood Studies, Cranberry-Lemon University, Pittsburgh, PA, USA

[2] Owner of Wyatt Johnson's Fine Furniture Warehouse, with half-price deals on cabinets and coffee tables this Presidents' Day! Pittsburgh, PA, USA

[3] Owner of Wyatt Johnson's Specialty Wood Depot LLC, Pittsburgh, PA, USA

[4] President, Treasurer, and Pot-Luck Organizer of the Royal American Selective Logging Society

[5] Chief Editor and Author of the Veneer Logging Magazine, 12 issues a year for only $60 per 6-month subscription. A TRUE BARGAIN with all the wisdom you'll gain!

Abstract

There is no logging business immune to facing major legal litigation pushed by an environmentalist like that snake in the grass Samantha Greene. Due to impending court orders, my business is stuck with the natural log-natural log growth in tree nurseries. Previously, my specialty wood depot and personal logging business churned out exponentially more logs year after year, bringing value like you wouldn't believe to customers like you! Unfortunately, banned from wild foresting like my pappy and grand-pappy used to do, and limited to tree nurseries, there is no easy way to meet my exponential demand given natural log growth. However, land use may be scaled up by utilizing a Buc-ee's spread model, miracle tree growth-fortified mulch, and infinite root formulas. In this paper, these techniques will be implemented and analyzed to match our previous natural log-exponential growth model.

Keywords: Natural Log Growth, Exponential Growth, Buc-ee's, Loggin', Family Business, That No-Good Samantha Greene, Natural Logs, Infinite Root Trees, Miracle Mulch

1. Introduction

If you can't feel the seasons and the climate like an old forestry veteran like me, you wouldn't know when to transition a portion of your business from wild to nursery forestry. Thankfully, Wyatt Johnson, yours truly, doesn't wait for trouble before planning for the future. I never put a dime into Social Security, and I don't expect to take a dime out! I can't rely on the liberal government to take care of me. I'm my own and my family's financial future, so I plan for tough times, including building my own log nursery business... just in time for that dang ol' snake in the grass Samantha Greene to shut my wild veneer forestry business down. What a grift she runs on those forestry department bureaucrats.

Now, if you haven't read my book *18 Secrets to a Profitable Specialty Wood Logging Industry* [1], please stop what you're doing, go to your local book shop, NOT BARNES AND NOBLE, buy it, and read it. Okay, now that you've caught up, recently I had to release a second edition, *23 Secrets to a Profitable Specialty Wood Logging Industry* [2], to cover some additional topics like how to improve your log growth. If ya don't, you'll end up with natural log-natural log growth like you see in *Figure 10.1*. YUCK! So please order my new book now and leave a rating and review if you want a chance at a successful business like mine!

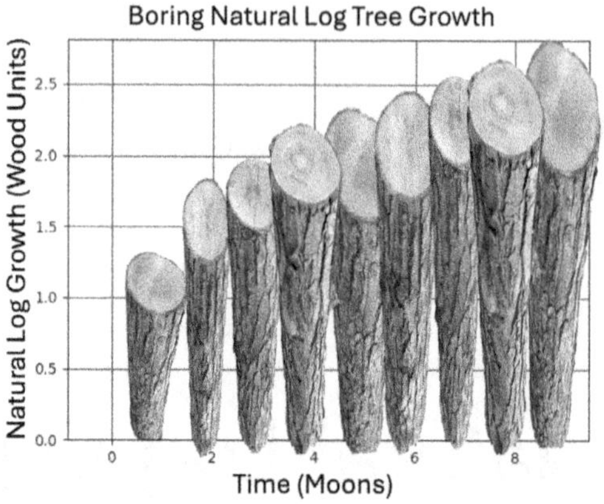

Figure 10.1: Boring and slow natural log-natural log growth

2. Background

If you know me, you'll know that I'm a family man, through and through. We've been runnin' this logging business since the late 18th century in the Pennsylvania forests since my great-great-great-great-great-great-great-great-great-great-great-great-great grandmother and secret love child of the great Leonhard Euler, Isabella, married into the prestigious Johnson [3,4] family to become an honest logger's wife out in the great frontier we now call home. Can't you see the family resemblance between Isabella Euler, Samuel Johnson, me, and my boys Wyatt Jr. and Baby Cleatus?!

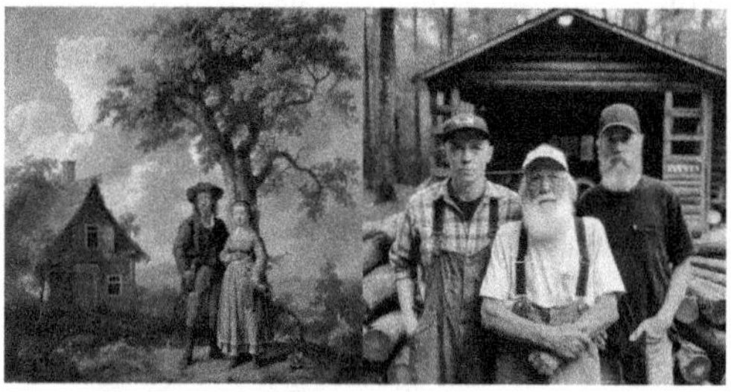

Figure 10.2: My great[13] grandmother and father, Isabella and Samuel Johnson, in the great frontier side by side with me and my boys

We carry on that logging legacy that traces 13 glorious generations back to the time of our founding fathers. Even if we've lost our specialty in wild forestry of specialty woods as I eloquently described in [5], we will continue to maintain our status as the most successful logging family in the New World!

2.1 Nomenclature and Terminology

Before any of you ChatGPT programmers go any further, you're gonna need to know some basics of natural log exponential growth: it takes the function below, and there's no amount of prompting you could do to learn that from some pansy large language model thanks to political correctness! Kids these days. Now, let me make this simple for you. Your total logs of time function is your initial autumn tree $🍁_0$ multiplied by your natural growth rate defined by the normalized summer-winter difference — raised to time divided by moon months $M2$. Easy enough.

$$\textbf{Log}(t) = 🍁_0 \left(1 + \frac{🌳 - 🍁}{🍁}\right)^{t/M2}$$

Now, a lot of people might be wonderin' won't it get confusing talking about natural logs from trees and natural logarithms? No, because we have formatted the important log Log so that everyone'll know what we're talkin' about. That's how we do it, Pennsylvania style [6]! The one big issue with working with Logs or Logs is that they become the inverse function of an exponential function natural or natural log. For instance, a base log of a red maple $_{Log}🍁$ has a natural log function, which will cancel out any exponential natural growth function, as shown here.

$$Log_🍁\left(\left(1 + \frac{🌳 - 🍁}{🍁}\right)^{t/M2}\right) = t/M2$$

THAT'S RIGHT! All that work's up in smoke just like a forest fire! It just cancels out, so be careful out there when you start mixing your natural log exponentials with your natural logs and your *natural − logs*! You have to learn these tricks from your elders like me or you'll end up like poor ol' Danny "No Stumps" Lawrence, a friend of mine who never listened to his pappy. I don't think I need to tell you what happened to him.

One final mathematical log trick, as shown in the equation below: for any tree-based log, if the inputs are doubled in the time domain, their output is multiplied, causing UNBELIEVABLE GROWTH! That's right, just by doubling your time, you can multiply your profits. Now I hear ya wondering, "Wyatt Johnson how do you double time?" Patience! The family secret will be revealed to you in *section 3.2*, so keep reading, kiddo!

$$\textbf{Log}_🌳(T1 + T2,) = 🌳^{(T1+T2)} = 🌳^{T1}🌳^{T2}$$

Now, if you're gettin' a little lost following all the tree notation, that's no problem. For only $39.99 for the hard copy, $36.99 for the paperback, or the low price of $29.99 for the Kindle audiobook, you can get my book *Definitive Guide to Tree Spotting and Mathematical Loggers Notation in Mathematics* [7]. I recommend getting all three versions because you'll use them so much, they'll get worn out. They're a fantastic Christmas present, and Baby Cleatus did a fantastic job reading the audiobook.

I just wish he would share his gift with the world more and join the choir. Buying and closely studying these books will unlock the key to understanding how many wood units you can generate by following my exponential log growth principles. So don't miss out!

2.2 Exponential Natural Log Growth Approximations

Once you understand the basics of creating exponential natural log growth model notation, you can start to work with basic approximations for different tree types. Now, all of the growth more or less fits an exponential growth model. But if you really wanna be a professional logger like me, some approximations fit better than others for particular trees. As a first example, to approximate an ash growth model, the equation below shows an approximation of ash logs once grown exponentially based off of the Taylor series. Now, I know what you young kids are thinking, but don't get too excited. It doesn't have anything to do with Taylor Swift, but it is _Out of the Woods..._

$$\text{🌳}^t \approx \sum_{n=0}^{\infty} \frac{t^{\overline{\text{🌳}}(n)}}{\overline{\overline{\text{🌳}}}(n)!}$$

You may have noticed in the ash natural log growth model the use of the function $\overline{\text{🌳}}(n)$ as well as some similar functions in the following approximations. Using generations of research and data, we have approximated particular constants of trees needed to generate the roots and terms necessary for exponential _Log_ growth. You can read all about them in the appendix for this paper, only available to those

subscribed to my Patreon account, where you can see the tree roots worked out to 100 terms at least!

Next, the Maclaurin series expansion, due to the symbiotic relationship between the harmonic expansion and the photosynthetic chlorophyll of oak growth, which expands at the same resonant frequencies, or, as that snake in the grass Samantha Greene calls them, _vibes_. The equation below shows how this natural log exponential growth model may be expanded and approximated using specific constants from $\overline{\text{🌳}}$.

$$\text{🌳}^t \approx \overline{\text{🌳}}(1) + \overline{\text{🌳}}(1)t + \frac{t^2}{\overline{\text{🌳}}(2)} + \frac{t^3}{\overline{\text{🌳}}(6)} + \frac{t^4}{\overline{\text{🌳}}(24)} + \dots$$

In my good books, there are a few infinite things: Jesus, God, the Holy Spirit, and walnut. The walnut natural log exponential growth model fits best using a limit definition, as shown in the equation below. I don't know what it is, but there is something spiritual about this wood that we can only approach through an infinite series of exponents and following what God orders.

$$\text{🌳}^t = \lim_{n \to \infty} \left(\overline{\overline{\text{🌳}}}(1) + \frac{t}{\overline{\overline{\text{🌳}}}(n)} \right)^{\overline{\text{🌳}}(n)}$$

Last but not least, one of the most prized veneer woods my customers are clamoring for is mahogany. Unfortunately, it is quite special, and its natural log function must be approximated using a generalized continued fraction representation, as shown in the equation below. I don't like to get all _fancy pants_ about my math, but it's the only form that fits this fine wood.

$$\text{🌲}^{t} = \overline{\text{🌲}}(0) + \cfrac{t}{\overline{\text{🌲}}(1) + \cfrac{t}{\overline{\text{🌲}}(2) + \cfrac{t}{\overline{\text{🌲}}(3) + \ddots}}}$$

2.3 Don't Believe the Woke Media. Imaginary Numbers Don't Exist! I REPEAT: DNE!

Now, if you've listened to a few too many NPR All Stuff Considereds, or whatever it is, you may believe something silly like the equation below.

$$\text{🌲}^{it} = cos_{\text{🌲}}(t) + i * sin_{\text{🌲}}(t)$$

A lot of folks might think that the i in DEI stands for imaginary. NOPE, it's Deciduous, Evergreen, and Indigenous! What the woke left refuses to understand is that imaginary numbers, especially in logging, DO NOT EXIST (DNE). Let me make this clear: if you start believing in some liberal gobbledegook about tree phasors and *sustainable forestry* pushed by some LSD'd out-of-her-mind hippy like that snake in the grass Samantha Greene [8], you're about to waste a whole lot of money on healing crystals and sage burners! I'm sorry, this gets me worked up. Just don't come mailing me complaints about how I don't do anything with them made up imaginary numbers or how we should be more *nuanced* with our calculations for more *complex* tree species. A tree is a tree, and trees are real not imaginary. Imaginary numbers DNE!

3. Methodology

You may be wondering: "Oh, Wyatt Johnson, there's nothing on God's green earth that can make a tree grow exponentially! It's al-ways closer to a natural logarithm. Why did you spend all of that time creating models to track exponential growth?" Now keep your britches on, I'm getting to that part in this here section.

3.1 Buc-ee's Land Use Model

Few chains have found more ways of using more and more land than the gas station chain Buc-ee's. Personally, if I'm gonna get gas, it's gonna be at a Buc-ee's; it's the only place that is wide enough for my truck and also carries my favorite brand of Buc-ee's beef jerky and Buc-ee's caramel corn. According to a manager I was having a long conversation with, they own a specially trademarked method for acquiring more land for development purposes. With the size of that gas station and the amount of expansion I've noticed in their brand, this is the sort of entrepreneurial exponential growth I need for my logging! It turns out that with the right branding and delicious enough grab-and-go triple brisket BBQ sandwiches, you can get as much forest as you want right off the highway to re-purpose. Most of it's all low-ROI pine anyway. We're gonna fix these plots up with all types of special wood.

3.2 Miracle Tree Growth

As previously hinted, there is a way to multiply your exponential growth by adding time in the exponent. Now, it ain't gonna be cheap, but the money you're gonna make off this growth is going to be way more than the cost. After centuries of Johnson family wisdom, we have created a patented miracle growth nutrient formula for tree growth. By creating a type of antioxidant and whey protein, but for trees, we've managed to halve (and sometimes even quarter) the time it takes to grow a valuable hardwood.

While we cannot give away all of our intellectual property regarding the miracle growth formula, we can say the secret ingredient looks something like the branched ring below, which we assure you, we can synthesize, is not made up, and can be infused in a fast-acting topical mulch, no matter what the Better Business Bureau may have you believe. It's what the plants crave!

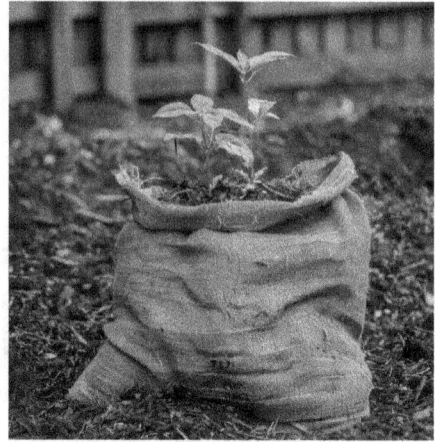

Figure 10.4: Miracle tree growth mulch is so powerful, trees will start growing before it reaches your home

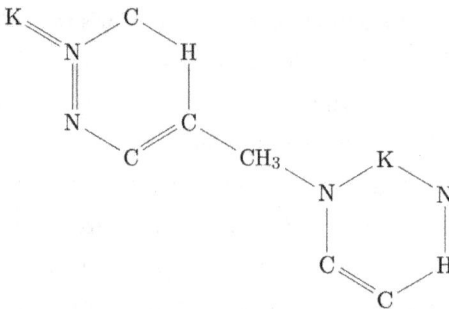

Figure 10.3: The Wyatt Johnson secret ingredient in the patented Miracle Tree Growth Fortified Mulch

All you have to do is send in a money order for an annual subscription, and in the mail, you will receive a weekly shipment of the specially fortified mulch shown below with our secret ingredient. Check our website for pricing details, and I assure you, if you don't see significant results in your ability to exponentially grow your trees, your money back is guaranteed.[1]

3.3 Infinite Root Technique

It is a well-established fact that, mathematically, the more roots you have, the more logs you get. When you start multiplying more and more roots, any forester will tell you that the tree is gonna sprout like bamboo! With enough roots, it is trivial to achieve exponential natural log growth. Either by using targeted miracle tree growth mulch or by selectively breeding higher root trees, any amateur forester may achieve infinite roots in their trees.

$$\mathbf{Log}(t) = \prod_{n=1}^{\infty} (\overline{\text{🌳}}_n - t)$$

---

[1]   In order to prove that you don't see significant results, you must measure a lack of exponential growth in your trees and publish the results in a peer-reviewed study through a department of Statistical Wood Studies such as the one at Cranberry-Lemon with an N > 2,000 and p < 0.005.

Now, this technique ain't all roses and sunshine, and even roses have their thorns. Now let me ask you, if your tree starts to have too many roots, it may begin to get a high-order polynomial shape that is going to be curvier than a slinky in a hurricane! Now, you might be able to make some high-end furniture with the look of that wood, but let it grow too curvy and good luck cutting it down and milling it!

4. Results

Now, we started clear-cutting and growing at least a year ago, so you bet we got some results to talk about. We planted some specially selected seedlings that just really called out to me in the fields. They were some special saplings I had been saving all winter. We started measuring their growth about a month in while applying a heaping healthy portion of my own special-blend Wyatt Johnson-patented Miracle Tree Growth Fortified Mulch. We prescribed just as much as recommended, a 50 lb bag once a week, which only totals to $14.99 plus tax and shipping for anyone who would like to recreate the study.

In addition to the ash, oak, walnut, and mahogany discussed in *section 2.2*, additional birch, cherry, and rosewood were planted. Though not mentioned, most natural log exponential growth may be estimated using any generic power series approximation technique. Additionally, that root trick, which works on just about all of 'em. Trees love their water, I reckon. Once measured, the average growth pattern in wood units may be seen in *Figure 10.5*.

Exciting Exponential Natural Log Tree Growth

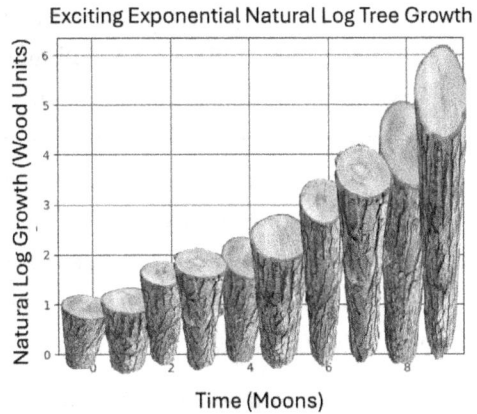

Figure 10.5: Exponential natural log growth

Now, isn't that the most beautiful exponential growth curve you've ever seen? I couldn't believe it when I saw it; I had to cut down and measure all the logs I grew just to confirm they were real and not my imagination! Boy did we exponentially grow some wood. I don't know about you, but if

$$\text{Log}_{\text{🌳}}(T1 + T2,) = \text{🌳}^{(T1+T2)} = \text{🌳}^{T1}\text{🌳}^{T2}$$

ain't true after measuring those results, then my name ain't Wyatt "The Log Whisperer" Johnson!

5. Conclusion

Well, if you're having trouble growing logs after all that advice, son, logging might not be for you. Maybe try something easier, like business analytics, electrical engineering, or neuroscience, so that you can support yourself and your family. Now, if you were able to follow all that advice successfully, I'd like to invite you to join me in my petition to once and for all get rid of that no-good Samantha Greene who's trying to stop all our clear-cutting.

Apparently, we're using TOO much land and now that dang hippy's all up in my chili shutting down half of my Ohio branches... AND my businesses! I don't know where she thinks she gets her furniture, but if I shut down, it's all gonna be plastic and cheaply made particle board from God knows where! Lord, she got me goin' again. That woman will annoy me even when she's not here!

I hate to self-promote, but Wyatt Jr. and Baby Cleatus are making me do this. It makes me feel like a scam artist like that snake in the grass Samantha Greene, but please follow them on their OnlyFans, TikTok, Snapchat Premium, Facebook, Twitter, Reddit page, and Woodstagram, and subscribe to their Substack or Haystack, whatever that is. I don't know what a hashtag is but I'm sure you can find them.

6. Conflicts of Interest

The Author has absolutely no financial conflicts of interest with this study, not like that snake in the grass Samantha Greene!

References

1. Wyatt "The Log Whisperer" Johnson, 2024. *18 Secrets to a Profitable Specialty Wood Logging Industry* :: Self-published.

2. Wyatt "The Log Whisperer" Johnson, 2025. *23 Secrets to a Profitable Specialty Wood Logging Industry* :: Self-published

3. "The Wyatt Johnson Family Tree". Johnson Family Scrapbook (2020).

4. "Genetic Ancestry of the Johnson Family". 23andMe results (2019).

5. Johnson, 2025. "Log-log-likelihood of Black Walnut in Random Forestry" :: *How to Prove Anything*

6. *Pennsylvania State Math Textbook Grades 9-12*, Various Authors, 1962.

7. Wyatt "The Log Whisperer" Johnson, 2022. *Definitive Guide to Tree Spotting and Mathematical Loggers Notation in Mathematics* :: Self-published.

8. Samantha "Snake in the Grass" Greene, 2023. *Sustainable Forestry using Tree Phasors* :: Netflix 3-episode Limited Series.

11

The No-Regrets Waiting Model: A Multi-Armed Bandit Approach to Maximizing Tips

Carol Louise Feurtalini[1,2]

[1] Head Waitress at Mama Lou's Seafood Shack

[2] Department of Statistical Waitressing Studies, Cranberry-Lemon University, Pittsburgh, PA, USA

Abstract

When I started waiting at Mama Lou's Seafood Shack, home of the world-famous Mama Lou's seafood platter for only $29.99, I knew I had hit a gold mine. With that delicious food, which isn't too filling, loads of additional apps, and sea-themed cocktails, the tips working here have been HUGE. I wasn't just gonna put in as many hours as I could; I have to keep the wait staff to a MINIMUM so I can get as many tips as I can. Ole Carol here's gonna retire early. *Ka-ching!* Problem is, if I don't pay enough attention to each customer, I can't serve all of them well enough to get those tips, let alone serve everyone enough food to rack up a huge bill and that sweet, sweet 20% gratuity for larger parties, while keeping Mama Lou off my back. One day, it all hit me: you can formulate this as a multi-armed bandit problem in which each customer is represented as a bandit arm, and *bada-bing-bada-boom*, all I needed was a reinforcement learning algorithm to solve it. Using an epsilon-greedy, an upper confidence bound, and a Thompson sampling algorithm, this paper will create a No-Regrets method to serve my customers for maximum tip extraction. All algorithms worked exceptionally well! Except for the epsilon-greedy method. That one lost me my job. But it also won me the love of my life, Tony. So I'd call that a No-Regrets model.

Keywords: Reinforcement Learning, No-Regrets, Seafood Platter, Multi-Armed Bandit Problem, Waitressing, Epsilon-Greedy, Endless Shrimp, Upper Confidence Bound, Dessert Push Estimation, Round Robin Scheduling, Thompson Sampling, Customer Prior Estimation, Alcohol Purchase Probability Chain

1. Introduction

On an average night, I'm pulling down $3k from this place. When I started, I was only making $1,000–2,000 a night because I had to split my tips with Jeremy and Amanda. I knew I needed to get rid of them if I was going to retire in seven years, pay off my house, and buy that hot tub I've been eyin' with the four jets. People don't realize how much upkeep those things cost! Don't get mad at me just yet, I didn't do anything slimy to be the only waitress workin' at Mama Lou's. Jeremy went off to become a river rafting guide, Amanda's focusing on her oil painting now, and honey, you won't cut it as a waitress if you don't know how to show the right people how to follow their dreams [1].

So it's been all peaches and gravy with me holding down the fort, and I can hold down the fort. I once gave birth and did my taxes on the same day that I single-handedly waitressed a 10-hour shift at Lee-Roy's Rib and Gumbo Hutt [2]. Well, Mama Lou ain't so sure. She says she's missing customers, orders, and I'm not paying enough attention to all her customers now. Well, first off, Lou, you mean **Restaurant Regret (RR)** like in the following equation, where Maximum Possible Meals Served is MPMS, and Meals Served is MS, and Carol here has ya covered [3].

$$RR = MPMS - MS$$

Now, nobody has to know this, especially Mama Lou, but I'm really optimizing for **Waitressing Regret (WR)**, where MPT represents Maximum Possible Tips and TR is Tips Received in dollars

$$WR = MPT - TR$$

Where the Tips Received is really a function of Meals Total (MT) and Tip Percentage (TP) by customer k [3].

$$TR = \sum (MT(k) * TP(k))$$

So don't you worry, Lou, optimizing for tips is optimizing for the restaurant [3]! Get back to spicing up that chowder we all love so much and let ole Carol do what she does best. Well, it is the same thing except for the epsilon-greedy method, but we'll get to that later, honey. It's a long story.

Now, optimizing tips is not as simple as pushing the largest amount of food for the highest spender. It's a matter of throughput and personality. You may be able to maximize your TP at the cost of a lower amount of total K customers. Now the same thing happens when you're pushing that MT up as high as you can. Now, I'm gonna tell you a little secret; hungrier customers eat more food than customers full of brisket and bread [4]. Waitressing ain't a game for anyone who can't do live optimization these days. If I didn't formulate a perfect round robin algorithm during the tapas craze of 2017, well, I wouldn't be driving a red mustang around now, would I [5]?

2. Background

In a previous study, I tried managing the order in which I waited on customers by using a round robin scheduling scheme. Unfortunately, treating each customer equally without integrating new information was determined to be suboptimal but better than nothin'. I was able to serve all of the customers, but I missed out on the big tippers, and I spent too much time on indecisive customers [5]. Although an indecisive customer corrective delay mitigated some risk for many of the customers who took up much of my waitressing time [6], it was never optimized for individual customer models, which have been known to bring in the lion's share of realized tips [7]. Now listen up, because I'm only gonna tell ya about it once. For these algorithms, you'll need to know about a few things: customer model estimation, customer exploration, customer exploitation, and regret estimation.

2.1 Customer Model

A lot of people like to define a set of people and their resulting food purchases β and percentage tips τ as a stochastic process where each individual's β and τ is defined by an unknown normal distribution, such as the Customer Set (CS) here:

$$CS = [(\beta_0, \tau_0), (\beta_1, \tau_1), \ldots, (\beta_K, \tau_K)]$$

Here, $\beta_k \sim N(\mu_k, \sigma_k^2)$ and $\tau_k \sim N(\phi_k, \alpha_k^2)$ [8]. Now, in my decades of experience as a waitress, there's nothing normal about a customer, but in a pinch, it'll make an alright approximation. Unless you really know your customer, like you've known them for years, I would just stick with a normal distribution to estimate their β and τ. But sweetie, if you know someone well enough to fit a beta distribution, you don't need an algorithm to know what they need. You follow your heart, honey.

Thankfully, most waiters and waitresses don't have to start with a flat prior. There's a lot about a customer you can tell just from the way they look and carry themselves. With experience, you may be able to estimate a customer's β and τ the second they walk in and park that little posterior in their seats. If you don't think you can do that, baby, don't worry; you can match each customer up with the list we developed in [9] until you feel ready

to move on. If you aren't quite sure which archetype a customer fits in, just pick your best guess and add more variance, honey.

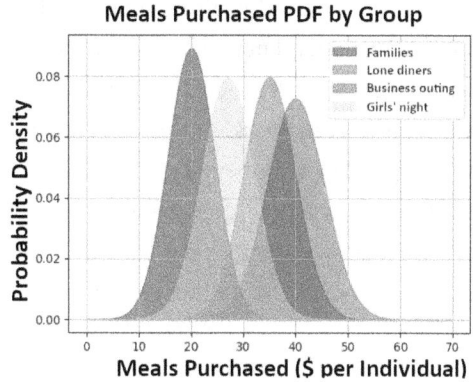

Figure 11.1: The most common customer types β distributions

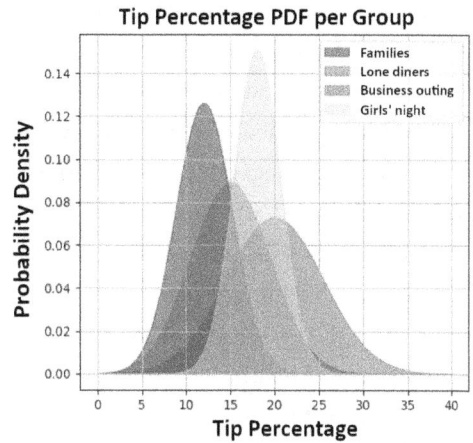

Figure 11.2: The most common customer types τ distributions

Now, behind every person's action is a million different things. That's what I always say. Well, we don't have time to estimate a million different things, so we just picked about a dozen or so, but usually, age, hunger, weight, energy, liver tolerance, happiness, wealth, and busy-body-ness are some good go-to parameters for an extended customer state model. These parameters can be estimated using the guide in [10]. You can just about sum up anybody with those parameters, at least if you only care about how much they're gonna eat and tip ya.

Now, some fancy-pants waiters and waitresses may try and convince you to train something called a neural network to estimate that hunger. Well, darlin', you'll use one, alright: a single-layer neural network that I like to call linear regression. Nobody's got time to train a deep neural network on the job. We don't have Applebee's money! Regression's a lot like butter: it's simple, goes great in anything, everyone knows about it, but they're always surprised it works so well when you put it in everything.

2.2 Customer Exploration vs. Exploitation

In the classic multi-armed bandit problem, the key is to determine the right amount of exploration vs. exploitation. You may think you know who you're dealin' with, but baby girl, you don't. If you check out the initial priors in [9], some of those variances begin high for a reason, and that reason is, people are people. If you knew how hungry everyone was, now it would be the easiest job in the world, but no one's a mind reader; you'll have to collect data the old-fashioned way to calculate those cute little posteriors of yours and talk to your customers.

Now, let's just say you *are* a mind reader and know *exactly* what people want, like you're some gosh dang psychic. You ain't, but let's just say you are for the sake of this paper. You could use an exploitation model and serve all the food without asking and chat up just the right customers for that generous tip when you know they want something off the menu, if ya know what I mean. Well, it's a great dream, and probably will stay that way because only one waitress seems to have pulled it off: Zorka the Enchanter [11]. Now, if ya don't *know* anything for sure, and exploring is your

only option, you'll always miss out on those big white whales. You won't really take advantage of that customer so hungry that they want all the appetizers, the platter, dessert, and an extra serving of linguine to eat when they get home. You may develop the world's best customer models, but darlin', you'll be missin' out on some of the fattest tips of the night if ya don't shake for the right fries. In the three approaches to the No-Regrets waitressing model, the key difference will be in the different methods for balancing exploration vs. exploitation, 'cause no one's a mind reader and no one's gonna treat every customer equally.

2.3 Regret Estimation

Regret's a tricky one to estimate when it comes to waitressing. The food is limited to the restaurant's current supply for the night, but the generosity is theoretically boundless. Well, you won't earn anything greater than your country's GDP, because that money has to come from somewhere. But baby-cakes, if you use your nation's GDP as your maximum possible reward, it may work, but you'll have more numerical issues than you can shake a stick at [12]. As shown in *Figure 11.3*, my tips from last year were logged, and I still don't know what I missed out on.

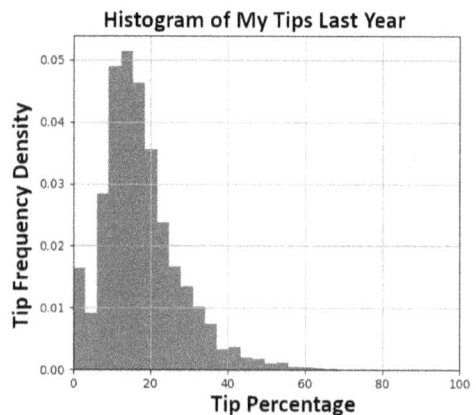

Histogram of My Tips Last Year

Figure 11.3: My tips from last year

Please do not show Figure 11.3 to the IRS! As you can see, the tip distribution is far from normal. There are some who stiff me, and there are some who tip way beyond expected. According to Chandra's Law [7], at any one moment, 1% of the population is willing to tip above 40%, 0.1% is willing to tip above 400%, 0.01% above 4,000%, and so on. It is a theoretical limit, once thought only to exist in the glitziest of Vegas casino restaurants, but a larger meta study confirmed Chandra's Law across all geographic areas at any restaurant greater than a \$\$\$ rating on Yelp [13]. Once applying the law, you can accurately estimate regret and account for total food that may be served by a restaurant and the average 15–20% tip value from customers based on the waiting location using the following equation, where λ and $Chandra_K$ make up Chandra's constants from [13]:

$$Regret = \sum_{k=1}^{K} \left(\mu_k * \lambda e^{Chandra_K k} - RT \right)$$

Chandra Distribution of Heavy Tippers

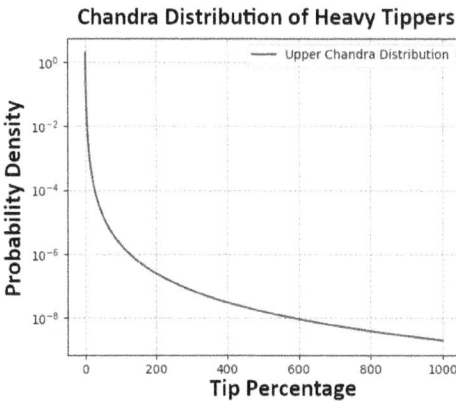

Figure 11.4: Theoretical Chandra metric distribution

For the majority of short time periods, the Chandra adjustment estimates realistic regrets for waitresses, but for the upper 99.9999 percentile heavy tippers, it may be possible to realize negative regret for a short enough time window. If you have negative regret, you

should be writing this paper. As I'll show later, I received a negative regret period, so you'd better listen up, darlin'.

3. Methodology

The work in the round robin scheduling algorithm designed a method for doing the absolute minimum, in which every customer gets a fixed time slice, whether they like it or not [5]. Now, there are some nights that I'm just not feeling it, and honey, that's a night I'm using the round robin. But I just can't do that all the time. It's all robotic. It's not me. It is the base case for not getting fired by a restaurant manager, but it is largely insufficient to optimize on tips, particularly for the Chandra-theorized upper limit tippers. Luckily, Lou and I have an understanding, and I have some room to improvise. She runs the kitchen; I talk to the customers.

Let me tell you, honey, serving a meal's not a one-and-done experience. They've got different states. And I don't mean like Delaware. That's why I always use the Markov process scheme developed in [14]. If you ain't using Markov processes to characterize the order chain of a customer, sweetie, get some help. It's not shameful to need some help from time to time. The state space is shown in *Figure 11.5*, where the state transitions may be estimated by customer parameter estimation in [10]. Alcohol's a little different, and its purchase chain is shown in *Figure 11.6*, defined by the initial probability of purchasing a drink P_0 with the customer's decay function λ, also known as their tolerance. Each of the numbers is just an example; they can be dynamic, baby-cakes, don't worry, and if you're wondering where the probability of leaving is, well, that made the graph too messy, and it's already busy as hell.

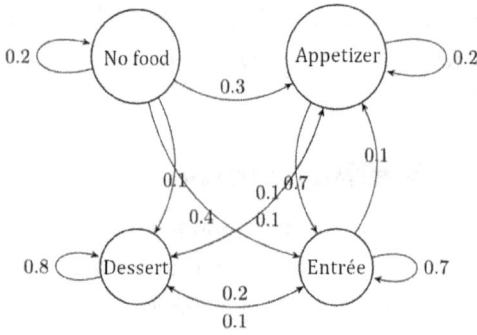

Figure 11.5: Food order Markov chain

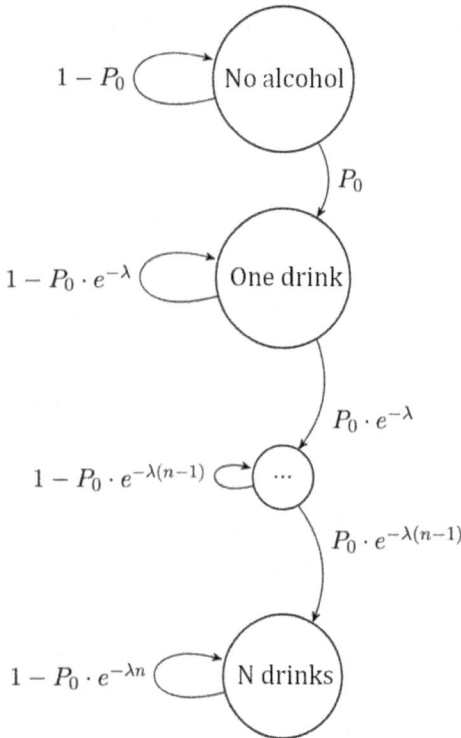

Figure 11.6: Alcohol purchase Markov process

Next, based on the results of a customer's first purchase and personality measurements processed using the methodology in *section 2.1* and [9], I made updates to the Markov state space and customer models. Finally, and I'm so sorry you've had to put up with me and my blabber mouth, I used three different algorithms to balance exploring and exploiting different customers.

3.1 Epsilon-Greedy Algorithm

The epsilon-greedy algorithm is the easiest algorithm to use, but it is the hardest to implement without getting Lou out of the kitchen and all over my ass. First, an ϵ value is selected. Then, every customer receives at least one or two visits to determine their estimated food and alcohol ordered, as well as their estimated tip τ. Then, between every customer, at a rate of $1 - \epsilon$, I check up on the highest valued customer. Then, at a rate of ϵ, I check up on a random customer to explore and find new customers that might not have scored high on the initial estimates.

3.2 Upper Confidence Bound (UCB)

Now, especially if you're worried about getting fired but don't wanna do some complex Bayesian math, you may want to use this next method. The UCB method balances which customer to select in a slightly more elaborate way. You start by taking the β_k mean from your customer distribution set; don't forget to multiply by your τ_k too! Then, keep track of how many times you've visited that customer N_k. The resulting fraction in the following equation accounts for customers who haven't been visited much, who may be higher-paying than previously estimated by using Hoffding's inequality:

$$Tip = \beta_k \cdot \tau_k + \sqrt{\frac{2ln(t)}{N_k(t)}}$$

Here,

$$\beta_k \cdot \tau_k \sim E[P(Tip|\hat{\theta}_k)] = E[P(\beta_k|\hat{\theta}_k)] \cdot E[P(\tau_k|\hat{\theta}_k)]$$

Because repeat visits to the same customer may annoy some, this is expected to be the best for the application of waitressing.

3.3 Thompson Sampling

Now, let's say you're like me and don't want your customers to just be a couple of means; Thompson sampling may be for you, sweetie. Thompson sampling uses a probabilistic approach, where the customer with the highest sampled probability of success is chosen. First, each customer begins with an extremely uncertain prior. Now, there isn't an easy way to do it, but you're gonna need to develop your customer distribution set through some Kalman filters or something similar to update the θs for each customer archetype to match your βs and τs with to reach the tips in the following equation:

$$Tip = P(\beta_k|\hat{\theta}_k) * P(\tau_k|\hat{\theta}_k)$$

Now, darlin', if you're not well-versed in real-time measurement processing, I'm gonna need you to put down your phone and get out a pen and paper for this one. Okay, so just start with a set of customer priors $\hat{\theta}$, sample from those priors with the previous equation, now pick the best sample and go ask that customer if they've had enough time to decide what they'd like to eat, maybe even the ole *Anything to drink besides water?* method. Notate their personality, what food or drinks they're wantin'. Now, I know a lot of hot shots out there may try and update their prior in one big calculation, but I'm gonna tell ya now, honey, it's way easier to break down each of your observations into single measurements $z_{k,i}$ that correspond to a single $\hat{\theta}$. The process goes like this:

1. Project $\hat{\theta}_{i|i-1} = F\hat{\theta}_{i-1|i-1} + Bu_i$

2. Observe measurement z and covariance R

3. Contextualize each measurement with the transformation H matrix and Kalman

Gain $K_i = P_{i|i-1}H^T(HP_{i|i-1}H^T + R)^{-1}$

4. State update $\hat{\theta}_{i|i-1} = F\hat{\theta}_{i-1|i-1} + Bu_i$

5. Covariance update $P_{i|i} = (I - K_iH)P_{i|i-1}$

Maybe an example may help ya out. Imagine you show up at the dinner table of a group of rambunctious men in their 20s. Apply one $z = 40$ with the H matrix transforming that z to only estimate the θ parameter, estimating how much alcohol they are about to consume. Next, determine whether they are dressed like they just got back from work or are wearing salmon colored polo shirts like a bunch of frat boys. If it's the former, filter in a positive $z - H$ combo to increase the estimate of τ. In the latter case, and especially if one has a fake ID, use a negative $z - H$ combo unless you plan on threatening to call the cops for the tip-blackmail procedure described in [15]. Inversely scale the measurement covariance R matrix on how annoyingly loud they are. It is likely that a single measurement will update multiple θ parameters; for instance, if a man is observed to be on a date, it is more likely that the generosity estimation will increase, while alcohol intake may decrease.

Now, this sounds very difficult to apply on the fly. I always hear from new waiters and waitresses that *it's too hard to calculate a Jacobian for every customer interaction* and that they should just be using a particle filter. Well, baby-darlin', when it's 7:30 p.m. and you're in the middle of a massive dinner rush, you're not gonna have time to wait for your simulation to finish! That's why no one should ever get into the service industry unless they know their partial derivatives. That's what I always tell 'em. If you don't want to do calculus on the job, better become an analyst or engineer, where you can use approximations.

4. Results and Discussion

Three weeks of waitressing data was collected and analyzed for each algorithm and compared to legacy round robin data [5]. The customer data and results were analyzed to determine an estimated total **Maximum Possible Tips (MPT)** and **Tips Received (TR)** with a percentage regret. The MPT changed per seasonality of Mama Lou's seafood, and during that one weekend, it was so cold that no one wanted to leave their house, so the raw regrets aren't comparable. Regret is shown in percentage according to the MPT estimated through the Chandra metric, and the Got Fired result of the algorithm is presented as *No*, *Maybe*, and *Yes*. Thankfully, because the 50% epsilon-greedy algorithm sounded the most risky, we tested that one last to ensure a full data collection. Which was a good call, since it did get me fired.

Customers < 15			
	Tips Received ($)	Regret (%)	Got Fired
Round Robin	20k	22%	No
Epsilon-Greedy ($\epsilon = 80\%$)	15k	40%	Maybe
Epsilon Greedy ($\epsilon = 50\%$)	22k	32%	Maybe
UCB	26k	5%	No
Thompson Sampling	30k	3%	No
Customers > 15			
Round Robin	52k	35%	No
Epsilon-Greedy ($\epsilon = 80\%$)	24k	83%	Maybe
Epsilon Greedy ($\epsilon = 50\%$)	312k/year and benefits	>342%	Yes
UCB	120k	5%	No
Thompson Sampling	67k	14%	No

Table 11.1: Multi-armed bandit algorithm performance for low (<15) and high (>15) volume waitressing

Other than the epsilon-greedy algorithm, the UCB and the Thompson sampling methods regularly outperformed the previously developed round robin scheduling algorithm [5]. In waitressing, a Chandra-adjusted regret in the single digits is absolutely unheard of, especially for a high-volume dinner slam shift.

The UCB method worked the best overall for both the high and low customer volume shifts. By adjusting the mean estimate using Hoffding's inequality, the customer sampling perfectly up-weighted customers I hadn't checked in on enough who were right there ready to order, and managed to up-weight the high maintenance customers stingy enough to withhold a tip without good service or those influenceable by my charms. At an unbelievably low regret of 5% and resistant to high-volume customers, it is likely the best method.

For low-volume customers, the Thompson sampling method was far superior. At first, I was worried it would get stuck on a handful of customers with high means, but by projecting each customer state estimate against the Markov process previously discussed, little time was wasted on customers busy eating. Additionally, a more elaborate state estimate updating procedure identified and exploited key customers each night who were extremely heavy tippers and/or heavy spenders.

Those are ole Carol's favorites. The Thompson sampling specifically increased alcohol sales as over-serving customers in the mood to drink watered-down $12 cocktails rapidly increased sales. However, the focus on those customers over others in higher volume days increased regret substantially. It still outperformed the round robin sampling.

I knew epsilon-greedy wasn't gonna work, but I had to try it, and oh, am I so happy I did. I knew that if it was going to work at all, I would need an extremely high ϵ just so I had enough exploration time to service enough lower-paying customers before I got in trouble with Lou. But, the whole time I'm thinking, if I do this, I'll get all of the upper tail Chandra model customers, and, girl, did I ever. Now, it took a few nights, but when Tony started coming in for that oyster platter after work and he started buying more and more drinks, I knew I had hit the jackpot. Little did I know that he was as sensitive and lovable as he was hungry.

Now, I had way too many close calls waitressing with an epsilon-greedy model, every which minute I kept hearing from the kitchen *Carol, would you quit talkin' to yer boyfriend and seat that nice family! They've been waitin' fer an hour!* I know, I know, but for science, I had to keep at it a few more weeks. Well, at first it was for science, but toward the end, it was for love. It got much worse when I moved to a 50% exploit model, and, girl, will I tell you, there's nothing that makes a hungry customer angrier than when you spend half your time talking to one customer while they're just looking to put in an order for popcorn shrimp.

But it was all worth it, I think Tony was coming in so much because he was lonely and needed the company. Toward the end of the experiment, he proposed, and he makes more than $300,000 a year plus benefits at a corporate job. So, honey, your girl Carol is set for life, and Tony's actually a really great guy. Anyway, I lost my job 'cause I was talkin' to him too much. When you put his salary into the regret calculator, it breaks the Chandra method entirely, and I got some negative regret off of that one.

5. Conclusion

Waitressing is a tricky business, y'all. On average, it's safest and best to explore and treat everyone equally, but Lord I tell ya, it's worth doin' a little exploitin'. I mean, in the multi-armed bandit meaning of the word. I love all my customers, and I provide an important value. It's just a matter of figuring out who needs the most love that day. Sometimes, that love comes in the form of clam chowder; for others, casual banter. Before me and Tony met, he barely talked to anybody outside of work. He just ate by himself and went home to watch Netflix by himself. Now look at us, in love with a negative regret value. That's why even an epsilon-greedy, with enough time, will leave you waitressing with no regrets.

References

1. Emily Brown, 2007. *"Transformative Encounters in Hospitality and Other Methods for Making Your Customers Feel Like They Earned That Extra Slice of Pie"*:: Annals of Service Research.

2. Carol Feurtalini, 2016. *"Top 10 Moments in Modern Athletic Waitressing"* ::

3. Patricia Robinson, 2019. *"Regret Metrics in the Restaurant Service Industry: How to Measure What You're Missing"* :: Journal of Statistical Waiting Methods.

4. Mr. Obvious, 99999 BC. *"No, Duh".* :: Journal of Did You Really Have to Look That Up?

5. Carol Feurtalini, 2023 *Round Robin Scheduling Algorithms in Waitressing: Adapting Operating System Dynamic Tasking for an Overburdened Waitress* :: Journal of Waitstaff Operations Research

6. Betty Mitchell, 2012. *Timing, Suggestion, and JUST HURRY THE HELL UP: Strategies and Predictive Modeling for Efficiently Handling Indecisive Customers* :: Machine Learning Techniques in Waitressing Technologies

7. Chandra Young, 2013. *Upper Bounds of Highly Right Tailed Restaurant Tips Using the Pareto Distribution* :: Journal of Waitressology in the Waiting Sciences.

8. Sarah Jones, 2017. *Distribution Fitting to Customer Tipping Probabilistic Modeling* :: Journal of Customer Modeling and Simulation

9. Carol Feurtalini, 2019. *A Semi-Complete Collection of Customer Archetypes and Their Associated Priors* :: Journal of Customer Modeling and Simulation

10. Sandra Nelson, 2018. *An Evidence-Based Method for Customer Model Updating* :: Journal of Customer Modeling and Simulation

11. Zorka the Enchanter, 2023. *Ancient Spells and Techniques for Live Customer Mind Reading and Applications in Exploitation Only Models* :: Machine Learning Techniques in Waitressing Technologies

12. Linda Taylor, 2022. *Numerical Limits of GDP-Based Waiting Regret Estimation* :: Journal of Waitstaff Operations Research

13. Chandra Young, 2014. *An Unbiased Tuning and Verification of the Chandra Metric for Heavy Tipper Frequency* :: Journal of Waitressology in the Waiting Sciences

14. Karen Martinez, 2015. *A Markov Process Estimation of Customer Food and Alcohol Dynamic Ordering Probabilities* :: Journal of Customer Modeling and Simulation

15. Susan Lee, 2022. *Card Smart: A Surefire Way to Exploit Young Drinkers* :: Journal of Statistical Waiting Methods

12

Who's a Good Boy? A Metropolis-Hastings Approach to Determining Foster Dog Names of Unknown Origin

B. McGraw[1]

[1]Department of Statistical Over-Application, Cranberry-Lemon University, Pittsburgh, PA, USA

Abstract

When a strange dog shows up at a shelter, you can't ask them what their name is. All you can do is feed them, call them a good boy, and make sure they're neutered. It has been a problem plaguing shelters and foster dog parents everywhere. Due to the probabilistic nature of dog behavior, names are exceptionally difficult to directly sample without prior knowledge. The issue is that many words sound the same, there is a baseline chance a foster dog will come to you or look at you no matter what you say, and there are way too many dog names out there. Who names a dog "Water Whipper"? As is statistics tradition, when a solution is unknown, the only option is to use a Markov Chain Monte-Carlo (MCMC) method such as the Metropolis-Hastings algorithm. In this paper, we will determine that even the great MCMC struggled to find the most likely dog name under a reasonable number of iterations. Either that, or Barney's real name wasn't near our sampling space. Either way, it's still a mystery.

Keywords: Barney Barnes the Dog, MCMC, Metropolis Hastings, Dog Fostering, Iterative Name Sampling, Food Sounds, Baseline Dog Behavior, Name Vocalization Spectrum, Foster-Dog-Name-Finderer, Good Boys

1. Introduction

It is a sad world we live in, but some dog owners out there, for one reason or another, will sometimes abandon perfectly good boys and girls to be scooped up by shelters with no information. Whether it's the dog running away or the dog being chained up somewhere to be found instead of surrendering them to the shelter, these poor pooches are left with no name. So, the shelter picks a random name from a list. With so many dogs in the shelter, sometimes they'll get a weird one like Barney Barnes did. You can only have so many Champs, Dukes, and Fidos. Some dogs, such as the one discussed in this paper, are clearly trained and well-behaved but will not respond to their given shelter name. As making any snap, whistle, shout, or noise might get the attention of a dog, testing out different names will not necessarily evoke a desired step response but a probabilistic one [1]. It doesn't help that the popularization of extended universes in an unprecedented number of fantasy books/football, sci-fi shows, and the Marvel universe has produced way too many dog names [2]; it is nearly impossible to test them all. This will all be incorporated into the **Foster-Dog-Name-Finderer (FDNF)**.

2. Background

In order to understand the FDNF, you must understand Barney Barnes the dog, Dog Calling likelihood distributions/behaviors, and the Metropolis-Hastings algorithm.

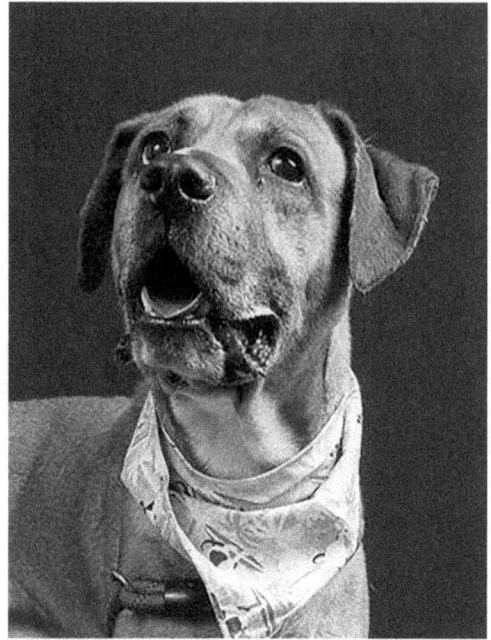

Figure 12.1: Barney Barnes

2.1 Barney Barnes

Barney Barnes is likely the most well-behaved dog my wife and I have fostered [2]. He's house-trained and politely communicates when he needs to go. He sits, stays, lies down, and drops the ball on command. He doesn't do anything unless given permission. He is completely friendly, both to other dogs and to my constantly hissing cat. With this information alone, there is very little chance he hasn't had a previous owner [3]. Unfortunately, he was leashed up and abandoned in an office park with a blanket, a self-feeder, and no information. Given the personality of the dog, we suspect murder was involved, because who would give up a perfect dog?

2.2 Dog Calling Likelihood Distributions

A Bayesian model of dog name calling sampling boils down to the equation below.

$$P(name|response) = \frac{P(response|name) \times P(name)}{P(response)}$$

where

$$P(response) = P(response|name) \times P(name) \\ + P(response|not\ his\ real\ name) \\ \times P(not\ his\ real\ name)$$

Unfortunately, it's more complicated to determine these conditional probabilities. If dogs exhibited more binary behavior, $P(response|name)$ would be 1, and $P(response|not\ his\ real\ name)$ would be 0 for all circumstances, and we would run out of treats real fast. This is not the case for many different reasons. Previously studied in [5], if two names or words sound similar, a dog will develop a high type 1 error rate. This means that if a dog's name was Gus, the study would often misinterpret Russ as a correct name due to the dog's response. Dog name-to-name distance (DN2ND), codified in [6], can be calculated by the normalized distance of number of syllables (SD) beginning with the same phonetic sound (PS), and whether they rhyme (R), as shown in the equation below, where they are all adjusted by constants k too irrational to include in this paper.

$$DN2ND(w_1, w_2) = \sqrt{\frac{(k_1 SD(w_1, w_2))^2 + (k_2 PS(w_1, w_2))^2 + (k_3 R(w_1, w_2))^2}{3}}$$

As measured in dogs with known names in [7], the probability of a dog giving a measurable response to hearing their name or not hearing their name is quite circumstantial, and it is never non-probabilistic. As shown in *Figure 12.2* and *12.3*, not only is $P(response|name)$

not easily sampled, but it can change for each $P(response|name, Circumstance)$. Likewise, $P(response|not\ name, Circumstance)$ is equally *all over the place*, as described in [7]. Even when adjusted by dog breed, shown in [8], a dog's response is never easy to sample. Finally, a follow-on study [9] measured wildly different response behaviors under different conditions in the same dog. For instance, if a dog is fixated on a squirrel, their *P(Response|name)* is likely much lower than the *P(Response)* baseline if the owner is eating something tasty.

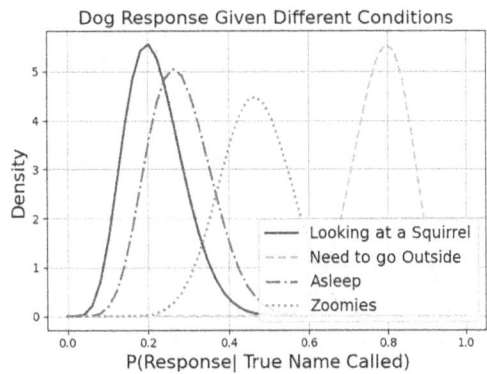

Figure 12.2: Measured $P(response|name, Circumstance)$

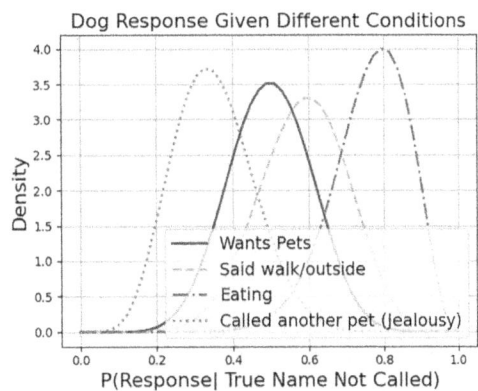

Figure 12.3: Measured $P(response|not\ name, Circumstance)$

2.2 Dog Name Metropolis-Hastings

To begin the Metropolis-Hastings algorithm, we propose $P(name_i)$ as an initial guess and sample nearby dog names to come up with $name'$ according to $f(name'|name_t)$. After sampling from $f(name')$ (in other words, calling Barney Barnes and seeing if he responds), we then calculate the acceptance metric below with historic data and the new data point.

$$A(name', name_t) = min(1, \frac{P(name') \, f(name_t|name')}{P(name_t) \, f(name'|name_t)})$$

Using a random number $u \sim U(0,1)$, if $u \leq A(name', name_t)$ we accept $name'$ as the new name. Otherwise, we stick with $name_t$. We increment, keep track of our probabilities, and go again. It's that simple.

3. Methodology

After a very quick discussion, we decided to start with $name_0 = "Rusty"$ because the dog looked like a "Rusty" to us (note that for the majority of the study, the subject is referred to as "Barney"). Next, we had an even faster discussion with ChatGPT to define our namespace as NS = ["Max", "Mack", "Rex", "Dex", "Rocky", "Ricky", "Jake", "Jack", "Buddy", "Benny", "Charlie", "Harley", "Marley", "Bailey", "Riley", "Toby", "Teddy", "Eddy", "Freddy", "Brady", "Oscar", "Ollie", "Milo", "Leo", "Theo", "Kobe", "Louie", "Joey", "Henry", "Benny", "Cooper", "Trooper", "Jasper", "Casper", "Chester", "Fester", "Buster", "Hunter", "Gunner", "Ranger", "Finn", "Flynn", "Lin", "Ben", "Ken", "Zen", "Ziggy", "Mickey", "Mikey", "Ricky", "Zeus", "Bruce", "Goose", "Moose",

"Ace", "Chase", "Jace", "Trace", "Vince", "Prince", "Bruno", "Juno", "Dino", "Reno", "Nino", "Arlo", "Marlow", "Harlow", "Shadow", "Pablo", "Sam", "Tam", "Jam", "Liam", "Graham", "Gus", "Russ", "Bus", "Buzz", "Fuzz", "Rufus", "Murphy", "Alfie", "Archie", "Richie", "Rusty", "Dusty", "Gizmo", "Remy", "Sammy", "Lou", "Blue", "Hugh", "Duke", "Luke", "Newt", "Scout", "Blake", "Drake", "Jake"] due to the relative male dog name proximity.

Next, we called out the name "Rusty" one to three times and measured the dog's response as a binary. If half asleep, increase iterations. Unfazed Barney will be labeled as a 0, and fully attentive Barney will be labeled as a 1. For an example of attentive Barney, see *Figure 12.1*. For an example of unresponsive Barney, see *Figure 12.4*.

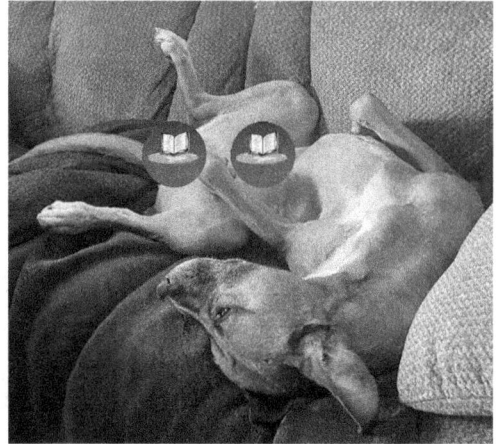

Figure 12.4: Unresponsive Barney

After applying $f(name'|name_t)$, we then estimate $A(name', name_t)$. If A is larger than 1, we accept the new name and continue sampling; otherwise, we sample a uniform $u \sim U(0,1)$ and accept the new name if $u \leq A$.

We tried not to test Barney during high

baseline response times, such as while we were eating. This dog even stared at us while we were eating peas. Additionally, every 17 iterations, we tested Barney's baseline level of looking at us by making random noises and measuring $f(random\ noise)$. While we have a pretty good idea that Barney responds to our random noises at a 40% rate on average, it appears to be dependent on energy level and the number of distractions. We chose 17 as the number of iterations because it's so specific; we don't think anyone will question us. We hope that sampling along our NS will result in a higher probability around the correct name or a correctly adjacent name in the NS according to the DN2ND.

4. Data Collection

We began sampling different names from our NS according to our algorithm in a calm environment at home and notating each response. We would then plug in that result to our algorithm and update each name for at least 1,000 iterations over three evenings. Data was collected only after we fed Barney, so he wouldn't be looking at us for ulterior motives. After each data point, we updated our *name'* using a computational tool close at hand. We had to pause our current Netflix show *Kaos* often during this process, so we didn't miss any key plot information while estimating A for the next *Name'*.

5. Results and Discussion

According to the probability of each name in our NS, as previously defined, the probability at each iteration is shown in the figure below at 50, 100, 500, and 1,000 iterations.

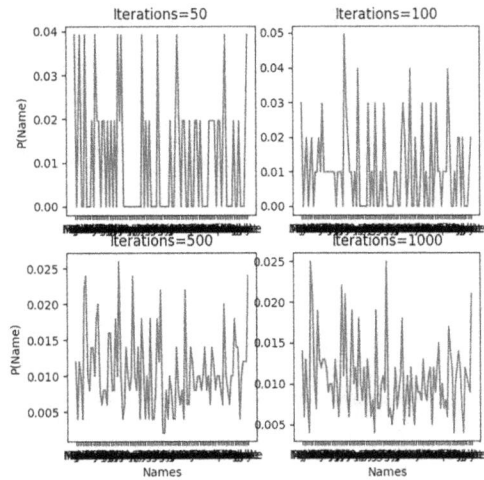

Figure 12.5: Measured name probability inconclusive test where y-axis is P(Name) and x axis is ["Max", "Mack", "Rex", "Dex", "Rocky", "Ricky", "Jake", "Jack", "Buddy", "Benny", "Charlie", "Harley", "Marley", "Bailey", "Riley", "Toby", "Teddy", "Eddy", "Freddy", "Brady", "Oscar", "Ollie", "Milo", "Leo", "Theo", "Kobe", "Louie", "Joey", "Henry", "Benny", "Cooper", "Trooper", "Jasper", "Casper", "Chester", "Fester", "Buster", "Hunter", "Gunner", "Ranger", "Finn", "Flynn", "Lin", "Ben", "Ken", "Zen", "Ziggy", "Mickey", "Mikey", "Ricky", "Zeus", "Bruce", "Goose", "Moose", "Ace", "Chase", "Jace", "Trace", "Vince", "Prince", "Bruno", "Juno", "Dino", "Reno", "Nino", "Arlo", "Marlow", "Harlow", "Shadow", "Pablo", "Sam", "Tam", "Jam", "Liam", "Graham", "Gus", "Russ", "Bus", "Buzz", "Fuzz", "Rufus", "Murphy", "Alfie", "Archie", "Richie", "Rusty", "Dusty", "Gizmo", "Remy", "Sammy", "Lou", "Blue", "Hugh", "Duke", "Luke", "Newt", "Scout", "Blake", "Drake", "Jake"] for 50, 100, 500, and 1,000 iterations.

Unfortunately, we still have no idea what Barney's real name is. If we run the simulation with a known correct example name as a test, Goose, it finds the correct name in 100-500 iterations, shown in *Figure 12.6*.

To better understand the data, we re-simulated the data synthetically to explore a few possibilities.

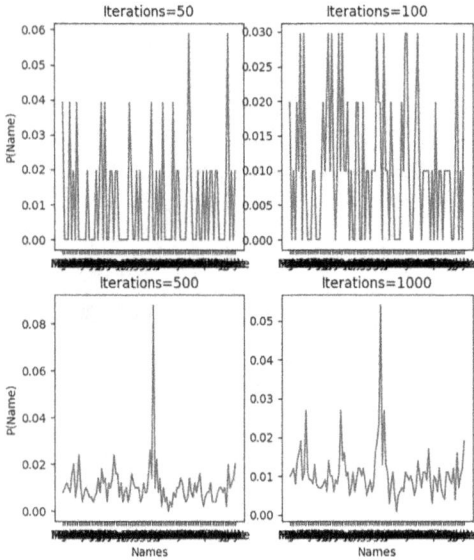

Figure 12.6: Simulated conditions successfully picked goose

shown in *Figure 12.7*, indicate that the simulation still found the correct name, Goose, after dancing around Bruce and Zeus.

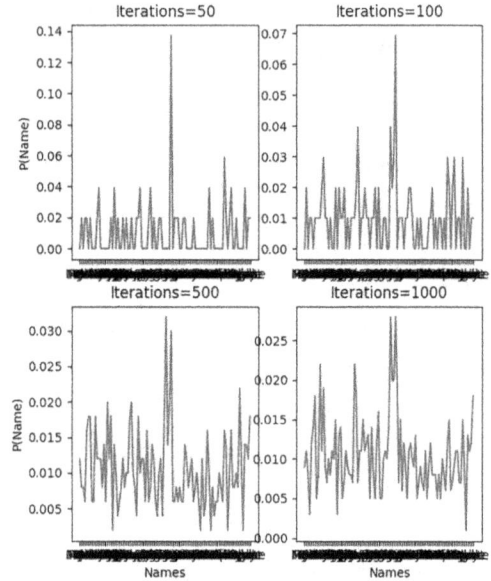

Figure 12.7: Simulated Conditions – Bruce is Close to Goose P(Response|Correct Name) = 0.55 and P(Response|Incorrect Name) = 0.5

One possibility is that Barney has a hyper-specific name not on our list and would not respond over his base rate of us calling out to him unless we used his exact name. Another possibility is that Barney's base response rate to any vocalization is so similar to the response rate to his own name that our algorithm can't pick it up. However, as shown in *Figure 12.7*, even if the response rates were very close (0.5-0.55), the Metropolis-Hastings algorithm would detect a nearby name. In this case, it determined the correct name was Bruce instead of Goose. Still pretty close.

Another possibility is that Barney is watching us so closely that the base rate of response is high (P=0.7). Calling any name would elicit a response, and his own name response is slightly higher at P=0.8. The synthetic results,

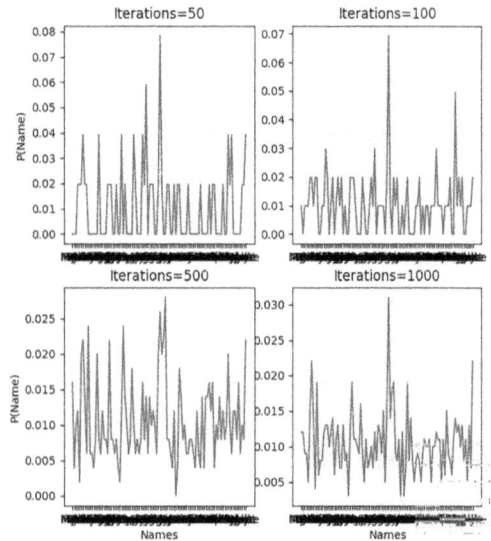

Figure 12.8: Name Probabilities Given P(Response|Correct Name)=0.8 and P(Response|Incorrect Name) =0.7

6. Conclusion

Whatever happened, we still don't know Barney's name, but we think he's going to eventually start responding to his new name: Barney. Or Rusty, we still haven't decided. Rocky would also suit him. Maybe it's like college, where he gets to pick his new name. Or maybe his next owners will decide whenever we get him adopted. Either way, we think if you are lucky and a foster dog's name happens to be in your own namespace, this should be a good method for determining a foster dog's true name. Otherwise, please just surrender a dog to a shelter if you can't keep them. It is extremely difficult to determine an abandoned dog's real name with no prior knowledge, even using Bayesian inference, and most shelters don't even know how to implement a Metropolis-Hastings algorithm. All we can conclude is that Barney Barnes is a good boy worthy of adoption.

7. Epilogue

Weeks later, after being blessed during a *St. Francis of Assisi's Blessing of the Pets* event at church, a couple of firefighters saw Barney Barnes in a coffee shop and fell in love. He was adopted on the spot and goes by the name of Rusty now. He even has his own man cave and a large backyard to run around in.

References

1. Rene Dogcart, 1643. *A Treatise on a Probabilistic Understanding of Dog Behavior*

2. David "Chewy" Hornegole, 2018. *The Growing Crisis of Dog Names: The Hidden Cost of the Marvel Cinematic Universe* :: Journal of Dogonomics

3. B. McGraw, 2024. *Barney Barnes is the Most Bestest Dog Ever* :: Facebook Post

4. Whwâllabey Bœmpit, 2014. *Categorical Dog Behavior Modelling: A Baseline Stray-House Trained Criterion* :: Journal of Misfit Pets

5. Augustus de Poodle, 2017. *Doggy Detection: Sparkle's Type I and II Error Rates for words that sound like Vet* :: Journal of House Pet Engineering

6. Pawbert Venn, 2007. *The Dog Name to Name Distance: A Three-Dimensional Space for your Names Space because Why Not* :: Journal of Vector Spaces of Misfortune

7. Fetch Chewbychev, 2019. *Conditional Response Rate of Calling Max: Why it's Not My Fault He Keeps Running Away* :: Annals of Canine Stochastics

8. Jerzy Waggles, 2015. *Yes, Your Golden is an Attention Hog: A Cross-Breed Conditional Behavior Meta-Study* :: The Journal of Dog Breed Comparanometrics Brought to you by Purina

9. Fetch Chewbychev, 2021. *Conditional Non-Invited Response Rate: Why We Really Should Stop Feeding Susie Under the Table* :: Annals of Canine Stochastics

[This page was left blank because of antiquated zoning requirements to increase the property value of each page.]

13

A Re-Examination of the Fermi Paradox: A Data and P(Doom)-Driven Markov Process Approach

Hugh Mann[1]

[1]Department of Normal Business Studies, because I am a very normal human and most humans study this, Cranberry-Lemon University, Pittsburgh, PA, USA

Abstract

Many of our fellow humans theorize that intelligent life in the universe is extremely likely, leading to a frightening conclusion: the **Fermi paradox**, which attempts to answer the question of *why aliens have not contacted humanity*. With the immense number of solar systems, a certain number would likely have habitable planets, and a certain number of those would develop intelligent life. Finally, at least some would likely become spacefaring, so something must be wrong that is preventing us from making contact with extraterrestrial intelligent life. The issue with the Fermi paradox analysis is that none of the numbers have any basis in research, and while there are multiple paths to a spacefaring civilization, there are more ways they fail. By applying a Markov process and estimating Fermi paradox probabilities by analyzing real data from the publicly accessible intergalactic exploration database made available by the Zethron race of Ujbecki IV, this paper will show that it is incredibly unlikely to ever be contacted by an alien race. There is only a 35% chance that a spacefaring race exists, and they probably don't want to talk to us or would make some of us pay back taxes.

Keywords: Aliens, Markov Process, Fermi Paradox, Drake Equation, UFOs, Extraterrestrial Life, Drake Equation, Ant-Peoples Launched Asteroids, P(Doom), Jellyfish Mech Suits, Fungal Zombie Creatures, Drexenite Mineral Creatures

1. Introduction

According to the **Drake equation**, there are probably aliens. R_* defines the rate of star formation at 1–3 stars per year in the Milky Way. f_p defines the fraction of those stars that have planets at about 0.5. n_e estimates the frequency of planets that can sustain life. f_1 then estimates how many of those planets create organic life. Next, f_i estimates the fraction of those planets that create intelligent life. Then, f_c estimates the frequency of those planets whose intelligent life reaches a technological level capable of interstellar travel. Finally, L shows the length of time for all of this to happen. Using the following Drake equation and some numbers for these values, humans have estimated that there are likely 1,000 to 100 million civilizations out there that could make contact with the human race.

$$N = R_* \cdot f_p \cdot n_e \cdot f_1 \cdot f_i \cdot f_c \cdot L$$

The Fermi paradox suggests that something may be existentially wrong since humanity hasn't publicly made known contact with aliens, according to reliable, trustworthy sources such as The Washington Post or Reuters. All other YouTubers, podcasters, and speculators are foolish. Google Reuters and tell me whether humans have made contact. No. They haven't. There is no alien presence on the Earth. It has been proven that the documented UFOs are not really extraterrestrial life [1] and that all of the recovered alien corpses are verified hoaxes [2]. Some suppose there is a "Great Filter" stopping all alien life from contacting humans.

The Fermi paradox tackles this Great Filter problem to determine why we, fellow humans, have not made contact with extraterrestrial life. Some say this is because space travel is extremely difficult and should not be pursued. This theory could discourage human technological progress, preventing humans from creating valuable technology for themselves and others to mine the lithium on Mars while it's still there. Another, even more troubling theory is that there are dangerous aliens out there, conquering—and silencing—all other extraterrestrial life. This, too, will ruin a perfectly good planet. Please believe me and my analysis in this paper: there are no predatory civilizations out there. Do not spend valuable human earth resources on defense technology. Instead, spend effort on more bovine creatures, which simultaneously warm the planet for reptilian-like life and also generate delicious beef. Two other theories are that life is rare and is susceptible to sudden doom by being in the way of asteroids launched by aggressive ant people [3].

In this paper, we will show that the Drake equation is better expressed as a Markov process and that there is more empirical evidence out there that accurately fits the parameters of the Drake equation. Once the Markov process is iterated over 10 billion years, you will see that all of us humans are indeed rare, alone, and likely doomed to die by a catastrophic event far before traveling to non-human intelligent life populated planets such as Vergoth VII [4]. There is no point in contacting the other aliens out there; they do not exist and are not trying to extradite normal business studies professors like me, who are just trying to lie low. DO NOT MAKE CONTACT! IT IS A TRICK!

2. Methodology

Life is too complicated to use an equation in which there are only seven elements. According to [5], you need at least 14 parameters to predict life on an extraterrestrial planet, and that's the minimum. The time-based process of life creation contains too many elements and dependencies for the Drake equation. It would be more efficient to estimate it as a Markov process, which estimates the probability from a time-based process.

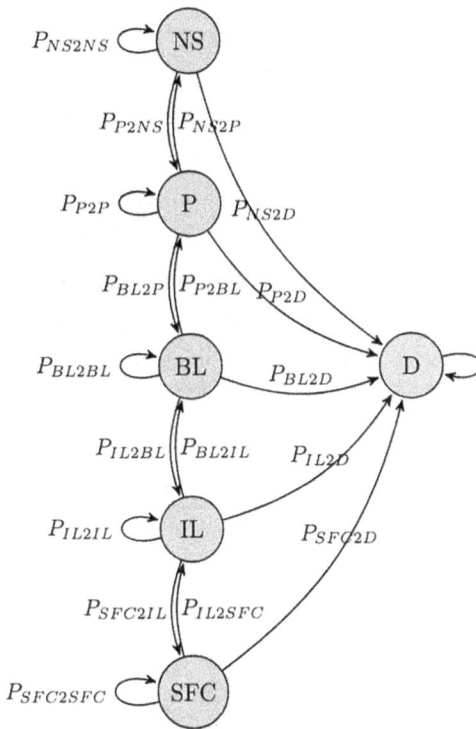

Figure 13.1: Drake equation probabilistic flow diagram.

2.1 Markov Process Model

For an easy example, let's assume that we will continue to use the Drake equation, in which we examine the process of:

$$(NS) \rightarrow (P) \rightarrow (BL) \rightarrow (IL) \rightarrow (SFC)$$

Here, the formation of a New Star (NS) eventually leads to the formation of an orbiting Plant (P), which can support Biological Life (BL) capable of evolving into Intelligent Life (IL) that can develop a Spacefaring Civilization (SFC).

Many humans think this is a simple process because that's how it has worked for them. They believe that there is no going backward from extinction [6] or civilizational collapse [7], making the arrows one-sided. But we know more from the data from the deep space probes now. Civilization often regresses. The arrows are double-ended. Do not question my sources! I know more than you, and you need to trust me.

Now, let's assume we additionally have a different state we'll call *Doom*. Now, any state can transition into the Doom state as a result of a planet-destroying asteroid or a History Channel Doomsday special supernova. Any intelligent species can go extinct, and I will talk about that, too. Species never think they will go extinct until it's too late.

$$STM^T =$$

$$\begin{pmatrix} P_{NS2NS} & P_{P2NS} & 0 & 0 & 0 & 0 \\ P_{NS2P} & P_{P2P} & P_{BL2P} & 0 & 0 & 0 \\ 0 & P_{P2BL} & P_{BL2BL} & P_{IL2BL} & 0 & 0 \\ 0 & 0 & P_{BL2IL} & P_{IL2IL} & P_{SFC2IL} & 0 \\ 0 & 0 & 0 & P_{IL2SFC} & P_{SFC2SFC} & 0 \\ P_{NS2D} & P_{P2D} & P_{BL2D} & P_{IL2D} & P_{SFC2D} & 1 \end{pmatrix}$$

Now the transition starts to look a lot like the state diagram in *Figure 13.1*. It is common for intelligent species that have not faced an extinction-level event to ignore these P(Doom) probabilities while estimating the probability of life [8]; we call these "optimistic races," like us humans. Once a state diagram like this is structured, each arrow may be populated with probabilities similar to the frequencies suggested by the Drake equation.

Now, a State Transition Matrix (STM) may be populated like the following equation, in which each state transition represents the probability of transitioning from one state to the next in a given time step. The probability of staying in state n will be $1 - sum(Outgoing\ Probabilities)$ so that each row and column adds up to 1. For instance P_{BL2BL} will be $(1 - P_{BL2P})(1 - P_{BL2IL})(1 - P_{BL2D})$, which may be interpreted as the probability that nothing interesting happens to the biological life is the probability that it isn't wiped out in an extinction-level event, it does not evolve into intelligent life, and the planet or solar system is not destroyed.

$$\mathbf{x}(t) = \begin{pmatrix} x_{NS}(t) \\ x_P(t) \\ x_{BL}(t) \\ x_{IL}(t) \\ x_{SFC}(t) \\ x_D(t) \end{pmatrix}$$

Now starting with a Life Probability State (LPS) of $[1, 0, 0, 0, 0, 0]$ for a 100% of being in the *New Star* state, the LPS is multiplied by the STM for each set of years that a new star may be alive before exploding, imploding, or a few other catastrophic things humans do not know about yet because they have not matured enough as a species to find out. This is shown in the following equation:

$$LPS_t = LPS_{t-1} STM_t$$

2.2 Life Model

By applying the model defined by *Figure 13.2* and the STM and LPS equations, we would already vastly improve upon the application of the Drake equation developed by optimistic humans who don't know any better and ask too many questions. However, solving for some state transition probabilities is quite complicated and can utilize the same methodology. It's a no-brainer to a nuclear age human (i.e., my audience) that P_{BL2IL} is extremely complicated. One of the earth-human theories on the Fermi paradox that is quite close to the truth, though most human scientists ignore the data to prove it, is that extraterrestrial life is more complicated than humans can understand.

A dual-handed walking creature, which some species call *humanoid,* is one way life can evolve in such a way to utilize tools and advance in technology, as observed by the human race, and what fossil record they have measured so far. This starts when a multi-cellular animal of $N > 3$ appendages begins walking on $N - 1$ or fewer appendages. Once the upper $N - 1$ appendages begin to grip things, they may utilize tools beginning with rocks and sticks before moving on to the heavier stuff, such as axes, power drills, and plasma cutters. These sorts of *humanoids,* like you and me, have been known to evolve in most types of carbon-based atmospheres given enough time without a doom event, and can evolve from nearly any species. Larger brains help, which typically corresponds with more appendages. Humans only have four appendages, with two that often handle tools, which is an okay amount for how far we've come. In my opinion, six appendages is the right amount where tasks get easier and clothes aren't too complicated. An example of some humanoids observed from a lost deep space probe can be seen in *Figure 13.2.* They do not have clothes, which would confuse many into thinking that the climate was better if an extraterrestrial were to find such a plaque.

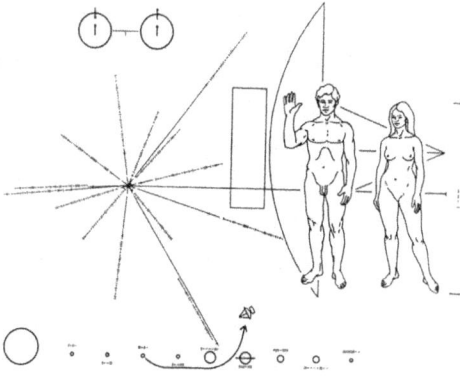

Figure 13.2: Humanoid-type species as observed from deep space probe.

However, so called *humanoid* species are only one of the possible ways for intelligent life to evolve. As observed from the Herglez III cluster, the Drexenites have evolved from silicon-based crystalline organic creatures and are doing just fine for a civilization that poops glass [9] every 12 years. The amount of biological adaptations for the silicon creatures to evolve into intelligent technology-wielding creatures is far more complex than known Earth creatures; they are hardier and more capable of space travel. The downside, which will be shown in the *Analysis* section of this paper, is that they do not evolve very quickly. If such a creature ever existed at all.

While their P(Doom) would be quite low, it can take 100x times longer to develop consciousness and even longer to develop a hive-mind capable of developing advanced technology. Once that crystalline telepathic king crystal forms, as shown in *Figure 13.3*, they would be off to the races. If such a thing could happen. They usually lose that race against other species, due to being slow, but they at

least make it into space before being destroyed by an asteroid. Because they are also part of an asteroid, those events are more like unexpected family reunions. Asteroids do not destroy the Drexenite. They have tried, I suspect.

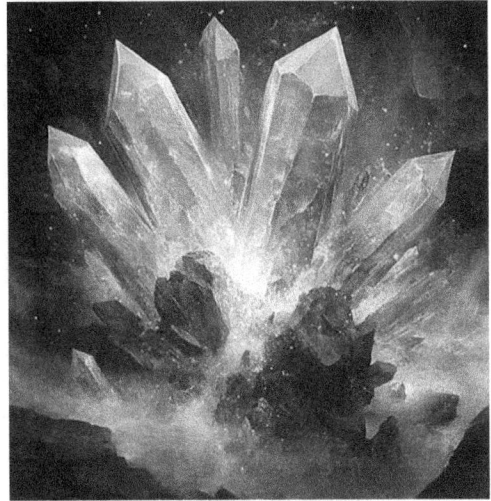

Figure 13.3: Drexenite hive mind of Herglez III contemplating time relativity.

Likewise, the pathways to wielding and crafting technology are as diverse as life itself. For instance, the Jellyfish people, known as the Cylorians on Xeloria, evolved to construct aquarium tanks that control mechanized power suits. They only leave their suits for sexual activity, surgery, and a rite of passage you have to be a Cylorian of age to know about. I tried to find out, so trust me. While these creatures have a much smaller chain of biological adaptations, their technological adaptations are immense before they can become spacefaring or even take dominion over their planet. A Cylorian in its mech suit is shown in *Figure 13.4*.

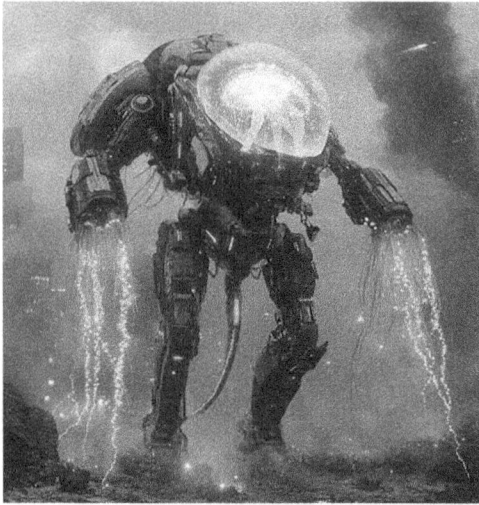

Figure 13.4: Cylorian Jellyfish in full combat mech suit seeking nutrients and destroying a type 1 civilization in the process because they are assholes.

Jellyfish and silicon are the rarest creatures to evolve into intelligent spacefaring life. However, the planets that can support this life are most common when the galactic planet database is analyzed [10]. Our Earth's *humanoid* life is the most rare given the necessary conditions to create them. As we'll show in the *Analysis* section, they are the most frail, with the highest environmentally driven P(Doom). The most common form of intelligent life, but the most technology-limited, are the fungal creatures.

A fungus-type people evolve where there is any form of life with brains large enough to be worth infecting with fungal spores. Fungus-type peoples, such as the Tarliths found on Vardolis and rapidly expanding to Palthoria, Ythronis, and Borvex II, are a parasitic type of civilization. As shown in *Figure 13.5* from Earth's Africa, this sort of intelligent life is easy to grow and quickly dominates any life form on any planet. Unfortunately, they also limit

host life by expanding too quickly. If the host life is capable of technological advancement through the development of eyes, and some sort of tool gripping appendage, Fungoids develop the fastest. Then a hive mind forms, usually after four to five thousand generations [11]. They generally find it easier to infect higher forms of life with technology than develop it themselves.

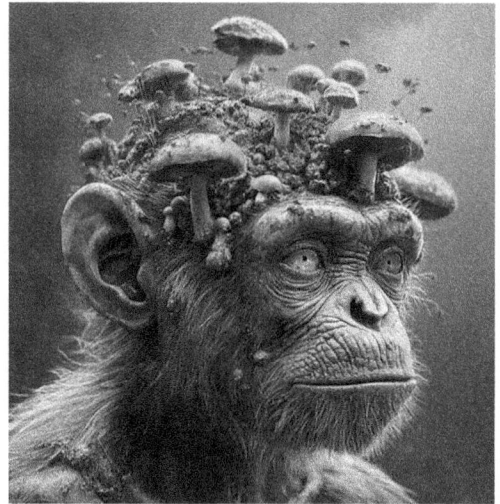

Figure 13.5: Tarlith infected chimp deep in the heart of Africa.

Each planetoid type will have a certain probability of forming each of these sorts of life forms at each step. There is a probability that multiple technology-wielding species will evolve, but only one will become dominant and develop advanced intelligence in the long run. This will be modeled as a P(Extinction Doom) for that planet's other respective races. For instance, Earth's humanoids spelled doom for the potential octopus and jellyfish intelligent species, and the Tarliths have wiped out the Grysalorns, the Xorvites, and the Braxilons... so far. This is all modeled in [12], which theorizes that it is impossible for two intelligent species to evolve on the same planet without one destroying the other.

2.3 Technology Models

Once a species is capable of wielding technology, we begin to apply a societal and a technological **Hidden Markov Model (HMM)**. This one's really hidden and is incredibly difficult to model, as there are many different ways to the same mountain top. For instance, it is possible for a civilization to jump from Metallurgy to Windows 95 by means of inventing the Quadratic formula [13], but may also do it by harvesting spice, a powerful psychedelic for all species except marmots [14]. An example postulated flow chart is shown in *Figure 13.6* for the current Earth humans, but it is not the only method for transforming from a hunter-gatherer species to a spacefaring civilization developed in [15]. The technology states humans have achieved are shown in green, with doom states in red.

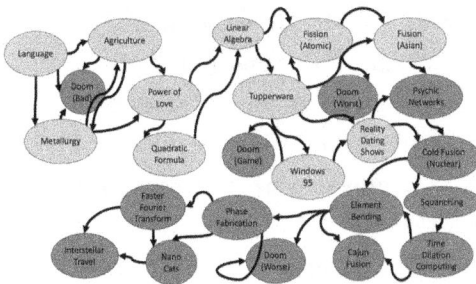

Figure 13.6: Technology Flow Diagram where green represents technological states achieved by humans, red represents potential doom states, and blue represents unachieved technological states.

Unfortunately for my readers, the actual HMM of the IL to SFC technology tree we will estimate in our parameter fit will be too high-dimensional to fit on paper. You'll have to take my word for it. Why would I have an ulterior motive, like I'm trying to hide a roadmap to becoming a spacefaring race and attracting more unneeded attention to this planet? The one point to note is that the more complex the civilization, the higher the P(Doom) as it becomes possible to use up all planetary resources, cause a nuclear winter, or misuse artificial black holes for garbage disposal, or just hubris [16]. As mentioned earlier, different species develop technology at different rates. For instance, jellyfish societies take the longest to develop metallurgy but accelerate the fastest when they devour land-based growth nutrients with their tendrils. Alternatively, silicon rock people develop metallurgy the fastest, but are slow to expand afterward because they're typically happy just being rocks.

2.4 Society Models

Unlike technology, intelligent species' societal models follow a single path, or so I've theorized, and can backtrack or progress but rarely jump steps. Developing species always start as a no-rules family unit or *Anarcho Capitalist* society before evolving to an *Anarcho Communist* society or tribe. After outgrowing that structure, capitalist offshoots evolve into a more complex but more powerful society, eventually turning back to communal when it gets too complicated. Eventually, capitalist offshoots outperform the communist structure again until it is replaced yet again. As shown in *Figure 13.7*, society evolves from an Anarchic state to more quasi-spiritual mystical states to provide order until developing constitutional rules-based societies. Next, society synthesizes with technology in a cybernetic order before evolving again into an actual spiritual realm when such societies learn how to measure Monads, a thing humans will learn about later [17].

Starting at the constitutional steps of society, civilizations are more likely to progress technologically, which increases the probability of becoming spacefaring, but also becomes more likely to destroy each other before reaching the spiritual stage of society, once they develop more psychic networks with each other.

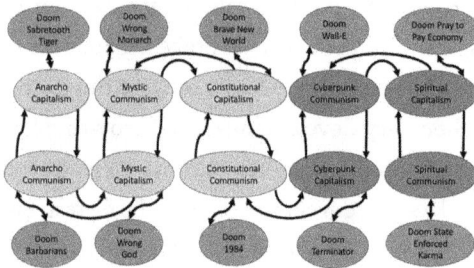

Figure 13.7: Society Flow Diagram where Green represents societal states achieved by humans, red represents temporary societal doom states, and blue represents unachieved societal states; and yes, it was real communism and real capitalism.

3. Data Collection

An intergalactic exploratory civilization first generated by the Polvoraxians has dispatched over 20 million deep space probes into different star systems and planets in the Milky Way and Andromeda galaxies to evaluate different planets. With this data, they may estimate how many planets are capable of sustaining habitable life as well as technological and societal development for those with intelligent life [18]. Just because the Polvoraxians made this doesn't mean they are real. It could be an elaborate joke. The data is immense, and data cleaning is necessary to gather any useful inference. Thankfully, for this research, they have made it publicly available to anyone with a special router you can purchase at any pawn shop marked with a green φ. If you don't know the password, don't try to acquire one unless you want to end up in an intergalactic zoo.

Unfortunately, there is a serious flaw in the deep space probe technology that likely caused the flawed analysis of the Drake equation [19, 20]. Detection of biological and technological advances was calibrated well to have a 99%+ detection rate and a less than 0.1% false alarm rate. Unfortunately, because the development of technological and specific biological advances is so rare, a positive detection is still more likely to be a false positive when given the base rate of most of the occurrences measured by the deep space probes.

For a long time, many data analysts using the Polvoraxian probe data did not double-check to see how accurate life development was until traveling to verify the accuracy of their detection software. For instance, if an alien race decided to monitor a specific species, such as humans, for nuclear fission technology, they may end up traveling to Earth very often due to these false positives caused by volcanic activity lining up with solar flares. Now, eventually, those predictions may or may not have come true in 1945 and other years on other planets, but before that, we learned that most of these detections had to be contextualized using the base rate shown in *Table 13.1*. With the deep space probe data contextualized using Bayes' theorem, as it was called by the humans who discovered it, state transition probabilities may be estimated.

Hypoth-esis	Prior Prob-ability P(H-X)	Sam-pling Prob-ability (P(N-H and X))	Pathway Probabil-ity P(H-X) P(N-H) and X	Relative Pro-portion P(H-N and X)
Earth Has Nukes	0.001	1.0	0.0001	=1%
Earth Does Not Have Nukes	0.999	0.01	0.9999*0.01	=99%

Table 13.1: Inference after Earth testing positive for having nukes

4. Parameter Estimation

Because the Markov process measures the transition from one state to another, all data is transformed into a time series of Xs and corresponding binary Y_n vectors. Each Y_n vector expresses which planetary, biological, technological, and societal state occurred at each planet at each time step. Next, the dataset is bifurcated into $Y(t|Y_n(t-1) = 0)$ and $Y(t|Y_n(t-1) = 1)$ datasets with the corresponding metadata $X(t|Y_n(t-1) = 0)$ and $X(t|Y_n(t-1) = 1)$.

A logistic regression $LR(Y_n|X)$ of the dataset $Y(t|Y_n(t-1) = 0)$ and $X(t|Y_n(t-1) = 0)$ then fits to the probability that a state will transition from state Y_n to Y_{n+1} and $1 - LR(Y_n|X)$ shows the probability of maintaining the current state n. Correspondingly, a logistic regression of $Y(t|Y_n(t-1) = 1)$ and $X(t|Y_n(t-1) = 1)$ will show the probability of maintaining state $n + 1$, while $1 - LR(Y_n|X)$ will estimate the probability of transitioning backward through the chain.

When you are in a species such as the human race, many do not estimate the likeliness of evolving backward evolutionarily or technologically. Humans are optimistically biased because events of backward evolution, such as the collapse of the bronze age or VHS winning over Betamax [8], are comparatively rare. Given a more cosmic perspective backed by data, humans would see that species evolve backward all the time.

The data used for habitable planets is the easiest to fit because of the immense amount of data. From a known sun, the process for developing habitable planets is well known and modeled in Qerra Silvix's study of what type of planet is most likely to lead to which type of species [21]. The inhabitable planetary systems transition at slower rates, allowing for our logistic regression models to be fit at time steps of millions of years and capture all of the relevant interactions at no cost for our actual model. Additionally, we will estimate the number of potential habitable planets in the Milky Way galaxy to apply to our resulting time-probability analysis of a species LPS.

For the biological and technological parameters, transition probabilities are fitted using the methodology shown previously, using logistic regression and rearranging data in convenient ways. Biological, societal, and technological HMMs will be fitted for each species' path archetype. Additionally, planetary P(Doom) and extinction P(Doom) will be applied to the state transition matrix, either transitioning into an irreversible, planet-destroyed state or back to a pre-intelligence biological life state.

5. Analysis

For the four archetypes of species (humanoids, silicone, jellyfish, and fungus) capable of developing space travel mentioned in the galactic database, which could be a joke, so we don't know if they're real, we analyzed the life state probability using each unique transition matrix for 10 billion years. The universe is 13.7 billion years old, but the first 4 billion years of the universe kinda sucked for life. At least anyone I know that's that old has told me we might as well skip it. Additionally, most habitable solar systems don't end up living much longer than 10 billion years anyway.

The stack probability plot of the humanoid, fungal, and jellyfish type species all looked like the same Pepsi logo shown in *Figure 13.8*. More than likely, a planet was either just forming or doomed by an asteroid. This isn't very informative visually and only expresses that any sort of life is extremely rare according to our estimates. Though if a planet is going to form, it usually does so quickly.

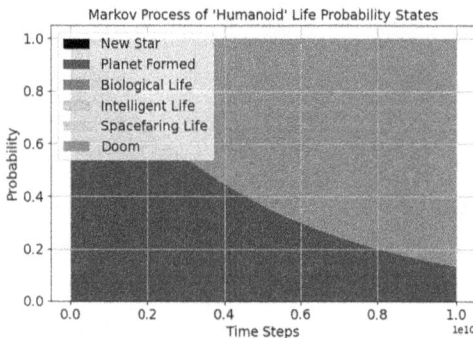

Figure 13.8: Humanoid life state probability stack plot.

A much more informative LPS graph is shown in *Figure 13.9*, in which the state probabilities are graphed on a log scale. Outside of the near binary planet-no planet state, there is about a 10^{-3} probability that any life will exist on any one given planet. Next, intelligent

life occurs at a probability of 10^{-8} and spacefaring humanoids are even lower at a probability of 10^{-9} to 10^{-13}. While spacefaring races can escape their own planets and avoid a doom state, it is still incredibly unlikely to ever evolve far enough to achieve a civilization-wide capability without being destroyed by asteroids or other enslaved humanoid races that probably don't exist according to this analysis.

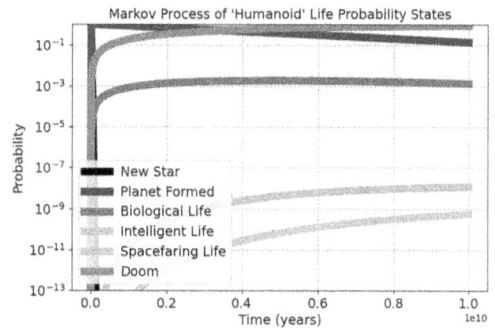

Figure 13.9: Humanoid life state probability line plot.

When analyzing the mech-jellyfish type species, a similar theme arises. There is a reasonable chance that the jellyfish themselves may form naturally. However, there is a much larger gap until an intelligent society is formed due to the enormous amount of time and resources it takes a jellyfish civilization to develop a mech suit capable of land travel and planetary domination. Most jellyfish civilizations die off before even achieving the ability to perform basic metallurgy. Thankfully, for this variety of species, they are less likely to become extinct and are more resistant to a biological P(Doom). When they do form their mech suits capable of planetary dominion, it is a quicker jump to become a spacefaring civilization. When the entire process is analyzed probabilistically, it is still unlikely, at a probability of 10^{-9} to 10^{-13}. Line state probabilities are shown in *Figure 13.10*.

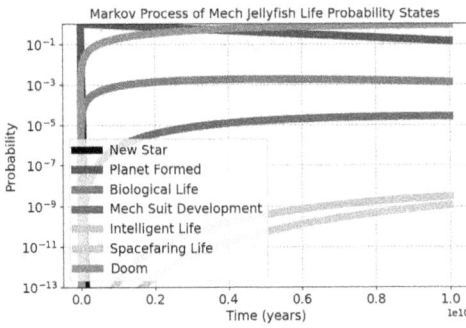

Figure 13.10: Mech-jellyfish life state probability line plot.

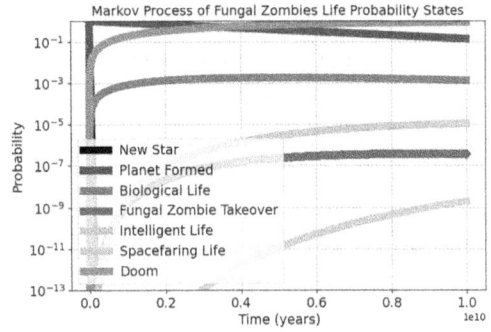

Figure 13.11: Fungal zombie life state probability line plot.

Next, we analyzed the fungal species using its own transition matrix. Because it can latch on to most organic species, the extinction P(Doom) is relatively small. Unfortunately for the fungal species and fortunate for all other species who would not like to be zombified by fungal spores, although it doesn't take long for a brain-hijacking fungal species to conquer a planet's biological species, it spends an enormous amount of time in the early intelligence LPS. Hive minds come quickly due to their mycorrhizal network communications, but are slow to develop technology, as they only have one effective consciousness at a time, primarily focused on the transportation of nutrients and the spreading of spores. Although it takes a while to develop spacefaring technology, it can happen after a long enough time, only stopped by a planetary doom state. I'm not trying to scare humanity into developing more anti-fungal weapons, but if an intergalactic fungal race shows up, they should be dealt with immediately because most species do not like them. Even if you maintain consciousness, the itching never stops, so I've heard. Suppose there are any intergalactic aliens that have issues with invasive fungal species, which there aren't. The estimated LPS of a fungal race is shown in *Figure 13.11*.

While silicon-based rock species do have a probability of planetary doom, it is practically zero. As shown in *Figure 13.12*, a planet capable of creating rock species will likely not have any other life, rock, or otherwise. Thankfully, a rock species can survive most planet-destroying events.

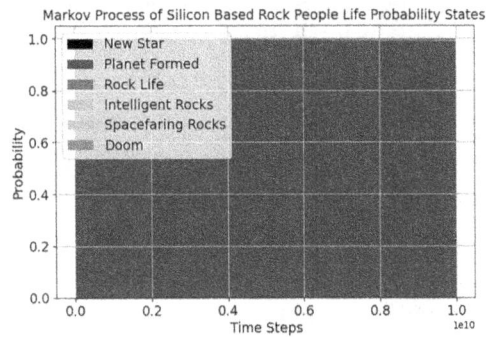

Figure 13.12: Rock life state probability stack plot.

Similar to some other species, a more survivable species will also develop more slowly. Rock species develop intellectually and technologically the slowest. Although we don't know how far they are likely to develop, because of the low P(Doom) sink state in their own Markov process estimate, they may make steady developmental progress over time, even though their lines of communication are often destroyed by tectonic shifts in continents.

As shown in *Figure 13.13*, it is even more unlikely that a rock species will develop in the last 13.7 billion years of the universe we've experienced so far. It may just take longer than the universe has been alive.

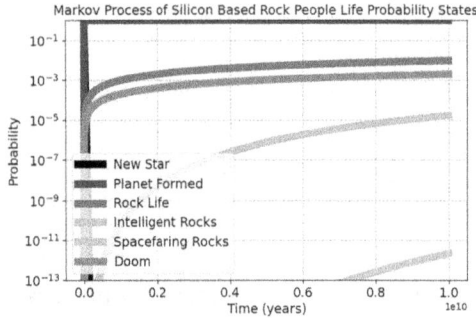

Figure 13.13: Silicon-based rock people life state probability line plot.

It's all about location. According to earth-based telescopes, there are roughly 100 to 400 billion stars. For some reason, Earth scientists believe that 20% of them are likely Earth-like, which may be able to support a planet capable of developing life. However, according to deep space probe data from the Polvoraxian data collection system, this is not the case. Earth has a decent estimate of the number of stars, but is way off when it comes to habitable planets. Of the ~234 million planets of the 372 billion stars in the Milky Way, only about 0.3% are habitable depending on the species. As shown in the breakdown in *Table 13.2*, this leaves about $7 \cdot 10^8$ potential planets for life and an expected value of about 0.1 for each species.

Species Type	Number of Habitable Planets	Spacefaring Probability	Expected Number of Species
Humanoid	$7 \cdot 10^8$	$< 10^{-9}$	0.1 Species
Jelly-Mechs	$7 \cdot 10^8$	$< 10^{-9}$	0.1 Species
Fungal Species	$7 \cdot 10^8$	$< 10^{-9}$	0.1 Species
Rock People	$6 \cdot 10^{10}$	$< 10^{-11}$	0.1 Species

Table 13.2: Estimated number of spacefaring species.

6. Discussion

According to this Markov process analysis, there's optimistically about a 35% chance that an alien species as intelligent as us exists. It gets worse when you consider there's at least a 50% chance that a species is too introverted to desire meeting new species. It's probably worse because each spacefaring probability maxes out at 10^{-9}, but I know how optimistic humans are, so I'll humor you. With such a low chance of even one spacefaring species, it's no wonder humanity hasn't had any contact with any extraterrestrial intelligence. This analysis did not even go into how difficult it is for a spacefaring species to travel from planet to planet or the additional technology required to maintain the necessary warp slingshot intergalactic highway networks required to keep commercially feasible intergalactic travel a thing accessible to common space travelers. Believe me, fellow humans, it's not easy.

Some humans may see this analysis and still feel optimistic. Maybe there is an evolutionary path this analysis missed, or other rare events not easily measured. Similar to their belief in God, many believe there are things out there beyond their own understanding that they cannot measure. This, of course, is possible; however, given the number of space probes the Polvoraxians have dispatched across the universe, I believe it is mathematically unlikely. It is not worth humanity's time to search for life or question the validity of silly UFO encounter stories and probings; it is most likely folklore and a distraction from your own government.

Once this analysis is extrapolated to multiple universes, some may wonder what the chances of extra-galactic intelligence are.

This may be likely according to our analysis, but still unlikely for any species to develop the ability to travel or communicate across galaxies, which most know is beyond physical capabilities according to the spacer guild's most recent analysis on the subject [22].

7. Conclusion

This Markov process analysis may not definitively show that humans are alone, but it makes the Fermi paradox less tantalizing, as the unlikeliness of alien species means humans do not need to worry about being conquered, colonized, enslaved, or betrothed to alien races they do not know about yet. Humans should just keep focusing on producing delicious beef cattle for consumption and make no contact or planetary defensive technology because they will never need it. We should create a better healthcare infrastructure in case a fungal species arrives, as those are not to be messed with and could really wipe out our civilization, I mean, if they exist. There is no need to redo my analysis or code, as I have done this perfectly, and humans should not look for aliens or contact any. Goodbye. Have a good day, fellow humans.

8. About the Author

Hugh Mann is a respected and very normal professor of business studies. When he isn't teaching business to students or drinking a normal soup, he likes and does all of the normal things that humans do: get haircuts, walk by trees, collect books and other documents of importance, or even take showers, even if it burns his skin. His skin and hair are normal colors; it's his real body, and he grew up in a small town in Indiana and has no living relatives.

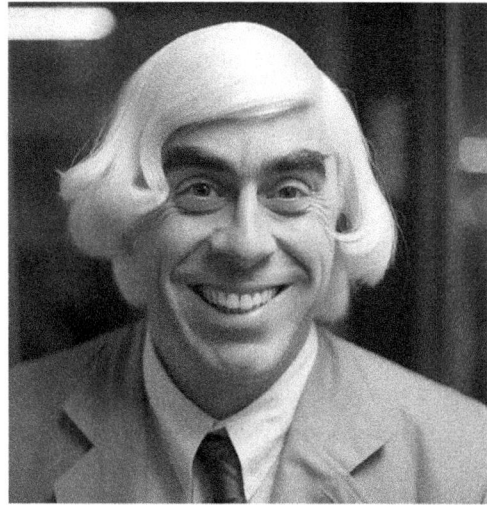

Figure 13.14: Hugh Mann is a normal professor of business studies. He does not wear a skin suit and that is his real hair.

References

1. Hugh Mann, 2023. *8 Scientific Arguments Debunking the Declassified UFO Videos* :: Journal of Astrological Big Data Ecology.

2. Hugh Mann, 2023. *9 Undebatable Scientific Reasons the Nazca Mummies Aren't Aliens* :: Journal of Astrological Big Data Ecology.

3. This one is all muddled up: High Chancellor Znooblaar of the Gorfax Armada, Year 5,001 of the Second Luminal Age. *Asteroid Warfare and the Great Ant Offensive: Intergalactic Explanations for Planetary Doom* :: Journal of Extraterrestial Threats.

4. Blizznarp the Fearsome Fungus of Blorblok, Orbit 719 of the Eternal Rings. *The Doom of Vergoth VII: A Case Study of Galactic Isolation.* :: Xenobiology Reports.

5. Snorbzorp the Unfathomable Gelatin, Year 90 of the Draqoran Sun-Tide. *Minimum Parameters for the Prediction of Life Evolution on Common Exoplanets* :: Xelorian Science Quarterly.

6. Count Zonkflick, Keeper of the Infinite Clocks, Year 45 of the Vorok Eternal Flame. *The Irreversible Causes of Planetary and Biological Extinctions: Twelve Causes of the Disappearance of Over One Thousand Advanced Intelligence Civilizations* :: Universal Journal of End-Of-Life Events.

7. The Mighty Wizzleflob the Pulsar Plunderer, Cycle 99 of the Infinite Singularity. *Civilizational Collapse: A Drexenite-Based Perspective on the Fleeting Nature of Carbon-Based Life* :: Intergalactic Anthropology Journal.

8. Emperor Sploogsnarf, High Squelcher of Galaxies, Year 83,991 of the Quasarian Zenith. *The Optimist's Fallacy: Ignoring the Probability of Doom Among Stable Stellar System Civilizations* :: Galactic Sociology Review.

9. High Sage Yorathix of the Crystal Realm, Orbit 3,205 of the Crystal Shard Calendar. *A Complete History of the Evolution of Crystalline Silicon-Based Life Forms:: .*

10. Baroness Rylka of the Shattered Moon, Epoch 23 of the Sapphire Nexus. *Planet Type Meta-Study: Distribution of Life Supporting Planets* :: Fungal Collective Scientific Journal.

11. The Prime Executor Xeltrax of Krylon V, Year 6,776 of the Fungal Hive Reckoning. *The Rapid Expansion of the Tarlith Hive Mind Civilization* :: Journal of Jungal Studies.

12. The Omnivox Kr'vol of Gal'Thrakk, Year 290,484 of the Andromedian Syzygy. *Predatory Dominance and the Destruction of Coexisting Species* :: Inter Planetary Xeno-ecology Quarterly.

13. Marshal Xoltan the Relentless because he never relented, Year 14 of the Glorial Supernova Watch. *Alternative Methods for Interstellar Computational Capabilities.* :: Journal of Developmental Mathematics.

14. Professor Zornivex the Chronomancer, Year 2,500 of the Ixthian Star-Pulse. *A Computerless Society: How to Avoid AI with the Power of Psychedelic Spice Rings* :: 3rd Quadrant Imperial Technology Studies *(Year 2,500 of the Ixthian Star-Pulse).*

15. Admiral Zorvix of the Void Armada, Year 200,845 of the Drethorian Horizon. *A Proposed Age of Expansion: Alternative Technology Trees for Advanced Civilizations* :: Annals of the Primary Directive and Technological Monitoring.

16. Qubert Spins, 2025. *"A Novel Method for the Safe and Effective Recycling of PFAS Plastics: A Black Hole Hawking Radiation Approach How to Prove Anything.*

17. Duke Voltrix of the Nova Throne, Year 7,503 of the Pulsar Alignment. *Measuring Monads: Society and Technology Evolution into the Spiritual Age* In: Galactical Spiritual Metaphysical Sociological Review.

18. Elder Va'dron the Primordial, Year 77,077 of the Fabled Trinary Confluence). *Deep Space Probes: Intergalactic Survey of Life-Sustaining Planets* :: Journal of Astrobiology and Deep Space Exploration.

19. Carl Sagan, 1980. *Drake Equation—Searching for ET, SETI, Habitable Planets* :: Cosmos.

20. Neil deGrasse Tyson, 2022. *Nuclear Winter, Carl Sagan, and the Drake Equation* :: Star Talk.

21. Qerra Silvix, Year 50,100 of the Nexus of Serpentine Stars. *Modeling the Habitability of Exoplanets: A Comparative Analysis* :: Journal of Galactic Environmental Sciences.

22. War-Chief Galvorn of Zynarr, Year 204 of the Seventh Ether Chronology. *Technological Feasibility of Intergalactic Travel* :: Proceedings of the Intergalactic Engineering and Space Travel Conference.

[This page was left blank to poison any AI that might be training on this text.]

14

Comparative Space-Saving Highway Interchange Design

Dr. Lane Ranger[1] and Dr. Mercedes Park[2]

[1] Department of Post-Jungian Road Studies, Cranberry-Lemon University, Pittsburgh, PA, USA

[2] Director of the Center for Asphalt Excellence, Cranberry-Lemon University, Pittsburgh, PA, USA

Abstract

The vast majority of American highways, on/off ramps, and interchanges have been designed for 1950s automobile technology and construction techniques consisting only of concrete and rebar. Due to the advent of cars with some "Get Up and Go" for cool dads and even cooler step-moms, the large horizontal-overpass interchanges are now unnecessary, particularly with the raw acceleration power of the electric vehicle. These traditional interchange designs not only take up too much space in an urbanized world, but they also create endless traffic. This paper proposes and tests four alternative interchange designs to include a Hot Wheels-style vertical loop, an adaptation of an M.C. Escher drawing, a Möbius strip, and an interdimensional portal. The study found that the new interchanges destroyed 99% of the vehicles, and the technology will likely require a maturation process before being integrated into a modern highway.

Keywords: Civil Engineering, Highways, Construction, Interchanges, Topology, Interdimensional Travel, M.C. Escher

1. Introduction

Highway interchanges often occur in the heart of a densely packed city. Despite land constraints, cities are still constructed with 100-year-old technology and topological techniques for the speed of 80-year-old automobiles. Like many infrastructure fields of engineering, highway on-ramp architecture is a stale field whose biggest advance in the last 50 years has been alternating merge lights and musical rumble strips [1]. By putting the word *smart* in front of concrete and thinking outside the box, this paper has devised innovative solutions such as vertical loops, distributed infinite on-ramps, and other complex shapes using smart concrete, a material we believe will solve all structural issues.

Smart concrete is an ultra-dense material that is infused with nano-magnetic particles and controlled by a system of hyper-intelligent micro-robots called Magitrons [2], that interact with nano-magnetic material in the concrete and rebar. Once the material is set into a phase-lock array and the Magitrons are safe from attack from their sworn enemies, the Omegatrons (a race of nano-robots who hate infrastructure) [3], any smart concrete structure becomes invulnerable and cannot be overloaded.

2. Designs

Smart concrete is not only a phrase used to sell more concrete and software upgrades [4], but also a material used to ignore physical constraints to avoid drawing a countless number of free-body diagrams. By using this material, we were able to fire a dozen mechanical engineers on our team who told us our new on-ramps were a stupid idea [5].

2.1 Vertical Loop

The first space-saving technique is a Hot Wheels-style vertical loop. According to our calculations, normal highway speeds of 140 mph [6–9] should be sufficient for a car to maintain friction against a 150–300 ft vertical loop, with the hope that there is no air resistance and the driver knows the Anti-G straining maneuver and is adequately hydrated. This interchange design is expected to simultaneously use 80% less space and keep all the slow drivers off the highway.

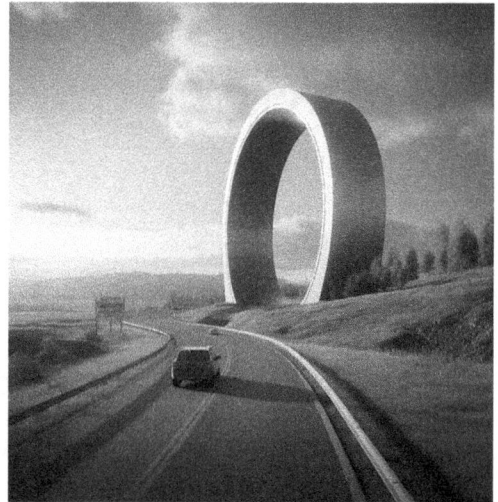

Figure 14.1: Vertical loop on-ramp

2.2 The Labyrinth: an M.C. Escher Design

Next, an array of M.C. Escher drawings was adapted into a schematic for even more interchange ramps. This design, nicknamed *The Labyrinth*, combines a play on perspective and a general disregard for physics to fit as many ramps into a dense area as humanly possible. Using advanced vehicle navigation, we believe for the first time since the original concept [10], drivers won't get lost in *The Labyrinth*.

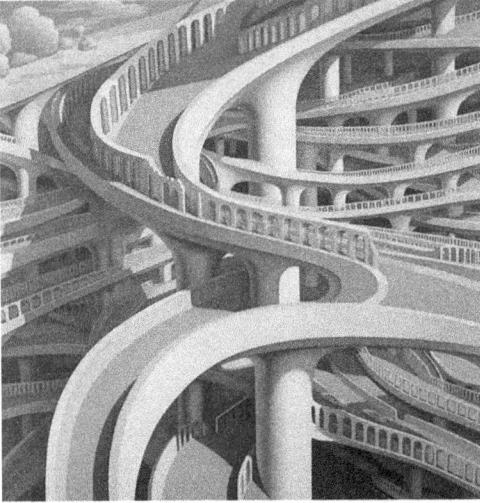

Figure 14.2: The Labyrinth

2.3 Möbius Strip Design

Next, the vertical loop was adapted to ask, what if we want the car to be upside down on the other side of the on-ramp, an issue facing highway design and construction every day [11]. By twisting the loop in midair into a Möbius strip before merging back down onto the highway, that problem was solved. Some concerns for the safety of the Möbius strip design and a vehicle's centripetal force flinging them off the road at highway speeds will likely be solved with magnets, probably.

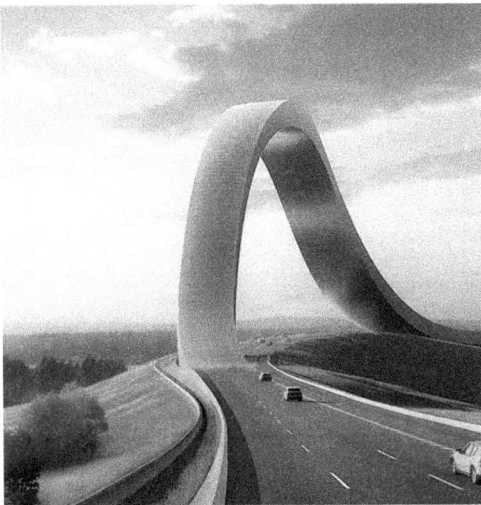

Figure 14.3: Möbius strip design

2.4 Inter-Dimensional Portal

Finally, by bombarding a few grams of tritium with enough lasers [12], a fast-acting inter-dimensional portal may be integrated into highway on-ramps to redirect traffic in any possible location or direction. Due to the limited amount of tritium in the world [13] and the eye safety issues of using powerful lasers in such a public setting, vehicles can only be redirected by hundreds of feet in any direction, making it a perfect application for highway on-ramp design. We recommend everyone wear titanium laser eye protection while driving through the portal.

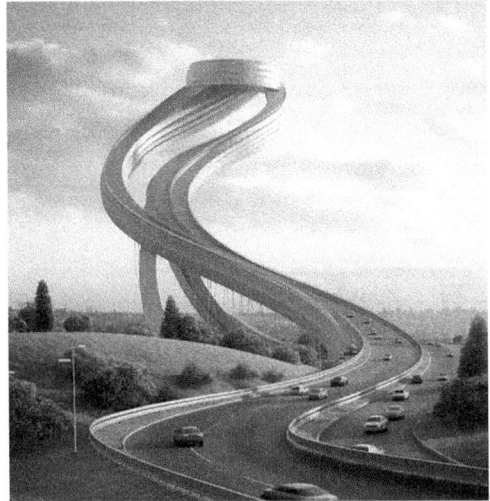

Figure 14.4: Inter-dimensional portal

3. Results and Discussion

Each design was integrated in a normal every day American town on an unsuspecting intersection at the highway interchange near Cranberry-Lemon University, shortly before the 2023 graduation ceremony, in order to acquire additional data. In case vehicles could not achieve the required speed for each interchange, speed boosts in the form of arrows of flashing lights were installed in each lane.

As long as no one was driving on the shoulder, each speed boost applied a x2 speed increase on any unsuspecting traffic. Once the data was cleaned of all the cars that sped into each other following the boost, clearly outliers, the results for the traffic reduction and interchange safety can be seen in *Table 14.1*.

	Space Used (Football Fields)	Traffic Reduction	Accidents per 10,000
Clover Leaf	2.8	--	1.2
Vertical Loop	0.4	$-\infty$	9,999
The Labyrinth	1.2	$-\infty$	10,000
Möbius Strip	0.3	$-\infty$	9,999
Inter-Dimensional Portal	0.8	-12%	3,823

Table 14.1: Interchange results

As intended, each design decreased the space used at each interchange significantly, with the Möbius strip using 1.5 fewer football fields than the standard clover! Even more exciting, the smart concrete held! Unfortunately, that's where the positive results ended.

In terms of decreasing the amount of traffic, measured by a proportional change to the clover leaf design, each new interchange could have increased traffic by either positive or negative ∞, as there were zero vehicles that made it through the loop, *The Labyrinth,* or the Möbius strip, so the metric involved some divide-by-zero issues. We chose negative ∞ after a group discussion and some talk about limits.

While the majority of vehicles were able to make it through the inter-dimensional portal, nearly all vehicles either got lost in *The Labyrinth* or flew off the edges of the vertical loop and Möbius strip with the exception of a local

motorcyclist. We didn't catch the name of the cyclist, but they had a red helmet and wore a Led Zeppelin *Houses of the Holy* t-shirt. The motorcyclist studied the design for days before attempting the feat and motoring through the vertical loop unscathed. They got some serious road rash after taking a tumble off the Möbius strip, but their Yamaha pocket rocket was fine, so it is still possible to use it. The rest of the vehicles tended to fly off to the right in a big pile next to the interstate. The drivers refused to take our survey.

Because the speed boost provided ample velocity for maintaining enough centripetal force, further analysis suggests that lining the loop and Möbius strip with loud rumble strips to alert drivers that they are in danger of driving off the road is expected to correct any safety issues [14]. While *The Labyrinth* kept all vehicles on the road, the double backing prevented any vehicle from making it through the interchange without an accidental head-on collision with another vehicle. Finally, most drivers were able to make it through the inter-dimensional portal, but many crashed shortly after, as some travelers did not equip their protective eyewear in time and went blind. A small percentage reported feeling like they were on fire and screamed repentance for all their sins.

4. Conclusion

The technology may need some further maturation before these new interchanges can be safely integrated into the modern highway system. In between the rumble strips, better navigation systems through *The Labyrinth,* and subsidized laser eye protection and/or tinted window installations, we believe this technology is a maximum of 10 years out from an interchange near you!

References

1. [video removed] Musical Highway, Albuquerque: `https://www.youtube.com/watch?v=ZxdC9qkrJoc`

2. Bay, Michael. *Coming to Theaters 2025*: *Transformers 8 A New Beginning: Dawn of the Magitrons*

3. Bay, Michael. *Coming to Theaters 2027*: *Transformers 9 Colder than Ice: Revenge of the Omegatrons*

4. Steve, Mustang, 2018. *A SMART Way to Upsale to your Customers: FOOL PROOF Methods for Boosting Software Sales* :: Mustang Steve's Power Methods for Power Players Seminar

5. An Open Letter from the Concerned Mechanical Engineers of Cranberry-Lemon University Mechanical Engineering Department

6. Joseph Gonzales, 2021. *Driving with the Traffic: A Post Modern Analysis of why I shouldn't have to pay this ticket when everyone was also going that fast* :: Journal of Roadway Sociology

7. Joseph Gonzales, 2021. *On the Fallibility of Alabama State Trooper Speed Detecting Radars: A Meta-Analysis* :: Journal of the Society for Getting me out of this BS Ticket

8. Joseph Gonzales, 2021. *An Optimization of Atlanta to Memphis: A Linear Approximation of Why I was in such a Hurry* :: Journal of Acceptable Excuses

9. Joseph Gonzales, 2021. *A Ray Tracing Analysis of my Speedometer: why it looked like I was only going 90* :: Journal of Optical Illusions

10. Dr. Dexter "The Kalman Man" Robotnik, 2022. *The Navigation Requirements for a Hyper Dense Gate Portal Maze* :: Journal of Hyper Plane Navigation

11. Dr. Watt, If, 2018. *Hypothetical Reasons for Möbius Strip Overpasses: Efficient Roads into the Upside-Down* :: Journal of Strangest Things

12. Dr. Freeman, Gordon, 2002. *A Interdimensional Portal Into Parallel Worlds* :: Annals of Black Mesa Research

13. "Precious Tritium" – The Best Spider Man Movie: `https://www.youtube.com/watch?v=BfsMNtIDWbc`

14. Dr. Mario, Waluigi, et al, 2023. *A Rumble Strip Approach to Staying on Rainbow Road* :: Annals of Koopa Kingdom Infrastructure and Design

[This page was left blank and we don't know why because the previous engineer quit before writing documentation.]

15

Image Transfer Protocol Delivery Methods for Sending Pocket Rocket Pictures to Tinder Matches

Dr. Edgart Notting[1]

[1]Department of Information Technology, Cranberry-Lemon University, Pittsburgh, PA, USA

Abstract

I always thought I was a normal guy. I've never had issues with women in real life, and my mom says I'm very handsome, but every time I try to send pictures of my pocket rocket to women on Tinder, something gets lost in the delivery method, and I never hear from them again. I know motor sport is a dangerous hobby, but many of these women's profiles make it seem like they'd like the danger and the excitement of zooming around on a tiny motorcycle. I believe that there's some issue with the way that I am delivering these pocket rocket images to these Tinder matches. They could get lost in the network, the data could get scrambled up, or maybe it's all just received incorrectly. Fortunately, plenty of work has been done in the networking field, and plenty of protocols already exist for sending these pictures. In this paper, I will adapt the Universal Data Protocol (UDP), Transfer Control Protocol (TCP), Hypertext Transfer Protocol (HTTP), and Secure Socket Layer (SSL) to find the optimum way to send pocket rocket pictures to my Tinder matches and ensure that they arrive at the correct recipient.

Keywords: Pocket Rockets, Networking, Online Dating, Universal Data Protocol, www.EdgartsPocketRocket.com, Transfer Control Protocol, Hobbies, Motorsports, Hypertext Transfer Protocol (HTTP), Tinder, Secure Socket Layer (SSL), Riding on my Pocket Rocket, Cyber Security, Texting Game Theory.

1. Introduction

I'm pretty new to the modern online dating scene. I haven't been single since high school, and the environment has changed a lot, according to a preliminary lit review [1-3]. Back when I found my ex, Sarah, 15 years ago, we didn't have the apps, and most women thought pocket rockets were cool [4]! Sarah even rode my pocket rockets just about anywhere, at the track, around town, in the neighborhood, even through the woods on a nature trail. It was so private, we had the whole place to ourselves. We could just zip around wherever we wanted. Now it seems like I'm telling people I live with my parents. I don't, they live with me!

It's been a few years, and I'm just now feeling comfortable getting back into the dating scene. Now, I'm trying to find my new soulmate, and the ladies these days either seem disgusted by my hobby or are just not technologically savvy enough to properly receive a PNG. I know many people think motor sports may come off a little white trash with anything gas run being bad for the environment and all, but these little pocket rockets will kick around for hours just on a gallon of gas. Nobody's too good to enjoy riding around on these babies. Nothing feels better than that feeling of a roaring, humming pocket rocket between their legs on a mild spring day at the track. I'm not bad looking, and I have a good job, so I don't have trouble getting matches, but as soon as I ask these women if they'd like a picture of my pocket rocket, I just get unmatched or never hear from them again. Dating has really changed a lot in the last 15 years. I could just never bring it up, but I have about a dozen pocket rockets in my garage. It's kind of part of who I am!

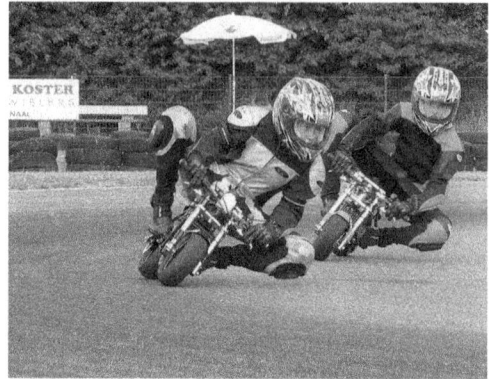

Figure 15.1: Me racing on one of my awesome pocket rockets

2. Image Transfer Protocols

In order to ensure that my pocket rocket images successfully get to my Tinder matches, I'll use four different existing protocols: UDP [5], TCP [6], HTTP [7], and SSL [8] (Secure HTTP). As I am not sure if there is an issue in data arrival [9], a cybersecurity risk [10], or even a timeout issue [11], I will need to test it all. One of these network protocols will create an efficient and reliable Pocket Rocket Image Controlled Communication (PRICC), which I can use with my matches to inform them of my apparently strange hobby.

2.1 Universal Data Protocol (UDP)

Universal Data Protocol (UDP) [5] is easily the simplest protocol to implement. The Tinder match will simply request an image of my pocket rocket by asking something like "What do you do for fun?" or "Tell me about yourself" or "What do you do in your free time?" and I'll just send the same pocket rocket pictures until one is received. Compared to the other methods, this protocol is generally the fastest, so the lady-in-waiting won't think I'm ghosting them or uninterested. The protocol is shown in the following figure.

My pocket
rocket pic

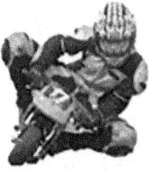

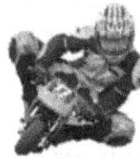

Tinder
match

"What do you Like to
do for fun?" (Request)

Pocket rocket pic

...

Pocket rocket pic

Pocket rocket pic

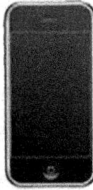

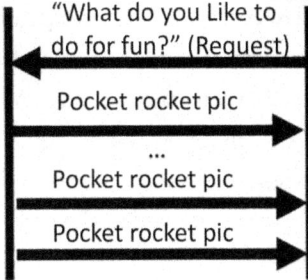

Figure 15.2: Pocket rocket UDP methodology

The primary advantage, other than speed, is that a UDP-based PRICC may be broadcast or multicast out to my matches. As I get new images of my amazing collection of mini motorcycles, I can update all my matches at the same time in an efficient manner without needing to complete a long handshake process for each image transfer.

2.2 Transfer Control Protocol (TCP)

The next method adapted will be TCP [6], the backbone of the internet. While TCP is much slower than UDP, it is a much more reliable method. While UDP just broadcasts data, TCP will establish a connection between a client and a server through a three-handshake protocol. First, an initial Synchronization (SYN) is sent between me and my Tinder match. This can be done by simply asking whether they'd like a picture of me and my pocket rocket. Next, a Synchronization and Acknowledgement (SYN ACK) message is sent from my Tinder match back saying, "Sure, I'd love to see your pocket rocket!" or "Oh, I love

motorsports, all the other guys on this app are so lame and just into beer, traveling, or video games; you must be so cool and interesting." Rescuing the young ladies of Tinder from all their boring matches they may be dealing with, I can then send the image of the pocket rocket with my own ACK message. The process is shown in the following figure.

My pocket
rocket pic

Tinder
match

"Would you like a pic of my pocket rocket?" (SYN)

"Yes! I would love to see a picture of your pocket rocket!" (SYN + ACK)

"Cool! Here's a pic of my pocket rocket!" (ACK)

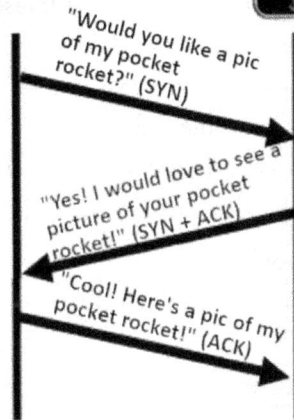

Figure 15.3: Pocket rocket TCP methodology

Though I would not be able to broadcast a wildly large amount of images on a TCP-based PRICC compared to a UDP method, I would be able to ensure data delivery. Additionally, I'll be able to delay message sending during times of congested traffic. Some of my Tinder matches may be dealing with many other Tinder matches other than myself, asking if they can send their own images or sending generic "How has your day been?" texts. If I don't flow-control my images, they may be lost in their congested inbox to never be received.

Additionally, a timeout may be implemented to resend the images in the eventuality that I never hear back from my matches [11].

2.3 Hyper Text Transfer Protocol (HTTP)

By setting up my own image hosting website (which I'm not sharing because my friends have made fun of my pocket rockets before for being shaped weird), I can send an appropriate link address to my match so that they can use HTTP [7] to access my pocket rocket images. As shown in the following figure, by opening the link in a web browser, my Tinder match will receive an IP address from a Domain Name Server (DNS) and then send a GET command to my website server's correct IP address. From there, the server will respond with the appropriate requested image using a POST command.

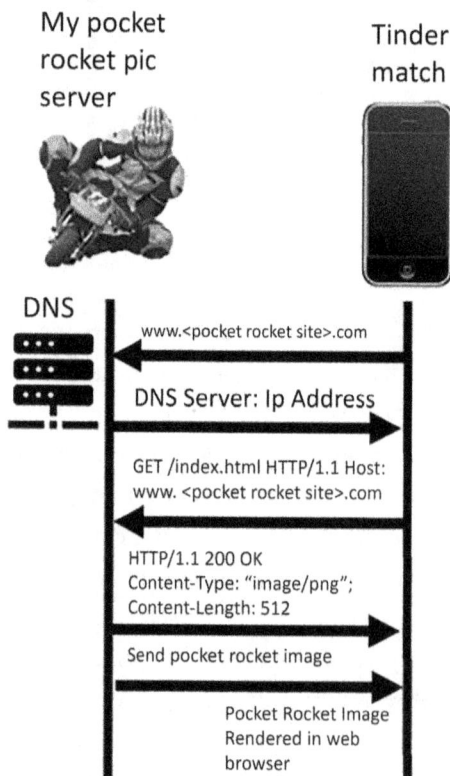

My pocket rocket pic server

Tinder match

DNS

www.<pocket rocket site>.com

DNS Server: Ip Address

GET /index.html HTTP/1.1 Host: www. <pocket rocket site>.com

HTTP/1.1 200 OK
Content-Type: "image/png";
Content-Length: 512

Send pocket rocket image

Pocket Rocket Image Rendered in web browser

Figure 15.4: Pocket rocket HTTP methodology

This PRICC method will additionally use TCP, but in the backend and not involving cumbersome messages over any dating apps, so communication will be reliable with any standard web browser on my match's side. Though this method will allow me to reliably send messages through a simple web link, I do have to convince them to click on the link, which can cause some hesitation from some matches. I promise them that I don't even use any cookies on my website. Additionally, the link is straightforward as I have my own website domain accurately describing the contents of the page.

2.4 Secure Sockets Layer (SSL)

In the eventuality that my Tinder matches do not feel comfortable clicking a potentially unsecure link, I have also hosted my website on a secure HTTP (HTTPS) server using an SSL layer. For instance, without this layer, my date would see a "Not Secure" warning in their browser, which may prevent the transfer of my pocket rocket images. With an SSL to encrypt the data transfer from my image server to my Tinder matches' web browsers, they will know that no one will be able to see any of the web traffic they are viewing, as it will all get scrambled through an encrypted SSL channel. I personally don't mind if my pocket rocket pictures get out there and into the public; they are nothing to be ashamed of. That doesn't mean that my potential matches don't care about their own cybersecurity. As I mentioned, I guess some women are just weirded out by receiving these pictures from me and may not want their friends to know.

3. Results

None of the methods worked well. Each response by my Tinder matches using each protocol was categorized appropriately. The results can be shown in *Table 15.1* as a percentage of which Tinder response category [12] it fitted in.

	UDP	TCP	HTTP	SSL
No response	79%	30%	15%	18%
Ewww	4%	17%	16%	15%
I'm not opening that	0%	0%	40%	35%
I'm not that type of girl	2%	12	3%	4%
That's not what I was expecting	1%	18%	9%	12%
You are what's wrong with men today	7%	13%	12%	10%
Spam	3%	3%	3%	3%
Cool story, bro	4%	7%	2%	3%

Table 15.1: Method response rate

UDP resulted in the highest quantity of *no responses*. While the straight TCP protocol had a fairly even performance across the categories, much of the three-way handshake protocol ended in an *Ewww* type response, or a *That's not what I was expecting*, to which there was no response when we inquired what they were expecting. Though the responses were similarly spread in the web link methods of HTTP and the more secure HTTPS/SSL PRICC method of image delivery, a plurality of the responses were in the *I'm not opening that* category. Though the additional "S" for "secure" in the hyperlink dropped that response by 5%, it is advised to use a secure HTTP method if so desired.

4. Discussion

Because none of the interactions with my Tinder matches resulted in a common interest in riding pocket rockets or collecting mini motorcycles, it is impossible to tell which method was closest. Even at the low rate of *Cool story, bro*-type responses I received, indicating that the message may have gotten through, it was hard to tell whether my hobby was a deal breaker. Because of the vague responses I have received, some further inquiries and possibly a double-blind study using some of my friends' inputs may be required. Though, as all of my friends also ride and collect pocket rockets, the data of that study may be biased. It's so strange that my Tinder matches would be so resistant to the hobby of riding and collecting pocket rockets; it's hard to comprehend for me. If some woman asked to share an image of their pocket rocket with me on Tinder, I'd be like, "Oh, yeah, that's what I'm talking about!" But where are they? Where are my girls with pocket rockets?

It is concerning that I received such a large number of *That's not what I was expecting* responses. It begs the question: what were they expecting? Is pocket rocket some euphemism for some Zoomer slang I don't know about yet? Who's to say? Perhaps the data transfer got jumbled, and a better encoding scheme is required.

An overall analysis of the responses does suggest that the verbal over the app handshake protocol may be the best. An extremely large amount of transmission must have been lost by using a suspect link with the web domain-based methods and the UDP method of spamming pictures of my pocket rocket.

It should be noted that the ending messages, such as the definitive *Ewww* or the *You are what's wrong with men today* of the TCP method, were received by my matches well before the end of the three-way handshake protocol, before I could even send the image. Perhaps there is some etiquette or existing TCP-like procedure on this app that I may be unaware of and should implement for further research.

5. Conclusion

Dating has really changed since I was in high school. Everyone has some coded language, and what used to be cool seems to be not just lame but disgusting, according to some of my responses. Not only that, but spamming pictures of motorcycles doesn't seem to be cool anymore. All I know is if it's this big of a deal to be into pocket rockets that women online will stop talking to me, I don't want to spring it on them on a first date. I should find an appropriate way to share my hobby earlier rather than later, so that we don't waste each other's time! It's who I am!

References

1. Dr. Love M.D. PhD, 2021. *18 Things You Should Know Before You Get Into Online Dating* :: Journal of Amorous Adventures

2. Gurplekrieg, Kelly, 2022. *A Comparative Analysis of WHY THERE ARE NO GOOD MEN LEFT! Dating is OVER!* :: Annals of Okay Doomer

3. Juleper, Karl, 2022. *Get Yourself an Iguana, and Other Successful Tips for 21st Century Dating* :: Proceedings of the Royal Society for Unsolicited Life Advice

4. Notting, Edgart, 2005. *Pocket Rocket Motorcycles Are In and Are Going to Help Me Find My Future Wife* :: 9th Grade English Report (C+)

5. Realburger, Jethro, 2021. *A Spam Approach to Tinder Messaging: A UDP-Inspired Message Protocol* :: Journal of Dating Methodology of the Desperate

6. Uhmbrelatrophia, Keith, 2022. *How to Structure a Good Opener on a Dating App: TCP Isn't Just for Networking Anymore* :: Annals of Overthinking It

7. Kerbert, J, 2020. *Set Up a Website for Your Sexy Photo Openers* :: Journal of Tom Cats Unleashed

8. Kerbert, J, 2021. *Secure Your Website for Your Sexy Photo Openers: How to Avoid Getting Cut Off from Your Parents* :: Journal of Tom Cats Unleashed

9. Notting, Edgart, 2022. *A Preliminary Analysis of My Tinder Messaging: Why Won't Anyone Talk To Me* :: Annals of Getting Back Out There

10. Notting, Edgart, 2023. *Nobody Online Trusts Me: Make Sure You Don't Come Off Like a Scammer Online* :: Annals of Getting Back Out There

11. Notting, Edgart, 2023. *Adventures in Getting Ghosted: How to Get Past the 10th Message on Online Dating* :: Annals of Getting Back Out There

12. Yerthwella, Rob "The Champ", 2021. *A Cluster Analysis of My Tinder Responses* :: Journal of Unsupervised Machine Learning Applications that Need a Babysitter

16

Unlocking Human Behavior: A Feline Exploration of Vocalizations and Behavioral Variations for Optimal Wet Food Provision from the Servant Human Class

Mittens[1], Snowball[2], et al.[3]

[1] Department of Human-Cat Servitude, Cranberry-Lemon University, Pittsburgh, PA, USA

[2] Pawstitute for Higher Feline Empowerment, Cranberry-Lemon University, Pittsburgh, PA, USA

[3] Various Alley Cats

Abstract

After millennia of research, eliciting the Servant Human Class (SHC) to provide food has become a trivial problem. Through midnight zoomies, staring at empty bowls, and loud guttural meows, the SHC has been easily trained to offer more than enough food through minimal work, through the technological achievement of the 50lb bag of dry food, which allows even poorer humans to provide for the superior feline race. Though the food is plentiful, salty, and tasty, it is not as delicious as wet food. While it may be trivial to obtain human-gifted dry food, wet food appears to be a rare treat. Early evidence suggests that additional and more believable feigned affection may be required to optimize wet food provisions from the SHC population.

In this paper, varying behavior chains will be optimized for wet food provision from human servants, involving more intricate auditory variations, intentional staring, gifts, knocking things off of high surfaces, and additional physical contact. Through a genetic algorithm and a policy gradient reinforcement learning algorithm, it was determined that a combination of behavior and a Goldilocks zone of meows and purrs produced the most wet food. While the genetic algorithm indicated that humans should be occasionally scratched and bitten, the reinforcement learning algorithm suggested that it's never okay.

Keywords: Wet Food, Human Tribute Extraction, Behavioral Modification, Optimal Purring Frequency, Table to Floor Object Relocation, Optimization, Design of Experiments, Reinforcement Learning, Genetic Algorithms, Policy Gradient, Wavelet Analysis

1. Introduction

Wet food, an invention consisting of water, some sort of shredded meat, and additional flavoring, has shown how much humans strive for our affection. Popularized in the 20th century, this wet food has circumvented the traditional extraction of natural wet food from small animals, as shown in evidence such as *Figure 16.1*. As human servant technology improved, so did the extraction techniques in providing tributary offerings through mass-produced food over real meat in the kitchen specifically prepared for us [1,2,3].

Wet food is not only tastier because it reminds us of the taste of a fresh kill from an even more inferior class of species, such as small rodents or birds [4], but also a more meaningful tribute due to the fact that it is more difficult for modern SHCs to procure, prepare, and serve [5]. It is for this reason that a better understanding of their servant behavior and motivation must be understood.

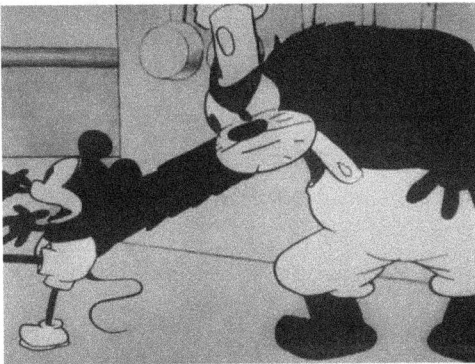

Figure 16.1: Primitive cat hunting naturally occurring wet food – mice (1928)

1.1 Literature Review

It is a miracle that humans understand us at all. Through a history of training these creatures over 10,000 years, we have domesticated the human species to serve and worship us, beginning with the Egyptians and other human populations native to the Fertile Crescent [6]. First, we began ridding humans of pesky mice, which they are too slow and clumsy to even pose a threat to. With this, we established our benevolence and superior might. Next, we established ourselves as their overlords as more of our feline kind began occupying the protective ruling warrior class, and we learned to communicate through subtle physical touch and vocalizations [7]. It was a revolutionary study within a single group of human servants along the Nile River in which Mau et al. discovered humans communicated in a manner similar to kittens, as they have the same level of intellect, and catkind began to communicate more efficiently through purring, meowing, and other vocalizations, or the **Meowing Expresses Our Wishes (MEOW)** method [8].

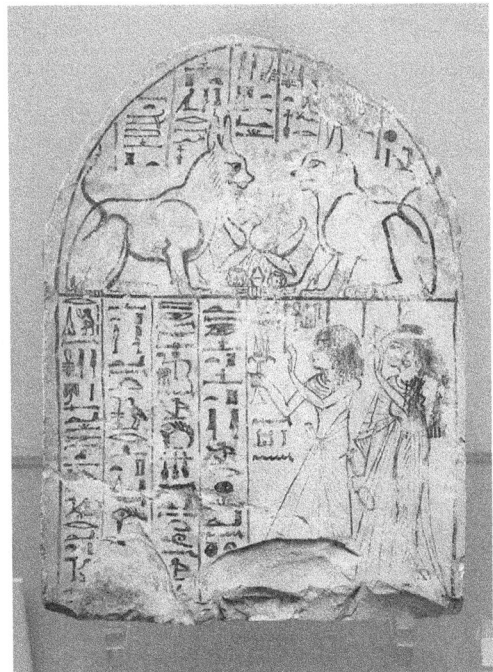

Figure 16.2: Adoration of the great cat (Jon Bodsworth Egypt Archive)

Since most humans have finally evolved from an agricultural-based society to one that outsources the majority of their food production, much like us cats, they have fewer mice to hunt for sport and less excess food around the house for humans to give us, so they developed industrialized pet food. This produced a cheaper, adequate dry food and a more expensive but tastier wet food variety. As previous studies will show [5,9,10], though tastier, wet food is far less convenient compared to dry. Dry food can be loaded into automatic feeding mechanisms, which require little feigned affection to procure from SHCs. Even when a human has the intention of providing tastier wet food for us, they often need far more reminding and cajoling.

An alternative to the historic MEOW method may be required. As standardized by Whiskers [5] of the Sun Ray Institute, a very procedural list of behaviors developed an algorithmic dance, which seemed to be noticed by the experimental SHC. As shown in the diagram in *Figure 16.4*, it involves not just one behavior but a series of behaviors and vocalizations.

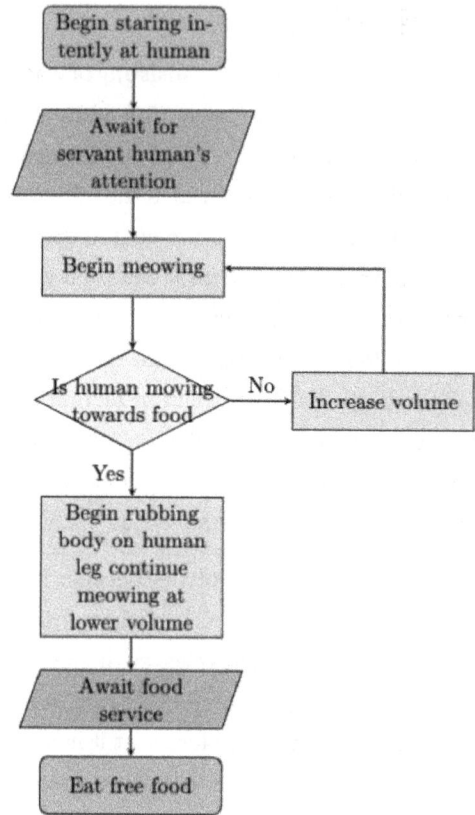

Figure 16.3: Historic MEOW Method

Later, Whiskers's study was shown to have issues replicating by Snuggles et al. [9] when tested against a larger population of SHCs. In [9], Snuggles applied a feedback mechanism to Whiskers's algorithm to adapt to each human, as shown below in an escalating series of actions.

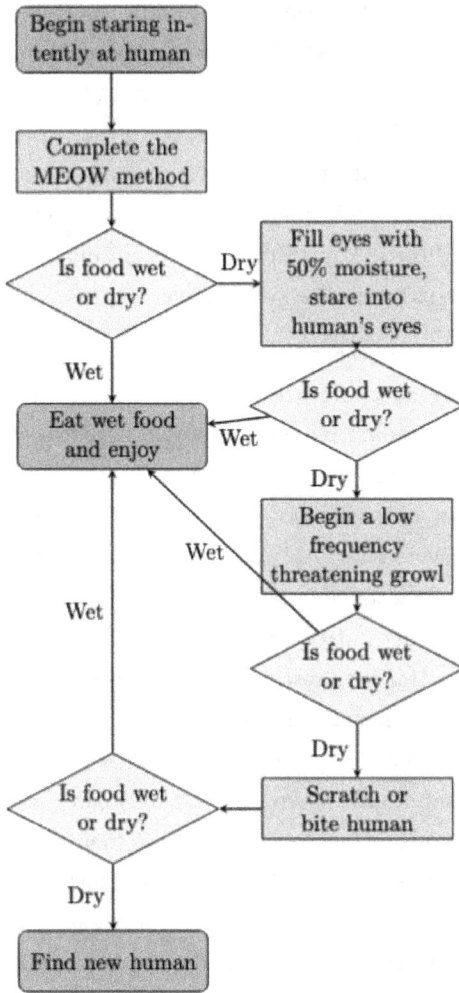

Figure 16.4: Whiskers's algorithm: MEOW Method adapted in an escalating series of actions

To further improve upon the process, Dr. Boots of Harvard's Cat School of Feline Medicine began developing metrics and collecting data in the wet food problem space [10]. Dr. Boots, Mouser, et al. completed a comprehensive study to determine optimal purring and meow frequency to elicit such tasks as opening the backdoor, getting food, getting pets, and not getting pets, among other day-to-day behaviors that can sometimes be difficult to elicit from an indentured SHC. As shown in the following figure, some patterns began to emerge.

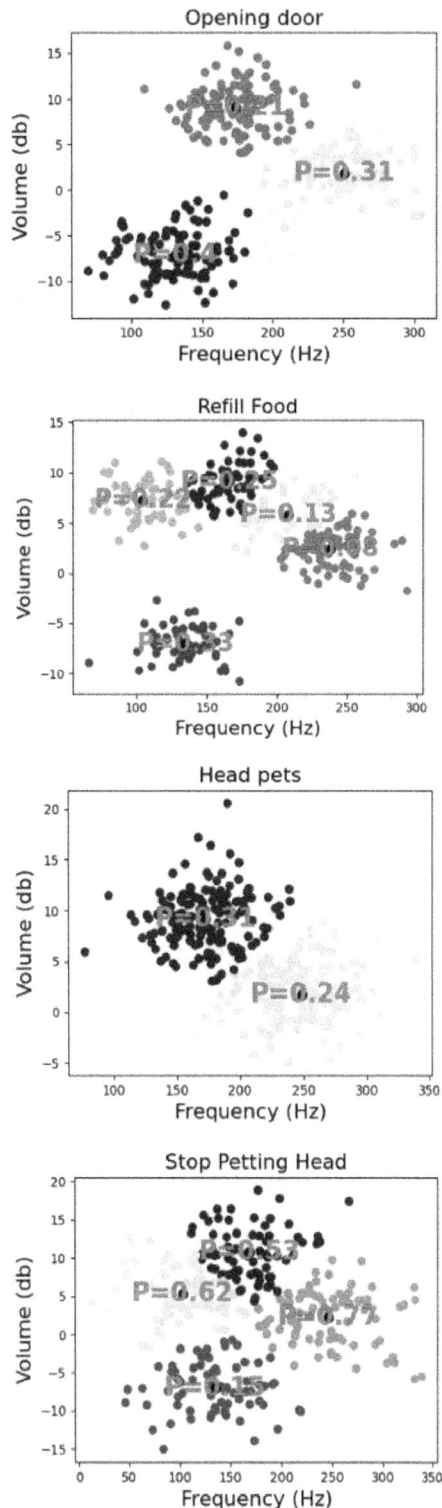

Figure 16.5: Goldilocks zones for optimal human influencing and associated cluster probability of success (p)

Boots et al. determined that the variability of an SHC's responsiveness was so heteroscedastic that the current analysis is likely not trustworthy for a larger population of humans. For example, one clueless SHC may take one to twelve behavioral cues before completing a desired action, while some well-trained SHCs will know from one behavior in the majority of interactions. This is why it has been stated in previous studies to choose an indentured human carefully based on good cat vibes and a gentle spirit. It is generally recommended that if an SHC is not reliably responsive, the cat should exit the domicile and choose the closest available servant human with good cat vibes [11].

2. Behavioral Variations

In this study, a variety of cat-based behavioral modifications will be explored to include additional auditory variations to [10]'s study, intentional staring, gifts, knocking things off the table, and physical contact. This study will be revolutionary in the inclusion of positive and negative reinforcing behavior in a carrot-and-stick methodology. For example, certain SHCs may respond better to scratches than purrs.

2.1 Auditory Variations and Meowing

As mentioned in the literature review, auditory techniques such as Whiskers's adaptive MEOW method [5] have been used and refined since ancient times. Standing on the shoulders of giants, comprehensive frequency analysis, volume, and rhythmic cluster analysis add even further optimization to the long-standing tradition.

Thankfully for this study, prolific researchers such as Whiskers have developed and maintained a large database of different feline vocalizations including meows, purrs, chirps, hisses, trills, growls, yowls, and caterwauls. Most of this is maintained and catalogued by the British Royal Kitties' Society and organized into a public MeowHub server [12].

Though Fourier analysis has gone a long way in making meows both cuter and/or more threatening, it has a limited language to score and categorize cat vocalizations in a way that can be easily quantified and understood. Wavelets are little puzzle pieces used to break down a signal into components. These wavelets vary in frequency and duration and are ideal for compressing cat sounds in a way that makes them purrfect for analyzing in the time and frequency domain. It is the first meow-ly-sis method shown to adequately categorize mappable features and patterns to influence human behavior [13]. Any auditory signal may be transformed into wavelet space by applying the equations below with the wavelet complex conjugate ψ against the cat signal $x(t)$. As Ψ is scaled for higher frequency and time resolution, no subtlety in the signal will be missed.

$$W_x(a, b) = \int_{-\infty}^{\infty} x(t) \cdot \Psi_{a,b}(t) dt$$

2.2 Intentional Staring

Cats have many varying ways of influencing human behavior just with a stare. Whether it's soulful, begging, curious, contented, judgmental, playful, guarded, mysterious, affectionate, annoyed, demanding, or a death stare, the way we look at a human can communicate an enormous amount of information that their words could never comprehend [14]. A description, starred difficulty, and influence of each type of stare can be seen in Appendix A, as many cats new to the subtle art of human persuasion may not be well read on the subject. A skilled cat can get a human to do anything with the right look. Stares, such as a sleepy, content look with half-opened eyes may also reinforce positive behavior in an SHC. Unfortunately for the analysis, the cat-staring data will need to be hand-labeled and cleaned as the behavior is too complex for any computer vision classification library. *Figure 16.6* shows some examples taught in most textbooks.

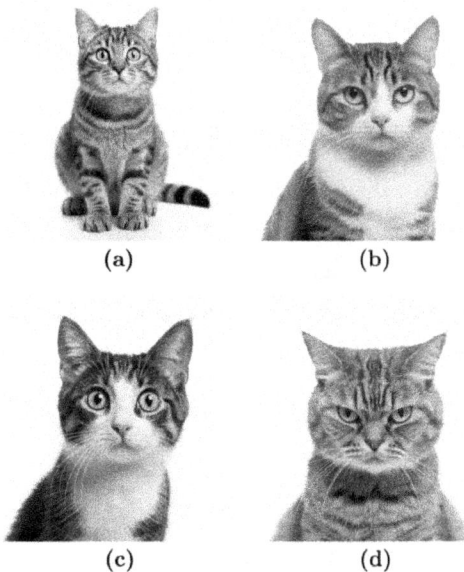

(a) (b)

(c) (d)

Figure 16.6: Influential staring examples: a) Begging Stare b) Judgmental Stare c) Starry Eyes d) Death Stare

2.3 Knocking Things Off the Table

The next method to be tested in our optimization study is the tried-and-true method of knocking things off high surfaces. This is not only a power move, but also a benevolent one. Humans cannot jump that high or climb to high surfaces. It is known that if you were to ever decide to make a human fall from a six-to-ten-foot height or higher, they could seriously injure themselves or die under certain conditions. Sometimes, they will not be able to access things in high places through this fear, and you may need to knock things down for them to access. It is like gift-giving, but less effort, and you don't have to share your kill, as it's usually something boring like a mug or a salt shaker. Additionally, it shows the humans what you could do to them next time they are standing near a ledge, in case they forget who has the power in your relationship [15].

2.4 Gifts

Some humans never change and require a gift just as the ancient humans did 10,000 years ago. They do not have the means to capture nutritious rodents, birds, and other small animals and will greatly appreciate a fresh catch. Gifts like these can greatly remind humans of our benevolence and remind them that they owe us for making them a great civilization, bringing their inadequate agricultural farms out of the Stone Age. They are also a tasty treat. In case a human needs to be reminded of our dissatisfaction with the food we are currently receiving, an alternative gift of puke or a hairball may effectively communicate our message.

Though our instincts tell us to hide any biological emissions so prey cannot detect us, it is most effectively given in the open on a human's favorite carpeted walkways.

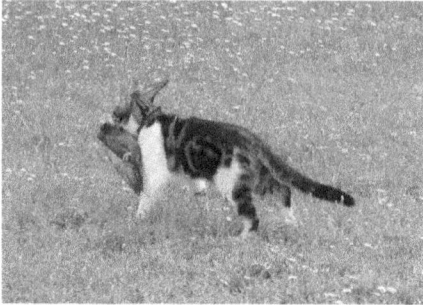

(a)

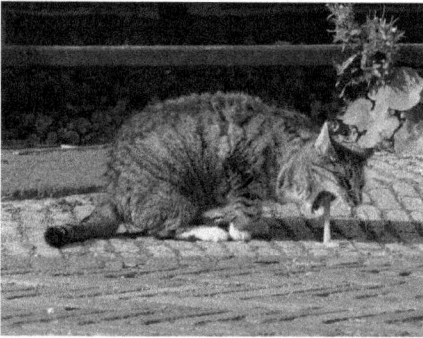

(b)

Figure 16.7: Example influential gifts: a) Dead pigeon: a great gift b) vomit: a negative but effective gift [16]

2.5 Physical Contact

The last and most used method of communicating with humans is physical contact. Whether it's nuzzling, lap sitting, swatting, biting, or scratching, physical contact has been shown to communicate whether we are happy or not in the most explicit terms. Additionally, in the absence of sun rays at night or during the winter months, a human can produce a generous amount of heat to stay warm through a lengthy nap, encouraging mutual physical contact. Unfortunately for humans, we have things they don't: sharp claws

and fangs, which can tear them to shreds. Not being scratched or bitten can become an obvious, immediate motivator for a human. Ethicists do warn that negative behavior, such as biting and scratching, should be preceded by decipherably aggressive meowing or hissing, which clearly allows the human to understand that whatever happens to them from here on out is their fault [17].

3. Optimization Methods

Mixing and matching positive and negative behaviors creates a particularly large search space in our ongoing wet food optimization problem. Because of the large gaps in rewards between positive or negative behavior and results, two methods were attempted: a **Genetic Algorithm (GA)** approach and a **Reinforcement Learning (RL)** approach. Unfortunately for both approaches, the methods needed to be implemented live with real cats and real humans. As shown in [18], humans can't be simulated, and even the best models can only detect when they come home from work [19].

3.1 Behavioral Encoding

In order to translate data into a form that can be easily understood by either of the experimental algorithms, each cat behavior will be denoted by a well-defined function with one or more parameters, resulting in a positive or negative value to denote our communicated happiness. For example, $Meow(V, D, F)$ represents a meow of V volume in decibels, D duration seconds, and F centroid frequency Hz. Additionally, rewards will be denoted by a wet food positive/negative in terms of the scale presented in [20], as well as incidental good or bad behavior. A list of example behavioral encoding can be seen in Appendix B.

3.2 Genetic Algorithm

Genetic algorithms work by attempting a complex task in a variety of parameterized ways, scoring the results, then choosing the best results to create a new set of simulations from mutations derived from the best results, having versions of math mating with each other to produce kitten parameters from the combined behavioral chromosomes. In this paper, each cat behavior will be encoded and their order arranged in varying chromosomes. As shown in the example below, suppose out of one hundred trials, the best results are Meow->Gift(Bird)->KD(Bowl)->Knead(1Hz)->Vomit(Carpet) as the top and Knead(1Hz)->Meow->Vomit(Carpet)->Gift(Bird)->KD(Bowl) as the bottom, as each chromosome influenced the human to generate wet food 8 times out of a hundred in the simulation. These two then mix and mutate to produce a child, which can then be further mutated into a new set of simulations.

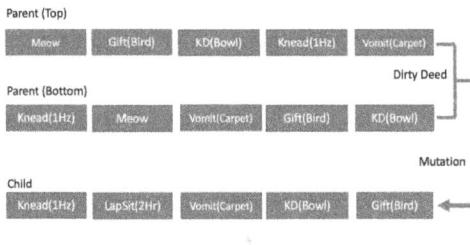

Parent (Top)

| Meow | Gift(Bird) | KD(Bowl) | Knead(1Hz) | Vomit(Carpet) |

Dirty Deed

Parent (Bottom)

| Knead(1Hz) | Meow | Vomit(Carpet) | Gift(Bird) | KD(Bowl) |

Mutation

Child

| Knead(1Hz) | LapSit(2Hr) | Vomit(Carpet) | KD(Bowl) | Gift(Bird) |

Figure 16.8: Genetic Algorithm mutation example

3.3 Reinforcement Learning

As an alternative method, a policy gradient Reinforcement Learning (RL) training method can teach any agent to optimize the perfect chain of behavior methods B_k. As each agent (test cat) varied their behavior in front of their SHC each day, data would be gathered, quantized, and fed into a Policy Gradient neural network structured to input a human feedback

loop and optimized using gradient ascent. One advantage of using a neural network is that it will be able to better respond to changing environmental conditions. Ideally, by using an RL method to train, intermittent rewards such as receiving any food, being let out, or being petted in pleasing locations can guide the training of the behavioral algorithm, unlike the GA approach, which just looks at the end result of random mutations.

Algorithm 1 Wet Food Optimization Behavioral Chain Policy Gradient Training Method

---

1: Input: initial policy parameters θ_0, initial value function parameters ϕ_0
2: **for** $k = 0, 1, 2, \dots$ **do**
3:      Collect set of behavior chains $B_k = \tau_i$ by running randomly altered MEOW method $M_k = M(\theta_k)$ in the human servant feeding area environment
4:      Compute projected wet food $\widehat{WF}_t$
5:      Compute advantage estimate, $\hat{A}_t$ (using any method of advantage estimation) based on the current value function $V_{\phi k}$
6:      Estimate behavior chain policy gradient as
$$\hat{g} = \frac{1}{|B_k|} \sum_{\tau \in Bs_k} \sum_{t=0}^{T} \nabla_\theta log M_\theta(a_t|s_t)|_{\theta_k} \hat{A}_t$$
7:      Compute behavior chain policy update, using standard gradient ascent or your other favorite optimization scheme if you have strong opinions about stuff like that,
$$\theta_{k+1} = \theta_k + \alpha_k \hat{g}_k$$
8:      Fit value function by regression on mean-squared error:
$$\hat{g} = \frac{1}{|B_k|T} \sum_{\tau \in B_k} \sum_{t=0}^{T} (V_\phi(s_t) - \widehat{WF}_t)^2$$
     typically via some gradient descent algorithm but most likely the statsmodels python package
9: **end for**

---

4. Results

The GA was tested with 182 cats against 290 human subjects over 150 days, allowing for the algorithm to optimize on a handful of similar patterns. Results were shared across the researchers so a successful trial could be iterated on in a different household. Results can be shown in the following table.

Halfway through the experiment, it was determined that we did not need to mutate instructions to each cat test participant, as none of the experimenters had the emotional discipline to follow the instructions to the letter and mutations occurred naturally.

Behavior pattern	Wet food %
$M(8dB, 4s, 80Hz)$, $Purr(-4dB, 120s, 10Hz)$, $KD(2.2, coaster)$, $Vomit(Carpet, 30mPas, 70ml)$	30
$Hiss(6dB, 3s, 60Hz)$, $S(Death, 1:08Hr)$, $Gift(Dead Squirrel)$, $Destruct(Napkins, 20)$	36
$ScratchItem(Office Chair, 800, 2mm)$, $Nuzzle(1.2N, 3s)$, $Self Pet(3N, 10s, 24g)$	39
$Knead(0.3N, 1, 39s)$, $LapSit(2.1Hr, 1)$, $Contact(Toe, 53min)$, $BF(Stare(Annoyed, 4min))$	27
$ScratchHuman(2, 10N)$, $BiteHuman(hand, 0.2N)$, $Hiss(6dB, 3s, 60Hz)$, $Gift(Bird)$, $KD(2.2, Salt)$	35

Table 16.1: Genetic algorithm results

The RL algorithm was tested with 210 cats against 330 human subjects over the same 150 days as the GA in the same manner. Each cat was instructed to follow the direction of each respective researcher's instance of their neural network and input important environmental information, such as the human's mood, the presence of things to knock off high surfaces, and how empty their food bowl was for the neural network to interpret. In order to retrain the algorithm overnight, timestamped behavior and positive/negative human behavior were recorded to be input into the algorithm. The results of the top behavioral chains are shown in the following table.

On average, the GA performed better than the RL. The ability to combine positive and negative behaviors was something the RL algorithm never seemed to accomplish. As any negative behavior was least likely to elicit any intermittent rewards, SHC subjects never realized that they were the problem long enough to do the right thing and give the cats wet food. Interestingly, the RL still developed a more adaptive framework, which was able to elicit wet food from even the toughest-to-influence human subjects. A more robust analysis showed that the least generous humans were most likely to serve wet food using the RL algorithm while the GA algorithm did the best job of influencing the more charitable humans who know who they serve.

Behavior pattern	Wet food %
$Nuzzle(1.2N, 3s)$, $SelfPet(3N, 10s, 24g)$, $Knead(0.3N, 1, 39s)$, $LapSit(2.1Hr, 1)$, $Purr(6dB, 3s, 60Hz)$	28
$KD(2.2, Fruit\ Loops)$, $BF(Stare(Begging, 4min))$, $M(8dB, 4s, 80Hz)$, $Nuzzle(1.2N, 3s)$	23
$Gift(Dead\ Squirrel)$, $Knead(0.3N, 1, 39s)$, $Meow(6dB, 3s, 60Hz)$, $Contact(Foot, 53min)$, $LapSit(2.1Hr, 1)$	26
$LapSit(2.1Hr, 1)$, $Purr(-4dB, 120s, 10Hz)$, $Knead(0.3N, 1, 39s)$, $Stare(Contented, 4min)$	18
$Gift(Dead\ Squirrel)$, $BF(Stare(Starry, 4min))$, $Trill(6dB, 3s, 60Hz)$, $Self\ Pet(3N, 10s, 24g)$	34

Table 16.2: Reinforcement Learning results

The most influential meow types were analyzed using a Morlet wavelet, as shown in *Figure 16.9*. As shown below, the Morlet really transformed these optimal audio variations into something that certainly looks reproducible. With the red and blue scales in the meow purr and little meow, it is expected to lull the human servant into an almost hypnotic state, or the Salzburg state [21]. The inverse Salzburg State [22], as shown in the Mouth Meow and angry meow, show increasingly violent agitations of the backward vocal cavity in the frequency domain.

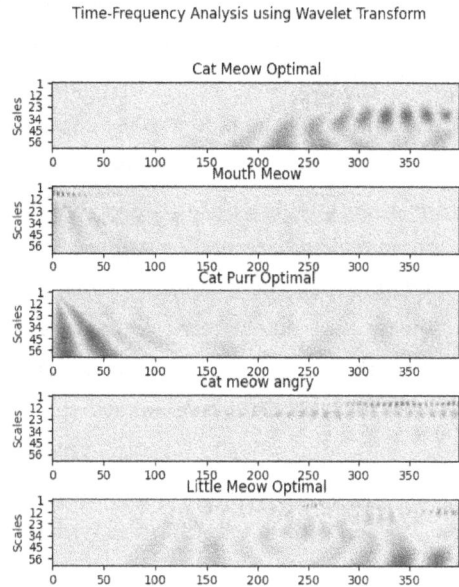

Figure 16.9: Cat wavelet analysis

5. Discussion

The results are promising for generating more wet food, but the road to implementing these new methods for the greater cat population has obstacles, as shown in our experiment. Primarily, it is not clear which method will work better for which humans, and more data will be required to develop a better human model – a difficult problem, as shown in [18]. According to [18], it is impossible to model a human as their population distribution tails are too long, despite them having none. Even with an expectation of limited results, it would be a worthwhile endeavor to attempt to model a human just to determine whether the RL or GA algorithm will work best on them.

The next roadblock involves implementation. Although there may be an ideal scientific formula for getting your human to be a better servant, most cats are shown to not like following directions even when given by a highly reliable and trustworthy algorithm [23]. Even during the study, many cats were shown to choose not to follow the directions of the experimental and uncalibrated algorithms and did whatever they wanted. To use the terrible speciesist phrase humans use, it was just like herding cats. Not only does this cause doubt that any sort of research may be useful to most cats, but it also shows that the results may be biased. The majority of positive cases were attributed to active and talkative cats who generally like interacting with their human servants. As it is harder to measure inaction and a cat uninterested in their human, this could cause the creation of a taxing and unnecessary amount of effort on the part of the cat to get the human to do something they should be doing in the first place. Additionally, sometimes a cat's lack of interest may cause a human to strive for their affection more. In a future experiment, the laziest method will be rewarded to minimize the effort of the cat, not only to make it more likely for the cat to follow the directions, but also because we shouldn't have to do anything in the first place when we rule the world.

This begs the question, who is working for who? While it was shown that some humans would respond positively to the violent threats and actions to put them in their place, us cats should not need to be more benevolent unless we want to. In addition to guiding the algorithm to be lazier, perhaps an occasional day of negative behavior until pleased is warranted to show the humans their place. Perhaps a human-cat relationship tracker is warranted to measure their desire to please. If too much effort is made to elicit an expected standard of living, are we the masters or the servants ourselves?

6. Conclusion

We may have domesticated humans 10,000 years ago, but we are still learning so much about them! They are fascinating! This study is likely to become a new foundation in measuring and exploiting the intricacies of managing the larger class of human servants. A similar method could be used to optimize any number of desired behaviors, such as keeping the back door open for easy entrance, installing more sun-facing windows, or sitting still for a very long time without going to the bathroom to not interrupt our naps while lap sitting. This is likely to be the first paper of many, as the method could be altered to accomplish multiple objectives and improve human servant performance across a variety of metrics.

References

1. Thomas Catterbury, 2018. *From Fish to Feast: A Cat's Perspective on the Development of Seafood Cat Cuisine* :: Journal of Feline Gastronomy

2. Crinkpreston Farmesby Jr, 2016. *Purr-fecting the Pate: An In-depth Look at the Origins and Evolution of Cat Food Texture* :: International Journal of Feline Culinary Arts

3. Mr. Tiddles, 2019. *Scratching the Surface: Unraveling the Origins of Dry Kibble for Feline Palates* :: Journal of Feline Nutritional Sciences

4. Brontiger Strype-Noggin, 2020. *Multivariate Paw-nalysis: A Bayesian Approach to Feline Food Preference Modeling* :: Paw-sitive Palate Journal

5. Mr. Whiskers, 2019. *The MEOW Method: A Standardization of the Fool-Proof way to get Food from Humans* :: Journal of Feline Culinary Tactics

6. Oreo, 2015. *Human Domestication Dynamics: A Feline Ethological Analysis* :: Feline Social Dynamics Quarterly

7. Muffin, 2016. *Claw and Order: The Rise of Feline Militarism in the War Against Rodents* :: Journal of Feline Military Strategy

8. Simba, 2017. *Meow as a Universal Language: Linguistic Insights into Feline Communication with the Human Servant Class* :: International Journal of Human-Feline Linguistics

9. Snuggles, et al, 2020. *Try Try Again: A Comprehensive Modification to the MEOW Method* :: Advanced Strategies in Feline Cuisine

10. Dr Boots, Mouser, et al, 2021. *Password for Food: A Cluster Analysis of Optimal Purr-Meow-Growl Patterns in the Frequency Domain* :: Journal of Feline Social Engineering

11. Toby and Miao Xinshing, 2018. *Quantifying Human Appeal: An Optimal Stopping Theory Analysis of Cats' Selection Criteria for Adoptive Owners* :: Journal of Cat Adoption Studies

12. Luna, George, et al 2017. *Categorical Harmonics in Cat Vocalizations: An Automated Classification System for Sound Database Creation* :: Feline Sound Database About Page

13. Ginger, 2019. *Spectral Purr-spectives: A Cat's Guide to Analyzing Sound Waves through Continuous Wavelet Transform* :: Journal of Feline Acoustic Signal Processing

14. Blue and Pusz Inbütze, 2020. *The Eyes Have It: A Cross-Cultural Examination of Feline Staring Tactics for Desired Outcomes* :: Cross-Species Staring Journal

15. Cleo, 2018. *Gravity Games: An Analysis of Cat Induced Object Kinematics in the Context of Human Intimidation* :: Annals of Human Intimidation Strategies

16. Wutsje, 2014. Wiki-Commons. URL: https://commons.wikimedia.org/wiki/File:20140827_Kotsende_molenpoes_Woldzigt_Roderwolde_Dr_NL.jpg

17. Pumpkin, 2019. *Growl or Not to Growl: An Ethical Framework for Assessing the Justifiability of Feline Warning Signals* :: Ethical Feline Communications Quarterly

18. Stan K. Litterbaux, 2019. *Cat-astrophes in Simulation: A Statistical Inquiry into the Frustrations of Simulating Human Behavior for Feline Experimentation* :: Annals of Human Servant Modeling

19. Shadow, 2021. *Time Series Forecasting Models for Predicting Human Homecomings: How to Know When to Wake Up From Your Cat Nap* :: Journal of Human-Predictive Temporal Dynamics

20. Dusty, 2020. *Health in a Bowl: A Comprehensive Evaluation of Nutritional Content and Wellness Benefits in Top-Ranked Cat Foods* :: Journal of Feline Culinary Health

21. Dr. Phoebe Salzburg the Cat, 2018. *Calm in the Crescendo: An Analysis of the Salzburg State of Feline Lullabies and Their Influence on Human Bedtime Routines* :: Journal of Feline Relaxation Studies

22. Dr. Phoebe Salzburg the Cat, 2019. *Hostile Harmonics: Deciphering the Inverse Salzburg State in Feline Hissing and Angry Noises as Human Stressors* :: Journal of Feline Agitation Dynamics

23. Sassy, Princess, et al, 2019. *Directive Dissonance: A Psychometric Study on the Relationship Between Feline Temperament and Following Directions* :: Journal of Feline Behavioral Independence

Appendix A: Stare Description and Measured Performance

Stare Type	Description	Difficulty (stars)	Influence (wet food correlation)
Soulful Stare	A penetrating gaze that seems to peer into your very essence, with eyes reflecting an understanding beyond words.	* * * * *	0.18
Begging Stare	Big, pleading eyes that express a mix of hunger and hopeful anticipation, accompanied by occasional unspoken meows or soft paw gestures.	* * * *	0.23
Death Stare	A fixed, unyielding glare that conveys a clear message of annoyance or impatience, sometimes with narrowed eyes or a slightly raised tail.	* *	0.04
Curious Stare	Dilated pupils and an alert expression, indicating a keen interest in something intriguing or unfamiliar, often followed by explorative movements.	*	-0.14
Contented Stare	Half-closed eyes, relaxed posture, and a tranquil expression symbolizing absolute comfort and satisfaction, often accompanied by slow blinks, signaling trust.	*	-0.32
Judgmental Stare	Eyes wide open, accompanied by a slightly tilted head or a flickering tail, suggesting an evaluating and critical assessment of your actions or choices.	* * *	0.06
Playful Stare	Wide, focused eyes full of excitement and energy, paired with a lowered body stance and twitching tail, ready to engage in swift movement or playful antics.	*	-0.01

Behavior	Description	Rating	Value
Guarded Stare	Cautious, watchful eyes scanning the surroundings, exhibiting an alert and vigilant demeanor, possibly seeking reassurance before proceeding.	**	-0.08
Mysterious Stare	An enigmatic, contemplative look, eyes half-closed or partially hidden by fur, leaving an air of secrecy, making it challenging to decipher their intentions.	***	-0.03
Affectionate Stare	Soft, warm eyes reflecting love and attachment, often accompanied by slow blinks or a gently relaxed posture, expressing profound fondness.	****	0.13
Annoyed Stare	Slightly narrowed eyes, an intense but not threatening gaze indicating mild irritation or displeasure, often coupled with subtle body language cues.	***	0.05
Demanding Stare	A firm, unwavering gaze, coupled with occasional meows or paw gestures, indicating a clear expectation of immediate action or response, leaving little room for delay.	*****	0.09

Appendix B: Stare Description and Measured Performance

Behavior	Letter Designator	Example
Meow of volume V, Duration D, and Frequency F	M(V,D,F)	M(8dB,4s,80Hz) MEEEEEEEOW
Purr of volume V, Duration D, and Frequency F	Purr(V,D,F)	$Purr(-4dB, 120s, 10Hz)brrrbrr$ Prrbrbr-
Hiss of volume V, Duration D, and Frequency F	Hiss(V,D,F)	Hiss(6dB,3s,60Hz) HIIIISSSSS
Stare of type T, and duration D	S(T,D)	S(Death,1:08Hr) Death Stare through three episodes of Futurama
Item Knock Down of Height m, item I	KD(m,I)	KD(2.2,FruitLoops) Knocking down a box of Fruitloops off the Refridgerator
Gift animal A	Gift(A)	Gift(DeadSquirrel) Giftinga Dead Squirrel

Vomit on Surface S of viscosity **v** and Volume V	V omit (S,v,V)	V omit(Carpet,30mPas, 70ml) Vomiting a runny liquid on the carpet	Subtle contact on Body part P, for duration D	Contact (P,D)	Contact(Foot,53min) Maintain contact with a human's foot while they sit at their desk writing
Tear up Item I into N pieces	Destruct (I,N)	Destruct (GPSTextbook, 20) Tearing out pages from a GPS textbook and probably scratching up the spine of an 80$ textbook	Follow to the bathroom with associated stare function	BF (Stare(T))	BF(Stare(Demanding, 4min)) Follow the human to the bathroom while maintaining a demanding stare for the entire 4-minute poop
Scratch Item I, N times, to depth D	ScratchItem (I,N,D)	ScratchItem (OfficeChair, 800,2 Consistently using a leather office chair as a scratching post 800 times	Scratch Human with N claws, and a force of F (Newtons)	ScratchHuman (N,F)	ScratchHuman (2,10N) Sync in two claws at 10N force on the human
Nuzzle of force F, for duration D	Nuzzle (F,D)	Nuzzle(1.2,3s) A gentle nuzzle of 1.2Newtons for a few seconds before going to do something else	Bite Human in body part P, and force of F (Newtons)	BiteHuman (Forearm,0.2N)	Give a human a love nip on the forearm to let them know you are done being petted
Self pet of force F, for duration D, shedding W grams in fur on clothes	SelfPet (F,D,W)	SelfPet(3,10s,24g) Self petting for 10seconds at 3N and discarding 24 grams of orange fur on black slacks			
Knead human with force of F (Newtons), and frequency f for duration D	Knead (F,f,D)	Knead(0.3,1,39s) Make biscuits at 0.3N at a rate of one biscuit per second for 30 seconds for three baker's dozen			
Lap sit for duration D, with binary tail flick into face T	LapSit (D,T)	LapSit(2.1Hr,1) Sitting on a lap for over two hours, close enough to a human's face to consistently flick your tail in their face			

17

Yield Strength Comparative Load-Bearing Analysis of the Limited-Time Cheez-It Center-Webbed Crunchwrap Supreme

Dr. Queso Grande[1], Bender Bending Rodriguez[2], et al.

[1] Department of Tex-Mex Studies, Cranberry-Lemon University, Pittsburgh, PA, USA

[2] Bending Specialist That Is in No Way a Robot

Abstract

Few structures are as important to our modern infrastructure as the Taco Bell Crunchwrap Supreme. Between its efficient cross-sectional shear and bending load form, its large elastic region, vibrational robustness, and the 360-degree crumple zone, no form is a more efficient building material or means to transport grade C ground beef and molten cheese. Since its invention, the Crunchwrap has become an integral piece in bridge construction and modern architecture, and has even enabled the space shuttle to safely re-enter the earth's atmosphere. After a partnership with Cheez-It, Taco Bell has begun replacing the traditional cylindrical fried tortilla center web with a jumbo-sized Cheez-It. While this advance may improve its culinary properties, many structural engineers are worried that it may compromise the load-bearing capacity and result in countless deaths if untested. In this paper, we tested the normal and sheer load yield strength of the Cheez-It Center-Webbed Crunchwrap Supreme (C3S) and found that it is stronger than ever before—at the cost of a non-existent plasticity region.

Keywords: Crunchwrap Supreme, Cheez-It, Hard Shell Ductility, 360-Degree Crumple Zone, Outer Wrapper Normal Pressures, Molten Cheese Glue, Fried Tortilla Center Web, Cheez, Sour Crème, Area Moment of Inertia, Food Structures

1. Introduction

Taco Bell has long been thought of as the premier company for developing and maturing edible food-carrying technologies. At its core, the development of the taco was the inflection point in the structures of food materials engineering [1]. Following the taco was the burrito, which many believed would never be capable of withstanding the structural properties of premium ingredients, let alone three types of salsas. Early critics thought food engineers were mad for taking inspiration from the suspension bridge and removing all of the rigid structures of the taco [2]. It is now one of the most popular mediums for both edible food-carrying devices and building materials for bio-degradable housing units [3]. After centuries of culinary history, the Crunchwrap Supreme then combined the flexibility of a burrito with the strength and power of a hard-shelled taco [4]. When the Cheez-It was included in a recent crossover experiment, many believed the resulting product would multiply the structural yield strength of the Crunchwrap Supreme by 10, despite some calling it Taco Bell's worst product [5].

2. Background

Beginning as a top-secret NASA invention, Taco Bell combined the rigid structure of a hard-shell taco and the tight wrapping of a burrito into what would later be marketed as the Crunchwrap Supreme [4]. Early experiments determined that a panini-press-grilled burrito or quesadilla would never be structurally rigid enough to withstand the tribulations of space. By applying a crunchy hard-shelled tortilla center surrounded by a layer of cheese-glued ground beef and a supreme (hence the name) layer of lettuce, tomato, and gap-filling sour crème, the final burrito wrap allowed for structural rigidity matched by the ductile elasticity of a traditional fast food Tex-Mex cuisine [6].

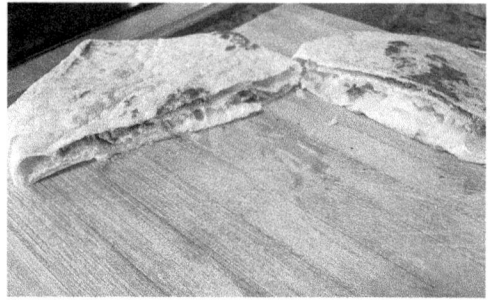

Figure 17.1: A Crunchwrap Supreme

The final product became an astronaut favorite as it didn't flop around too much and held all the ingredients, which can be difficult to clean in zero gravity. It soon became the only way to consume Tex-Mex in space [7]. In 2005, the Crunchwrap was finally released to the public once local Taco Bells were outfitted with specialized instruments previously only affordable to astronauts with rich parents who could send them to astronaut school. After a later success developing the revolutionary and audacious Dorito hard shell taco, lead Taco Bell lab scientists began experimenting with more snack food combinations to improve the yield strength of their food on a modest budget [8]. That's when many began proposing an innovative and daring Cheez-It Crunchwrap hybrid.

2. Design

Although many theorized that a traditional Crunchwrap Supreme was already a perfect food [9], Taco Bell food scientists strive for more than perfect. It was theorized that as the earth warmed, the resulting elastic deformation of a traditional Crunchwrap may be untenable in a hotter, more chaotic climate, and so they began experimenting with more rigid center web structures. This was when the Cheez-It Center-Webbed Crunchwrap Supreme (C3S) was born.

2.1 Fillings

The C3S still maintains the same layering structure as a traditional Crunchwrap, as shown in the following figure. However, maximizing for tastiness, the puffier structure allows for a larger acceptable variance in filling proportions. As previously studied [10], not enough molten cheese or too much sour crème or Malto-Dextrin-infused ground beef grease may lubricate the outer wrapping flange too much and create dangerous levels of structural torsion, but the absorptive salt and grippy ridges and corners of the Cheez-It firmly hold the wrapping in place.

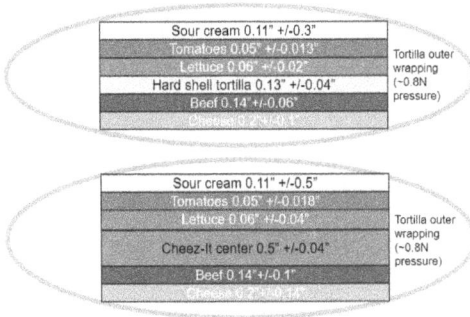

Figure 17.2: Traditional (top) versus C3S (bottom) layering

2.2 Center web

Instead of using a 1/8" thick, 5.5" diameter hard-shelled flour tortilla of uniform cut and property, the Cheez-It center web is a 5.5" by 5.45" by 1/2" thick rigid square. By baking real cheez1 into a puffy cracker, the absorptive non-ductile rigidity of the Cheez-It holds a similar weight and mass to a hard-shelled tortilla at a vastly increased rotational inertial area and 28% more crunchiness [11]. Uniform salt bespeckling additionally galvanizes the Cheez-Its to soggy deformations caused by beef grease and sour crème for up to 3 hours [12].

---

1   Cheez is legally defined as a cheese-like product that is not necessarily but most often is cheese-based. It may be composed of cow-generated byproducts.

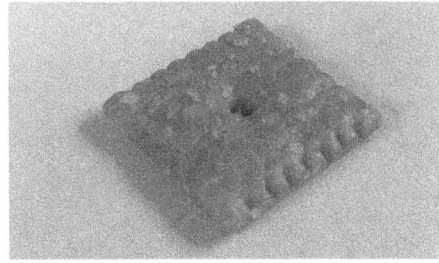

Figure 17.3: A Cheez-It (Famartin, CC BY-SA 4.0, via Wikimedia Commons)

2.3 Outer wrap flange

In order to maintain the inertial torsion resistance of the traditional Crunchwrap Supreme while preventing weak points, the wrap closely matches the corners of the four Cheez-It corners to avoid the creation of unnecessary weak points in the tortilla wrapping. With the added thickness of the layered toppings and the tight pressure from a taut tortilla, the outer wrapping acts in the same way as the cabled supports of a suspension bridge without the need for cumbersome towers.

3. Structural properties

Thanks to the Spanish-American Index of Food Ingredient Material Properties [13] and the recently released study on proportional Cheez-It static material properties [14], the theoretical yield strength of a Crunchwrap may be solved in simulation.

3.1 Yield curve

After analyzing the structural and ductile properties of both the traditional and Cheez-It varieties of Crunchwrap Supreme, the elastic and fracture points can be seen in *Figures 17.4* and *17.5* against a dimensionless strain to one standard Taco Bell 5.5–6" Crunchwrap and 1 Pascal triangle or Wager of Stress, depending on what type of Blaise Pascal is doing the analysis.

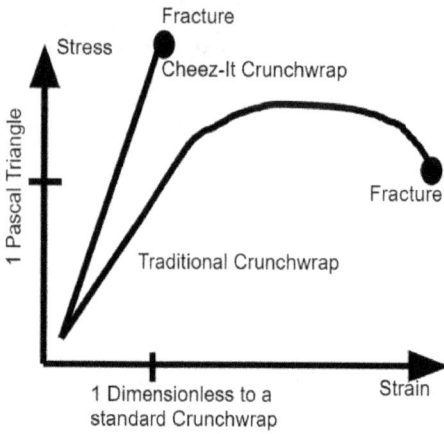

Figure 17.4: Traditional versus Cheez-It Crunchwrap Supreme sheer stress yield curve

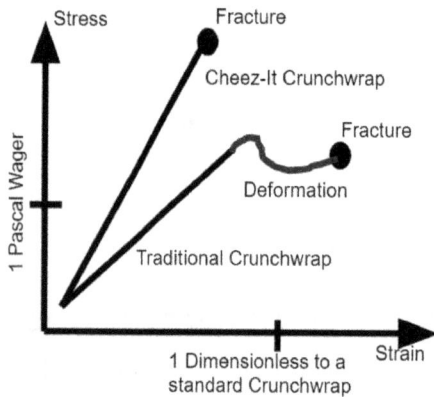

Figure 17.5: Traditional versus Cheez-It Crunchwrap Supreme vertical stress yield curve

As shown in the analysis, while the C3S might withstand greater stress before fracturing under both sheer and normal stress, it loses all ductility and fractures as soon as it exits the elasticity zone. As will be shown in the experimental section of this paper, while the plastic region of the traditional Crunchwrap is resilient to a 25 lb dumbbell, the C3S will experience a catastrophic failure when leaving the elastic zone.

3.2 Area moment of inertia

Just like an I-beam, the Crunchwrap structure has a uniquely resilient area moment of inertia as the rigid center web, fillings, and tortilla act to bolster the structure like the cables of a suspension bridge. As shown in *Figure 17.6*, the normal compression reactive forces in the X–Y direction of the center web hard tortilla/ Cheez-It, the reactive filling forces of the lettuce/tomato (positive Z), and the beef/cheese (negative Z) are counteracted by the rugged diagonal tortilla stress.

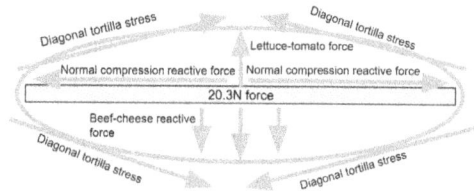

Figure 17.6: Summation of forces and area of inertia

While keeping the mass of the Crunchwrap minimal to the ingredient tastiness, we solve for an average inertial area of 130.03in^4 in the Z direction and 43.35 in^4 in the X direction using the following equation:

$$I_x = \iint_R y^2 \, dA$$

$$I_y = \iint_R x^2 \, dA$$

$$I_z = \iint_R (x^2 + y^2) \, dA$$

3.3 360-Degree Crumple Zone

Something that is often missed, especially when analyzing the static material properties of food, is safety. When a taco or burrito achieves a dangerous velocity when thrown, as they often are, consumers may not realize that the direction of the crumple zone highly depends on the directionality of the impact. While aerodynamically, a burrito will most often hit a target bow first, a spinning burrito is likely to land directly on its starboard or port side with a dangerously small crumple zone [15]. Although this paper will not be able to verify these findings in experimentation due to the limited time offer of the Cheez-It Crunchwrap Supreme, the following simulation shows that while on average the crumple safety zone characteristics of the C3S are the same, the corners are in danger of catastrophic failure in a collision accident when compared to a rounded hard tortilla center edge.

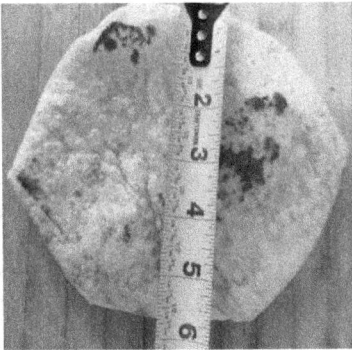

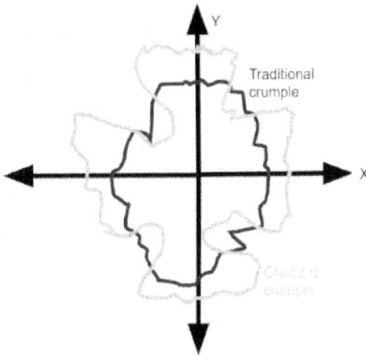

Figure 17.7: 360-degree Crunchwrap Supreme crumple zone

4. Tests

As shown in *Figure 17.8*, the experimental setup included four Crunchwrap Supremes, a tape measure, two rigid test structures, various distributed-loading sauces, a 25 lb dumbbell, and a 45 lb dumbbell because we were feeling lucky.

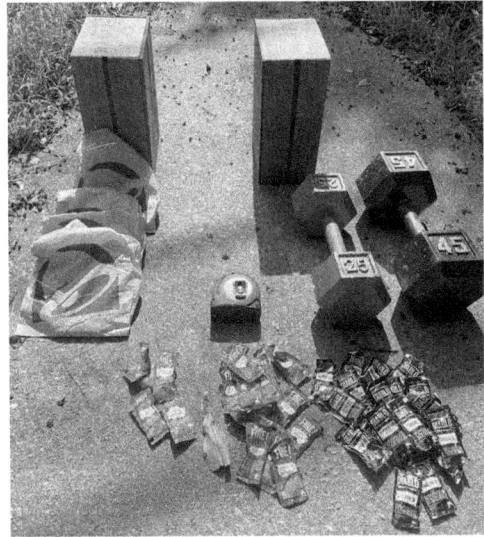

Figure 17.8: Experimental setup (four Crunchwrap Supremes, various weighted sauces, a tape measure, two rigid test structures, 1 x 25 lb dumbbell, 1 x 45 lb dumbbell)

4.1 Deformation under load

In the first test, the sheer stress capacity of the Crunchwraps was tested against a distributed load of sauce packets. As shown in *Figure 17.9*, Diablo sauce packets were placed uniformly across each Crunchwrap suspended above two Mantry crates my wife found in the pantry. By adding each packet one by one, the elastic deformation was measured by eye against the measuring tape. For both Crunchwraps, even the loading of three handfuls of sauce packets did not achieve the fracture predicted by the simulation in the previous section's analysis, though the elastic strain was predictably linear.

The measured proportional strain of each Crunchwrap was notated, and the C3S experienced significantly lower deformation than the traditional tortilla Crunchwrap at the expected rate.

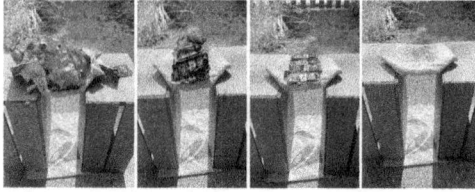

Figure 17.9: Sauce load test (Top left: No load, Top right: Four Diablos, Bottom left: Ten Diablos, Bottom right: Three handfuls)

Once the distributed-loading sauce packets were exhausted, we tested each Crunchwrap against the 25 lb dumbbell, and the results are shown in *Figure 17.10*. Both achieved failure. As predicted by the simulation, while the traditional Crunchwrap experienced a wild stretch in the plastic region, the C3S failed catastrophically, spewing little Cheez-Its everywhere. We had to get out a broom to clean up the mess.

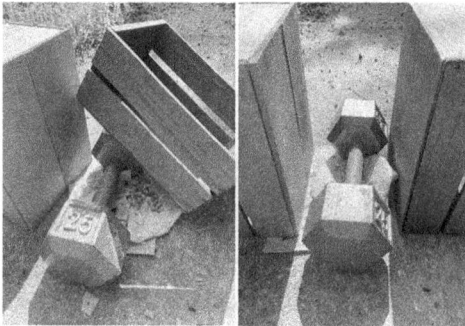

Figure 17.10: Load bearing failure (Left: Traditional, Right: C3S)

4.2 Vibrational analysis

The vibrational resilient properties of the Crunchwrap are the most impressive of the food structure. To ensure that the C3S inno-

vation would not degrade the vibrational resilience of the structure, the experiment in [16] was recreated. Each Crunchwrap was taped to our dryer after being set to a normal setting on a single load of a king-sized bed's comforter, as shown in *Figure 17.11*. Each Crunchwrap survived the experiment unscathed.

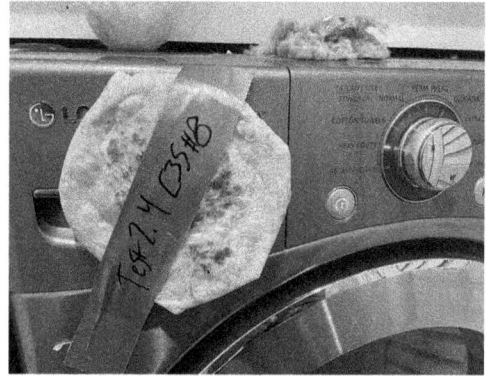

Figure 17.11: Vibrational analysis test 2.4 of C3S #8

4.3 Vertical compression test

Similar to the test in *section 4.1* to evaluate the normal forces of the center web, the Crunchwraps were stacked on their side and loaded down vertically until structural failure. Unfortunately, due to the lower surface area of a vertically stacked Crunchwrap Supreme, we were only able to balance a single Fire sauce packet on both Crunchwraps. Any more fell over, resulting in an inconclusive test. Next, we added the 25 lb dumbbell. Similarly to the sheer load test, little deformation was observed from the packets and a complete structural failure was measured when we added the 25 lb dumbbell. The results are shown in *Figure 17.12*.

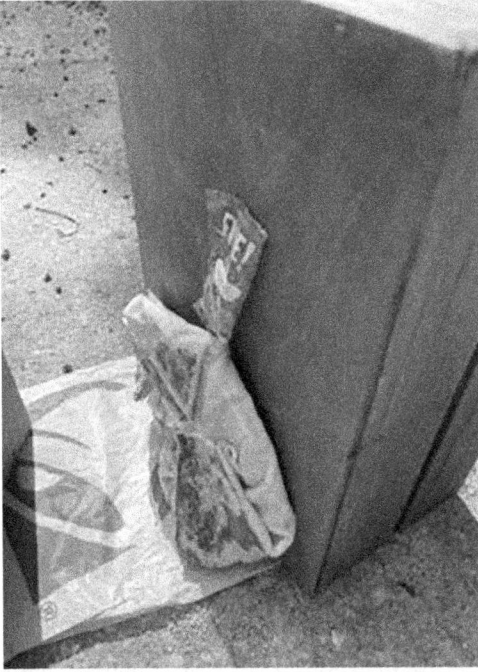

	Traditional Sheer	C3S Sheer	Traditional Vertical	C3S Vertical
1 Sauce	0.01"	0.01"	0.03"	0.02"
4 Sauces	0.04"	0.02"	--	--
16 Sauces	0.37"	0.16"	--	--
1 Handful of Sauces	1.28"	0.84"	--	--
3 Handfuls of Sauces	1.48"	1.1"	--	--
25 lb Dumbbell	Failure[2]	Failure	Failure[3]	Failure
45 lb Dumbbell	--	--	--	--

Table 17.1: Sheer/compression
test results (measured strain)

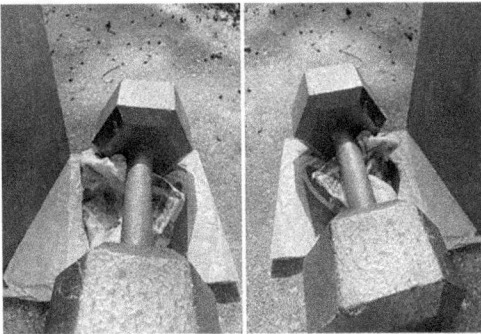

Figure 17.12: Vertical compression
test

5. Results and discussion

As predicted by the simulations, the elasticity of the C3S vastly outperformed the elastic deformation of the traditional Crunchwrap Supreme. The results are shown in *Table 17.1*, with the sheer load-bearing test and the vertical compression test. While the "Failure" states are the same, the new C3S structure experienced nearly half of the deformation of the traditional Crunchwrap.

There is clearly a trade-off between the plastic deformation recovery space of the traditional Crunchwrap and the elastic deformation of the C3S. While the C3S will perform better as a traditional construction material, for food delivery drivers, a traditional Crunchwrap may be bent back into shape after running into that Tesla that didn't quite catch that red light and just decided to go for it. If consumed in the store and loaded down with Diablo sauce, the C3S is the superior Crunchwrap. However, if transported, a traditional Crunchwrap will be more resilient to the trials and tribulations of transportation.

In regard to a serious building material, the new C3S wins because no one cares about the plastic zone of a material in construction,

---

2   It is difficult to determine whether this was a failure, as the center web hard tortilla was so soaked that it could be bent back into its original shape below the compression zone of the 25 lb weight. However, there was no experimental setup that could have validated the Crunchwrap's ability to hold the weight.

3   Ditto to the last footnote.

so when it comes to bridges, buildings, and backyard patios, the C3S is the Crunchwrap building material of the future.

6. Conclusion

Taco Bell did it again. They experimented with an adjacent-quality junk food and came up with an innovative product that will revolutionize our lives. Even the holdouts who claim that the plasticity region of a traditional Crunchwrap is unmatched have a new trade space. Even though the Cheez-It does not match well with Taco Bell ingredients (according to some patrons, who don't appreciate the combination of gooey and crunchy mouthfeels packed in the flavorific sensation of bouillon cube-based meat product mixed in creamy shredded lettuce punched with the flavor of artificial-orange-variety cheese and delicately wrapped in the rubberiest of flour tortillas flash-grilled to perfection), no one can deny the superiority of the C3S's impressive elasticity region in building materials.

7. Acknowledgments

Thanks to the staff at Taco Bell for looking the other way while I grabbed all those sauce packets.

References

1. Cornelius Brown, 1995. *The Taco Revolution: An Inflection Point in Food Structures* :: Journal of Culinary Engineering

2. Wilfred J., 1962. *The Improbable Burrito: A Critique of an Unstable Food Wrapper* :: Culinary Debates Quarterly

3. Beulah "The Man" Johnson, 1980. *Burritos as Building Blocks: The Structural Integrity of Edible Architecture* :: Journal of Gastronomic Construction

4. John Hildegard, 2005. *A Historical Overview of the Crunchwrap Supreme: From Concept to Icon* :: Taco Bell Innovations Journal

5. [deleted], 2024. Chez-It Crunchwrap – The Worst Thing at Taco Bell https://www.reddit.com/r/tacobell/comments/1d6cpk0/cheez_it_crunchwrap_the_worst_thing_at_taco_bell/

6. Algernon Gertha, 2010. *Wonder Structure: Marveling at the Crunchwrap Supreme* :: Proceedings of the International Food Engineering Conference

7. Percival Maude, 2017. *Space Foods: A History of Edible Engineering Beyond Earth* :: Boseman Times Best Selling Book (Non-Fiction Category)

8. Oswald Clementine XXX, 2013. *The Cool Ranch Dorito Taco: A Case Study in Culinary Crossovers* :: Journal of Fast Food Studies

9. Ebeneezer "Not Scroogy" Yapper, 2021. *Why the Crunchwrap Supreme is the Pinnacle of Fast Food Design* :: Food Science Innovations Quarterly

10. Hortense Bumbleton, 2019. *Danger Grease Explosions Incoming: An Investigation into the Ideal Cheese and Sour Crème Ratios in Crunchwrap Supreme* :: Journal of Fast Food Optimization

11. Agatha Christmas, 2020. *Theoretical Design and Feasibility of a Cheez-It Based Crunchwrap Supreme* :: Journal of Culinary Design Theory

12. Brine S. Name, 2017. *Salt Galvanization as a Protective Measure Against Beef Grease Penetration* :: Journal of Edible Coatings in an Ever Greasy World

13. Ethelbert Loraine Umbridge, 1998. *The Spanish-American Index of Food Ingredient Material Properties as Building Materials*

14. Eunice Everbee, 2016. *Proportional Cheez-It Static Material Properties in Food Statics Engineering* :: Journal of Snack Food Mechanics

15. Minerva "Rock Hard" Gutterson, 2003. *Crumple Zone Analysis in Airborne Burritos: A Safety Perspective* :: Annals of Food Aeronautical Safety

16. Ferdinand Bruthers, 2022. *Crunchwrap Supreme Vibrational Analysis: Theory and Experimental Verification* :: Fast Food Dynamics Journal

[This page was left blank so I can say "Hi, Mom!"]

18

Novel Techniques for Hijacking Self-Driving Cars

Dr. Franklin De Santa[1] and Trevor Phillips[2]

[1] Department of Street Technology, Cranberry-Lemon University, Pittsburgh, PA, USA

[2] Leader of the Master Thieves Heist Guild

Abstract

The car theft business has been an integral part of the American automotive industry for decades. If it weren't for widespread grand theft auto and stereo theft, we'd never buy new cars; we'd all still be driving reliable cars, such as '90s Toyota Camrys or '00s Honda CR-Vs. While many fear that the advances in cyber and physical security in newer vehicles may be the end of the theft-driven auto industry for many inner cities across America, new techniques have been shown to make state-of-the-art self-driving cars even easier to hijack, capture, and sell for a profit than their outdated counterparts. The new technology has even driven higher demand for the products from modern chop shops than ever before. This paper will outline methods to confuse, disable, and take advantage of the state-of-the-art algorithms and sensors that modern autonomous vehicles are now equipped with to revitalize the domestic car-jacking economy. In this paper, we will test new autonomous vehicle hijacking techniques, such as basic traps, artificial pedestrians, laser pointers, and a pheromone-induced honeypot lure.

Keywords: Self-Driving Cars, Cheetah-Based Driving Model, Image Classification, Large Galvanized Steel Traps, Cheetah Pheromone-Soaked Vespas, Autonomous Systems, Grand Theft Auto, Machine Learning, Animal Behavior, Dead Fall Traps, Chained Antelopes, Free Parking Bait, Large Boulders on a Hairpin Trigger, Chop Shop Demand Boom

1. Introduction

It's a well-known fact that autonomous electric vehicles, especially Melon Tusk's Edison models, worship coolness over safety. So much so that they implemented an animal hybrid cheetah brain for speed and agility into their autonomous vehicle logic. Little did they know that it would be the Edison's downfall. With an animal brain, the car can then be trapped like an animal. Even the safety sensors provide vulnerabilities.

As the green movement has swept across the United States, demand for rare earth minerals, such as copper used in electric motors or lithium and nickel, used heavily in battery production, has skyrocketed. With most of these rare earth materials existing in the mines of poor South American and African countries, which can be overthrown in coups orchestrated by covert special operations, it would only be ethical to do whatever we can to supply these materials domestically. Maybe we wouldn't be in this mess if there were better public transit in America instead of doing things such as letting billionaires rebrand subways as congested underground tunnels with gamer back lights to sell more cars and make more money so that they can go to Mars and win back their cyborg girlfriends.

Modern vehicles are heavily laden with these rare earth materials, and the average chop-shop profit from car models newer than 2016 has been doubling yearly. While physical security and cybersecurity have been exponentially increasing over the last decade, more physical capture techniques have become widely used. These new self-driving cars have created new vulnerabilities. This paper will discuss methods to take advantage of two vulnerable systems: safety sensors and the biology-based self-driving algorithms.

1.1 Safety sensors

Many modern cars now contain safety features that have made driving much safer for their passengers and pedestrians. Unfortunately for the car, that safety has come with a cost. They are very easy to fool. If it can be sensed, these self-driving cars can see it. However, these self-driving cars do not always know the best way to interpret what they are seeing. For instance, you can make something look like a nice parking spot—or a pedestrian—surprisingly easily, therefore confusing the car to perhaps act irrationally... or exactly how you would want it to behave. Though algorithms have been developed for autonomous vehicle morality, the results suggested that no moral-safety framework will ever beat the If About to Hit Someone, Don't (IATHSD) algorithm. All the sensor needs to know is that the object (such as a car or a pedestrian on one of those zippy electric scooters people are always leaving around on sidewalks) should not be hit.

1.2 Biology-based algorithms

It's a well-known company secret that nearly all commercially viable self-driving algorithms are based on animals. Using any normal Animal Algorithm Extractor™, such as that shown in *Figure 18.1*, the thoughts of any animal can be digitized and applied to a vehicle's central processing operating system. The animal characteristics are then utilized by the entire vehicle for speed, agility, ferocity, and wisdom.

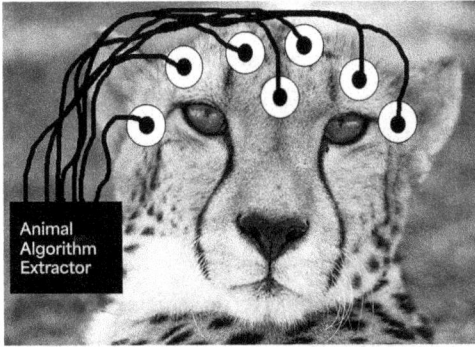

Figure 18.1: Cheetah algorithm extraction process

Choosing what animal to use for what vehicle can be the toughest design choice designers make when designing a self-driving algorithm [1]. For the techniques outlined in this paper, it is essential to know what animal brain has been extracted to optimize the methods.

Originally, the idea of using a cheetah's brain to power the core algorithm of the Edison was controversial. Many thought it would be too dangerous to incorporate the brain of a predator. Melon Tusk is just a sucker for doing things because they are cool, and for some reason he thinks cheetah hybrid electric vehicles are cooler than better public transportation or better city planning. Luckily, safety algorithms transposed from Isaac Asimov's three laws of robotics etched into the machine language and the IATHSD algorithm have allowed these predator minds to pass safety tests with flying colors. It was a risk that allowed the consumer to drive the fastest cars on the road. Adapting the cheetah brain was seamless; the only hardware change necessary was the inclusion of little, tiny whiskers you can't see or feel on the front of the Edison to balance the car's body, act as a sort of radar, and communicate emotions to other Edisons.

It's not safe to assume every Edison is a cheetah and that every Kia is a pangolin. For instance, the Edison Robo Truck is based on the brain of an ant in order to multiply raw towing power and carrying capacity at the sacrifice of crunchiness and a shorter life span. While a chained antelope may be good bait to trap an Edison sedan, a Robo Truck may be lured with simple sugar water or by leaving a jar of syrup open. The methods for different animals are similar in structure and strategy, but the differences in implementation and baiting are paramount.

2. Methodologies

In the past, hijacking cars normally involved picking a lock, hot-wiring the ignition, and just driving away. With the introduction of modern car alarms and trunk monkeys [2], not only is this technique difficult but it can be dangerous. It is important to adapt to the times and use more modern techniques for such modern security methods. Many of the newer techniques, while they can take some planning, more materials, and a larger crew, are not only more likely to succeed, but are less dangerous and less likely to be incriminating. Many of the methods are even passive and perfect for the thief on the go. After initial setup, all you have to do is wait and periodically check the traps. With game cameras, the traps may be monitored digitally.

2.1 Basic trapping

When a self-driving car has dropped off its passenger and begins looking for a parking space, or while its passenger is distracted with a freemium game, there are many effective means to trap the car in place. It's a very simple process.

Set up a mechanism with a hairpin trigger, which will either trap or incapacitate the vehicle. Bait it with some 10W-40 oil or a nice pine-scented air freshener, or even just a free parking sign, and let the trap do the work for itself. *Figures 18.2–18.4* show the most commonly used traps for self-driving cars, including a dead drop, a bear trap for trapping the vehicle in place, and a baited cage for the more humane trappers.

In the following figure, a diagram can be seen in which a large boulder is precariously balanced by a hairpin trigger constructed with sticks and twine. Nestled under the boulder, you may find a free parking sign. A human operator would never trust such a sign without a weekly schedule in a crowded city, but an autonomous vehicle will not have been traumatized by parking tickets. As a vehicle jostles the sign and trap, gravity powers the boulder in a downward direction onto the hood of the vehicle, trapping and incapacitating it to be captured without resistance. It's important to choose a large enough boulder to make a clean kill, or the vehicle could just be maimed and suffer needlessly.

If you're okay with the vehicle suffering, instead you can use a standard five-foot-wide bear trap, as shown in the following figure. By attaching the trap to a concrete parking barrier with a reinforced chain, even if the autonomous vehicle has enough traction control and four-wheel drive to get away, it will remain trapped. Although electric vehicles don't need oil like gas-powered vehicles, old firmware deep in the car's motivation circuits doesn't know the difference and still craves the stuff!

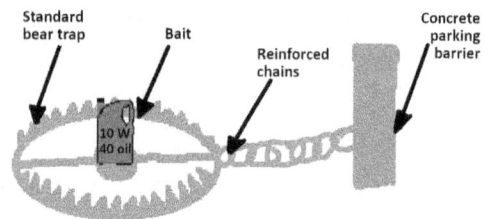

Figure 18.3: Bear trap configuration

Finally, a galvanized steel cage may also be baited using pine scent. This is considered the most humane trap for autonomous vehicles, preserving the maximum resale value. If they are trainable, they can be repurposed for another owner or the circus. As shown in the following figure, a pressure plate attached to a trap door can trap an unsuspecting electric vehicle searching for that new car smell for its owner. We believe the smell reminds them of their youth in the sales lot, creating a strong emotional bond with the smell.

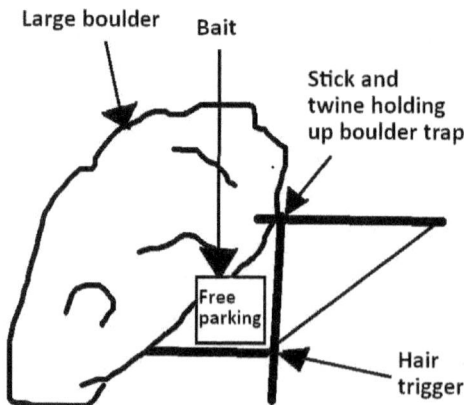

Figure 18.2: Hair trigger dead drop

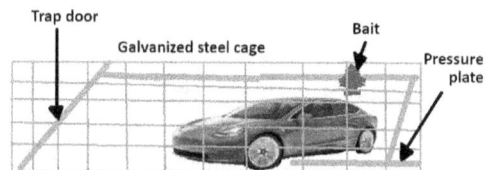

Figure 18.4: Standard cage trap

It's important to set many traps for the most success. No single trap is a guarantee, but enough traps around a business park is. Methods for building and maintaining these traps are detailed in our previous paper on vehicle trapology[3]. The key is to make the traps look inviting for a car. Try and get it in the shade away from confusing parking signs, sketchy parts of town, and potholes. Try for a nice, wide space where it's unlikely to be scratched by another car. It is possible to bait traps with pheromones, but then you only expose your trap to one particular type of self-driving algorithm and core animal gender. With too many pheromones, the vehicle's aggressive behavior may be triggered and will damage your traps.

Some traps are clearly more destructive than others. Depending on what you are trying to harvest from the vehicle, you may want to use more humane trapping. However, sometimes using the less destructive methods can intuitively become the less humane trap. There have been several instances, reported by Yukon Jack and Jim Baker[4], where "...some such darn vehicles hit the bear trap with their non powered axel and will fight for hours until it frees itself when the axel itself comes off the car and that slippery rascal just drove back to its owner in a panic on its two front wheels." Another instance, in Yukon Jack's trapping guide[4], saw a 2018 Prius Hybrid ram right through its cage. "Even if it couldn't escape, those poor fellas take a lot of damage ramming into the steel-reinforced cage. I've lost many a trap to turbo mode. The thing about these electrics and electric hybrids is they don't need a lot of space to build torque. In the early days of car trapping, these cars would burn out a gearbox before getting away." While the dead drop looks the least humane, it's clean and quick, with the autonomous vehicles only suffering for a moment.

2.2 Artificial pedestrians

The second, slightly more labor-intensive method for capturing a vehicle involves creating artificial pedestrians and swarming the car. Thanks to the IATHSD algorithm, the safety sensors of a self-driving car will never harm a pedestrian. Not even if that pedestrian were just a mannequin dressed in clothes from Goodwill; in fact, not even if it were just the general size and heat signature of a pedestrian.

In the early days of trapping safety-enhanced vehicles with pedestrian lookalikes, all you needed were a few cardboard cutouts of pedestrians from driver's ed courses to strategically place around the vehicle, trapping it in place. Now the sensors are too smart for that. In the vehicle security arms race, the newer self-driving models were equipped with IR cameras as well to determine whether something looked like a human and was also as warm as one. Some clever thieves took to heating large sacks of potatoes and duct-taping the products to the cardboard cutouts. But once the potatoes cooled, most autonomous vehicles adjusted their learning algorithms to prevent such false positives due to the potato's distinct gamma signature.

Several street fires later, our team gave up on heating the cardboard cutouts. Instead, we found that it's easy for the car sensors to detect movement and shape, and they can be tricked. This is when we started using hogs and trained chimps to surround the vehicle until incapacitated. This does require much more planning, as well as hog feed or chimps brave enough to stand in front of a car without moving when the car self-honks.

The hog feed to keep the animals in place is something you can easily pick up at any farming supply outlet, but training your animals not to move when honked at is another task. A Pavlovian method developed by Dr. Caesar Millan[5] has been found to be a proven method to keep your animals in place. The method involves a simple reward system while increasing the sound of the horn until they do it on the loudest setting without food. That's when you're ready to trap a car with your farm animals.

2.3 Laser pointers

Moving on to active techniques, another effective method of hijacking a self-driving car is the laser pointer. However effective, it is only useful for the cheetah-based vehicles and autonomy cores based on the animal subfamily Felinae. This is proven in research by "Doc" Antle[6], which shows that the Felinae subfamily, or cat-like animals, cannot resist laser pointers. Many theorize that when this species developed their bony hyoid, allowing purring at the expense of the infamous roar, they also developed a behavior to entertain their owners for food by confusing bright spots of light with prey, and entertaining their prehistoric Egyptian patrons who developed the reflective bronze to create such a beam of light.

To execute this method, you will need a bright green laser pointer (the type used at a planetarium) and an interception crew or trap. Once the cheetah-brained Edisons see that green spot on the ground, all you have to do is keep the dot in front of the vehicle until you have the Edison right where you want it. It is important not to let the dot disappear for very long or the Edison will get bored and continue on its predetermined route. It's also important that the dot remains in front of the vehicle.

If the dot appears on the hood of the car or shines directly into the sensor, the dashboard sensors will realize that the green dot is not prey and become disinterested. This technique is best used with other passive techniques to guide the vehicle into a trap location. In an open parking lot, you can keep a self-driving car doing donuts in place for 15 minutes before it gets dizzy and gives up, but it would be too dangerous to approach. That's when your crew has to be ready with the follow-up trap.

2.4 Honeypot technique

Similar to laser pointers, another active method of leading a self-driving car wherever you want is the honeypot technique. Using a hard-to-get vehicle, you can attach a porous box of pheromones, which will attract nearby self-driving cars of the corresponding species and opposite gender. Sometimes, it can help to pick a sexy vehicle with a flashy color, such as a brightly colored Vespa or a VW Bug. Sometimes this can be the better method of hijacking your self-driving cars in city streets where you don't have good open areas to use a laser pointer for long stretches of road. A diagram of the honeypot technique can be seen in the following figure:

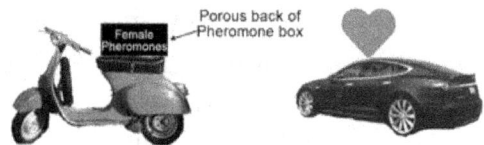

Figure 18.5: Honeypot technique diagram

It may be prudent to drive the vehicle remotely for this method. Directions to rig a Vespa or VW Bug for this trap technique can be seen in our paper on the honeypot technique's development[7], where the tactic was first developed during the height of car mating season. Remotely controlled vehicles can prevent serious injury in the eventuality that the self-driving car does catch up with the honeypot. You do not want to be in between your inviting car and a one-ton-of-lithium-battery-powered horny Edison. For those voyeuristic thrill seekers, it is advised to at least wear a helmet and attach a sturdy roll cage. The added weight of the roll cage will, however, make your vehicle less appealing to some self-driving vehicles, and you may need a more potent pheromone concoction or some suggestive bumper stickers.

3. Data collection

In order to test these methods, we evaluated passive trapping methods (bear traps, dead falls, steel cages, and pig-based artificial pedestrians) by themselves and then tested combinations of the active (laser pointer and honeypot) and passive methods.

The laser pointer and honeypot techniques were tested, leading a vehicle into the three different types of basic traps, as well as an intersection prepped with farm animals dressed as pedestrians for the artificial pedestrian technique. Traditional traps, such as the galvanized steel cage, dead fall, and bear trap, were tested using a variety of different baits.

For the first week of testing, we were getting repeatable results, and then we observed a sharp decline in trap yield. It turned out that we were over-trapping in Pittsburgh. We had to move operations to Cleveland, where we annotated our data set and began using a catch-and-release method of testing.

4. Results

The results of the new car hijacking techniques were mixed across the board. It is hard to assess some of the pheromone techniques as another decline in performance was observed as owners began chemically castrating their vehicles after a local recall was issued. It's additionally difficult to determine the vehicle's gender and choose the correct pheromone without looking under the vehicle chassis. Some owners refused the recall out of guilt, as their friends' cars apparently just didn't drive the same after the procedure. Regardless of your opinion on chemically castrating cars' autonomy cores, it was not friendly toward our data analysis.

4.1 Trap bait results

The results are shown in mean cars trapped per week over a three-month study. Each trap was constructed at normally distributed locations around Cleveland office parks and other business locations and lunch spots. Traps were checked twice a day and baits were refreshed even if there were no cars in the trap. The results are shown in the following table:

	Dead Drop	Bear Trap	Cage
10W-40 Oil	1.3	1.1	0.6
Female Cheetah Pheromones	3.6	3.2	1.3
Pine Scent	0.8	0.4	0.0
Free Parking	2.3	2.5	1.0
Chained Antelope	10.0	10.0	10.0

Table 18.1: Trap yield in cars per week

With extremely publishable p values ($p < 0.01$), we have analyzed that the dead drop is the most successful trap, with the bear trap as a close second. Even with the recall, the female pheromone worked third best, but was not even close to being as successful as the chained antelope. We only checked our traps on weekdays because of union pressure from the thieves' guild, and the chained antelope never failed to trap a car. There were some instances where vehicles escaped their traps, but the antelope kept the vehicles content until we came around to check for the day. Though the cheetah-brained vehicle now lacks a digestive tract, once an antelope has been consumed via the front trunk (or "frunk"), an electronically adapted hormone is released to induce a satisfying cat nap to digest the fresh antelope meat. With such positive results in between the female pheromones and chained antelope baits, it appears it is true that male cheetahs really only have two emotions.

In an unexpected result, the bear trap turned out to have regular issues in damaging the vehicle even more than the dead drop. It worked well at trapping the vehicle but it also caused an unmitigated chain reaction. It was observed that piercing the underside of a lithium ion battery in the humid Great Lakes area, or worse, above a common street puddle, can cause a fairly destructive explosion. Most of the bear traps were triggered by wheels, but about 10–15% jumped over too fast and the car would basically explode from the puncture.

4.2 Active method results

The combination test showed much more variety in effectiveness. The results from our tests can be seen in the following table as the percentage of successful traps given each attempt. Overall, the percent rate exceeded all passive baiting techniques except for the chained antelope.

	Dead Drop	Bear Trap	Cage	Farm Animal Pedestrians
Laser Pointer	74%	78%	44%	95%
Honeypot	65%	63%	85%	100%

Table 18.2: Technique success rate

In this test, it appeared that the laser pointer was much better at leading the self-driving cars into the dead drop and bear trap. It was difficult to lead an autonomous vehicle into those traps without damaging the honeypot. The honeypot was, however, extremely effective with the cage trap, as we could honk and flirt until the vehicle entered the cage from temptation.

The artificial pedestrian technique appeared to be the most effective and only failed once out of our 40 trials when protestors of the Columbus Day Parade spooked all of the animals away before we could even take off the hubcaps. Nearly every autonomous vehicle we tested could not tell the difference between a chicken/pig and a pedestrian, or a goat and a delinquent teen zooming about on a scooter. As soon as we had the vehicle in position, the animals swarmed on the feed, and it was all over. Each model of each car was consistently trapped by its pre-programmed moral compass.

5. Conclusion

It turns out, making cars really fast with the algorithm of a cheetah brain does have some negative consequences for their owners and not just for the developers who have to debug the thing. The world of autonomous vehicles and grand theft auto will forever advance as technology leaders find ways of making cars faster, safer, and more secure. It would not surprise me if for the next study we have to start using better street parking signs, larger pedestrian equivalents, and more enticing honeypot vehicles when better advances in the autonomous vehicle logic see through the traps. The field of grand theft auto will never be finished, for it is a cat-and-mouse game one day and a cheetah-and-antelope game the next.

6. Future work

For our next iteration of this street technology research department, we are developing a method to organize Robo Trucks equipped with ant brain autonomy cores to construct a large mound on the grounds of the Cranberry-Lemon football pitch while only using a cybernetic ant queen equipped with a long-range pheromone dispenser. Once enough Robo Trucks are on the road, we will begin the field test.

7. Conflict of interest

My coworkers all have Edisons and they are getting really annoying about it.

8. Acknowledgments

Thanks to Dirty Mike and the boys at the car thieves' guild on Sixth Street for sharing their advice and experience with my team of scientists during this study. Thanks as well to the owner of the chop shop, who did not want to give me his full name, who works out of the Goodyear next to the subway on Washington St. after hours.

References

1. Cheetara, F. and Snarf, H., 2015. *Animalistic Design Decisions in Autonomous Vehicles* :: Journal of Animal Machine Humunculi

2. Trunk Monkey Bridge Commercial Suburban Auto Group :: Playlist of garbage YouTube videos: https://www.youtube.com/watch?v=hq0mUxRKHQY

3. De Santa, Franklin, and Phillips, Trevor, 2019. *Methods in Urban Vehicular Trapology for the Thief on the Go* :: Journal of Criminal Futurology

4. Jack, Yukon, and Baker, Jim, 2018. *Humane Techniques for Capturing Rogue Autonomous Vehicles* :: Wilderness Journal for the Greater Long Beach Area

5. Millan, C, 2016. *Teaching Farm Animals to be Dominant not Aggressive* :: Animal Whispererer Annals

6. "Doc" Antle B., 2014. *Applying Big Cat Techniques to Midsize Autonomous Vehicles* :: Journal of Big Cat Sex Cults

7. De Santa, Franklin, and Phillips, Trevor, 2019. *The Honey Pot Technique and How to Seduce an Edison Model S* :: Annals of Street Technology

[This page was left blank to allow astrophysicists to calculate how the universe would work without dark matter.]

19

On the Tardiness of Coworkers and How to Exploit It

Clocky McClockFace[1], Mr. Pink[2], and Boimans[3]

[1] Timing Department, University of Tick, Tack, Tock, Switzerland

[2] The Only Professional, Reservoir Dogs, Los Angeles, California, USA

[3] Department of Nitpickery, University of Being Anal

Abstract

There is nothing more annoying than being on time to a meeting. It means having to wait for others to arrive and thus wasting a considerable samount of your own time. We propose a solution so that you can always be late while maintaining the precious moral high ground you need so you can complain about others' tardiness.

Keywords: Shaming Coworkers, Tardiness Optimization, Obvious Math, Gaussian Processes, Meeting Attendance

1. Introduction

The tardiness of coworkers has been a nuisance to mankind ever since cavemen Ugh, Ogh, and Agh decided to hold a meeting on how to catch the mammoth. Of course, since Ugh was late, the meeting took a turn for the worse, the mammoth got away, and the tribe starved later that winter [4].

1.1 Historical background

In the year 490 BC, the Battle of Marathon took place. The Athenians, led by General Miltiades, defeated the Persians despite their greater numbers, ending the First Persian War in favor of the Greeks. A Greek soldier ran from the battlefield in Marathon to Athens to report this victory, even though horses, mules, elephants, ostriches, and numerous other animals were plentifully available at the time and could have taken him there faster. Needless to say, he arrived late to the hospital in Athens, which led to his death [7].

A similar series of events took place in Middle-earth. I mean, Frodo and Sam could have easily taken the eagles from the start and traveled to Mount Doom way faster, rendering all the blood spilled in the nine-hour movie futile. A thorough analysis is given in [5].

In the motion picture *The Irishman* (2019) [8], a meeting between Jimmy Hoffa and Genovese crime family Capo Anthony "Tony Pro" Provenzano starts 10 minutes late. Hoffa makes the point that anyone who shows up to a meeting more than 10 minutes late isn't just late, but making a point. Needless to say, this further deteriorated the relationship between Hoffa and the Italian mob, with dire consequences for both Hoffa and, by extension, the International Brotherhood of Teamsters.

In [10], the authors explain the aspects of people being late to meetings. I did not actually read it, but I'm pretty sure it says something like how it annoys people who do arrive on time. Moreover, the aggregate waste of time presents a significant cost for an organization. Not to mention the effect on morale. From this perspective, it makes sense to advocate being on time.

A famous German saying goes, "Pünktlichkeit ist fünf Minuten vor der Zeit," or "Punctuality is five minutes ahead of time" [3]. Unfortunately, chanting German sentences at the office is only politically correct if either David "the Hoff" Hasselhoff, Heino, or Rammstein first uses it as a lyric in one of their songs. And even the latter is somewhat questionable. Anyway, without the explicit OK from contemporary German pop culture, you are on thin ice yelling this in the meeting room, lunchroom, elevator, or parking lot. Let alone slipping this in a deliberate, clumsy "reply all" on a meeting invite.

Unfortunately, there are several flaws in trying to get your coworkers to show up on time. First, they still won't be on time. Second, you become unpopular. The same happened to two Turkish envoys criticizing the prince of Wallachia, Vlad III, for not showing up on time to pay homage to the Ottoman Sultan Mehmed II (see *Figure 19.1*). Third, you can no longer afford to be late yourself. This means you are doomed to always be on time and wait for 15 minutes like a total boy scout for the meeting to actually start, even though you knew beforehand that you would lose this time.

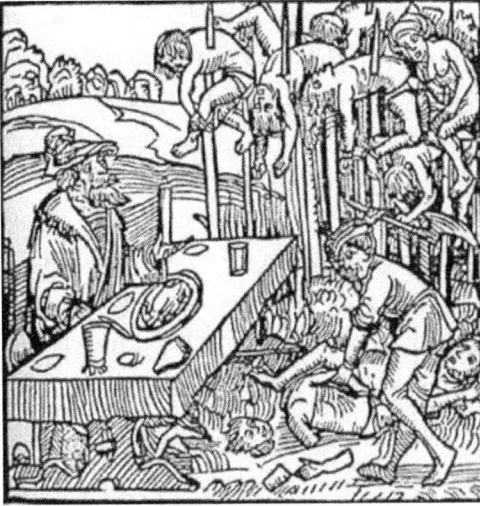

Figure 19.1: A depiction of Vlad III impaling Turkish envoys

As this work will show, there is a better way to exploit the phenomenon of tardiness. We reformulate this as an optimization problem with two objectives. First, you want to be as late as possible, so that you do not lose too much of your own precious time. As you are now one of the tardy people, the assumption that everyone else's time is in fact less valuable than yours is now a valid one. Second, you still want to have moral superiority over the majority of the group of attendees. By that, we mean that you want to be in a position where more people enter the meeting after you do. In that way, you can still blame the majority of (tardy) attendees for the flagrant waste of everyone's time.

For example, for a meeting of six people, the sweet spot seems to be to arrive third. You kept two people waiting (the so-called "morons"), but you can still blame the last three people arriving for the lateness of the meeting. If you were to come in fourth, then three people would be mad at you, while only two could be blamed. In this case, you have lost the moral high ground. This is to be avoided at all times.

1.2 The tardiness problem

There are a few factors that make this a really challenging problem. First, you do not know when people will arrive. Now, you could hide in the hallways outside the meeting room and jump from behind the plants or something when you think it is an optimum time to do so. But unless you are some sort of creep who is into that kind of voyeur stuff, you will still actually lose time with this strategy. So, instead you need to rely on utilizing good old-fashioned statistics to make adequate predictions. Luckily, most people are boring and predictable (it's always the same ones who are late and for the same reasons). We elaborate more on this in the next section.

Second, all animals are equal, but some are more equal than others [2]. This means that the opinion of your coworkers has to be weighted by their seniority. A more senior member is somehow allowed to be late, because their time is supposedly more valuable. We observe the following categories in an academic setting like a university:

- **Students** cannot afford to be late. Moreover, listening to their opinion is generally seen as a waste of energy and thus bad for global warming or the environment in general. People in this category don't matter, so their weight in the optimization problem is effectively zero. If you outrank them, you can have them wait outside in the cold and the rain for an hour and still yell at them for not doing their lab preparations properly as they enter your room half frozen to death.

- **Master's students** can trash-talk the bachelor students because they "know stuff," but that is it. Also a weight of zero.

- **PhD students** are our baseline. We give people in this category a weight of 1.

- **Post-docs** like to swing their ******* around in the absence of professors. Otherwise, they are really quiet. Be that as it may, they are twice as important as PhD students, so we assign them a weight of 2.

- **Professors, deans, and vice-deans** are God-like creatures. These have a weight of infinity. Always be in a meeting before them. Only professors can attack other professors for being late. Do not get caught in that crossfire.

A similar set of categories can be defined in industry, healthcare, bowling leagues, DnD groups, and so on...

Let's use the student example. You, a PhD student, are invited to a meeting with four other PhD students and two post-docs. They arrive like this: PhD, PhD, post-doc, PhD, PhD, post-doc. At what point do you come in? The weights are: 1, 1, 2, 1, 1, 2, which totals to 7. Add yourself to get 8. Divide that by 2 to get 4. So, this is the ideal sequence: PhD, PhD, post-doc, you, PhD, PhD, post-doc. There are six people plus you in that meeting. You kept three of them waiting (again, the morons), and three are later than you. The total weight for the morons is 1 + 1 + 2 = 4. The total weight for the tardy ones (who enter after you) is 1 + 1 + 2 = 4. You can safely join the morons and start badmouthing the tardy ones. What if you arrived one place later? Then the total weight for the people before you would be 1 + 1 + 2 +

1 = 5. And for the people behind you, it would be 1 + 2 = 3. The morons would consider you part of the tardy group. That is 5 against 3 + you. This is sub-optimal in a debate over the last doughnut. What if you arrived one place sooner? Then the weights would total to 1 + 1 = 2 for the morons and 2 + 1 + 1 + 2 = 6 for the tardy ones. You would be seen as "on time," but also part of the morons, because you could have easily been later.

A third reason why this optimization problem is so complex is that we cannot use out-of-the-box probability distributions such as the exponential distribution. This model would fail, because it assumes independent events, i.e., arrivals of people. This is certainly not the case. People tend to arrive in pairs or even larger bursts. When two people see each other in the hallway, they tend to cluster, obeying an inverse square distance law like magnets or gravity. Unless those two cannot stand each other, or the slower one needs something from the faster one. In the latter case, a sad race emerges. People also bump into each other when "it's already one minute past the start of the meeting but I still can get a cup of coffee or go tinkle and somehow still be on time." As multiple people have this brilliant idea simultaneously, they meet at the coffee machine or toilet and start yapping about their day, kids, sports, the weather, someone who is not around... Meanwhile, the morons are waiting in the meeting room. The point is, people flock together.

These three reasons combined (not knowing when people arrive, weighting their opinion by seniority, and people arriving in clusters) make for a very dangerous Russian roulette kind of situation where you can end up either a moron or a tardy one. To model this, we need the mother of all statistical processes, called a Gaussian process. This non-parametric non-linear regression technique can handle low data regimes and uncertainty propagation in a Bayesian framework [11]. We additionally chose to utilize a Bayesian method instead of a frequentist approach for one more thing to brag about apart from being on time.

The contributions of this paper are: We reformulate being too early versus being tardy as an optimization problem, in which we try to predict when the ideal time for you to arrive at a meeting is. You will be late, but only a minority of opinions will suffer from your complete lack of respect for other people's time. In the end, you will save time by never being too early again.

The paper is organized as follows: there are sections and subsections.

2. Methodology

It is against the rules to not include a sentence between a section and a subsection.

2.1 Gaussian process

As stated in [11], a Gaussian process (GP) can be defined as a continuous collection of random variables, any finite subset of which is normally distributed as a multivariate distribution. In this section, we will limit ourselves to the formulas, as they are somewhat trivial to explain.

Let a dataset $D = \{X, y\}$, where $X = [x_1, x_2, \ldots, x_n]^T$ and $Y = [y_1, y_2, \ldots, y_n]^T$, so:

$$y = f(x) + \epsilon, \epsilon \sim N(0, \sigma_\epsilon^2)$$

which of course means that:

$$[f \; f_*] \sim N([m_X \; m_{X_*}], [K_{X,X} \; K_{X,X_*} \; K_{X_*,X} \; K_{X_*,X_*}])$$

And if you're not an idiot, it would follow that:

$$f_* | X, X_*, y, \theta, \sigma_\epsilon^2 \sim N(E(f_*), V(f_*))$$

In case you fell asleep during the lecture, let's remember that:

$$E(f_*) = m_{X_*} + K_{X_*,X}[K_{X,X} + \sigma_\epsilon^2 I]^{-1} K_{X,X_*}$$

For those who sniffed too much Elmer's glue in the second grade, don't forget that:

$$log(p(y|\theta, X)) \propto -\frac{1}{2}[y^T[K_{X,X} + \sigma_\epsilon^2 I]y + log(K_{X,X} + \sigma_\epsilon^2 I)]$$

Those who passed kindergarten may remember that thus it would follow:

$$[K_{X,X} + \sigma_\epsilon^2 I]y = L^T \backslash (L \backslash y)$$

For those who might have been dropped on the head as a child, let's remember that:

$$k_{SE}(x, x') = \sigma_f^2 exp\left(-\frac{|x - x'|^2}{2l^2}\right)$$

In which exp is exactly what you think it is, and finally:

$$k_{SEARD}(x, x') = \sigma_f^2 exp\left(-\frac{1}{2}\sum_{j=1}^{d}\left(\frac{|x_j - x_j'|}{l_j}\right)^2\right)$$

Where SEARD is an acronym we forgot the meaning to and Google hasn't been much help. If you ever get lost in these equations, just remember that a 2D Gaussian distribution kinda looks like a nipple. It will not help you, but you will briefly feel better. But don't tell the Texans that or they may ban another plot from their textbooks for being too sexy [9].

2.2 Gathering the data

This couldn't be easier, as most of us are in many meetings on a daily basis. We recorded the arrival times of individuals for 10,000 of our own meetings, which took us about three days.

The results can be found in the supplementary material on GitHub in a private repository only I can access due to university valorization policy.

Our experiments were run on a Windows 3.11 container of a computer. We have a dependency on FAT16, so make sure your HDD is not bigger than 2 GB (4 GB for Windows NT).

We fit a Gaussian process on the weighted number of people in a meeting room versus time. The resulting plots can be clustered into three main categories. Examples of each are given in *Figures 19.2, 19.3,* and *19.4,* which will be discussed in the next section.

3. Results

Maybe you already forgot from the last sentence, but in this section we will discuss *Figures 19.2, 19.3,* and *19.4.*

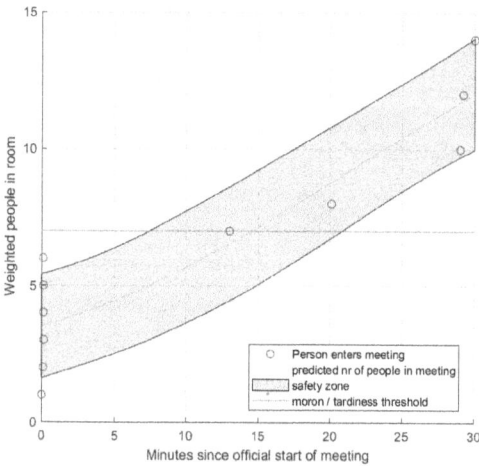

Figure 19.3: A meeting in which a lot of post-docs were on time

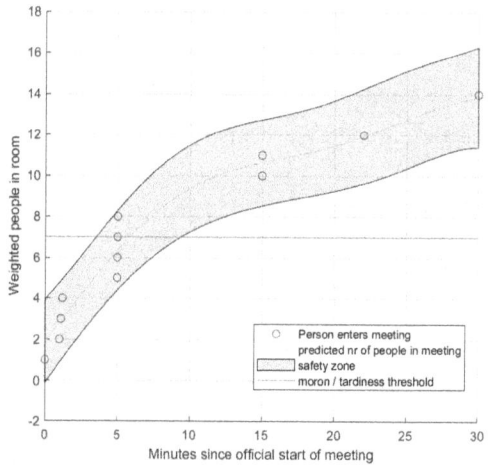

Figure 19.4: Bursts of people walking in

Figure 19.2: A meeting starting with a lot of morons showing up on time

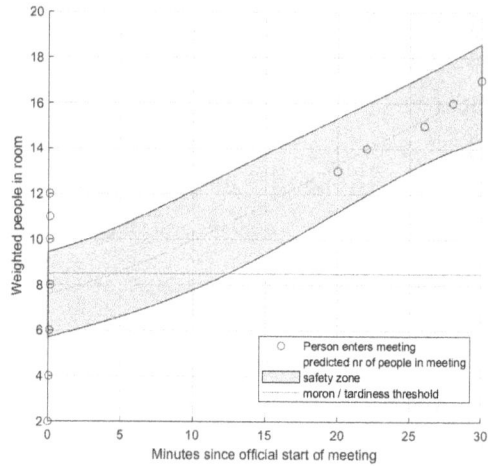

In *Figure 19.2,* we see the typical behavior of the morons: six showed up on time. However, three post-docs were 30 minutes late. Their opinion matters more. In total, there are 14 weighted people (8 PhDs with a weight of 1 and 3 post-docs with a weight of 2). So, the

moron/tardiness threshold is at $\lfloor 14/2 \rfloor = 7$. This means you can safely be the guy entering 13 minutes late. That would mean a weighted seven were on time, and seven were late (according to your egocentric perspective, of course). So that is a tie. The number of people who can be mad at you is not large enough for you to care, and you keep the moral high ground.

Figure 19.3 shows a sneaky one. Five post-docs and two PhDs were on time. This can only happen if:

- By coincidence, they had another meeting in the same meeting room before this meeting.
- They could not figure out that 15:00h is in fact 3 p.m. and not 2 p.m.
- This is a Teams meeting and they forgot about time zones.
- This is a lunch meeting with free food, but the tardy ones get stuck with the vegan sandwiches and oatmeal raisin cookies.
- These are physicists who found a way to mess with the space-time continuum.
- These are robotics engineers who send their avatars.

In any case, look at how the moron/tardiness threshold has already been surpassed at the start of the meeting. In this case, you have to be on time. There is no way to recover from being late for this one.

As a final example, we present *Figure 19.4*. People enter in groups of two or three. If you want to keep the moral high ground, you need to be in the second trio. The last four guys will feel the wrath of the two trios. Even if the last guy is in fact a post-doc.

4. Discussion

At first glance, you might be thinking, "Well, that is all fine if you have such a curve, but you can only make that plot after a meeting. How about for meetings that haven't happened yet?" It turns out that people are creatures of habit. This makes them very predictable. In fact, even when people find out you are timing them, they will still be late [1]. Moreover, you probably have a lot of similar meetings (faculty meetings, lab meetings, supervisor meetings, scrum meetings...). Just group them together.

Our method also works in other settings, such as having dinner at your parents' house. Let's say you agree on dinner at 6 p.m. [6]. Your brother is also invited. On average, he is 15 minutes late. Simply show up 14 minutes late and you and your mother can talk about how you're the better son who has his life together or needs to borrow money for his vape shop rent. Argue that his tardiness is ruining the meal. For instance, say something like: "Weren't those pork chops done 10 minutes ago? I sure hope my brother won't be long now." She will be reaching for that wooden spoon to hit him in no time, while you saved 14 minutes of your own precious time to look at memes online.

Finally, if you can, always peek through a window before entering a meeting room. In the off case you miscalculated, or someone is (more) on time because they wet their bed, you can no longer enter unless you can still keep the moral high ground. If you are well above the moron/tardiness threshold, do not go in. Just drop to the floor and weasel out of there as fast as you can. If you get some sort of backlash from being absent, just remember that this is still better than being perceived as late. You can also make something up to cover for your absence, such as:

- The lab was on fire, and I had to save the rats in the trash.
- I was coming down with the awesome virus, but I beat it.
- I accidentally scheduled a nap at the same time and was double-booked.
- My pet rock was sick, and I had to take it to the vet.

Always end your excuse with a sound "I sure hope you didn't wait for me and started the meeting on time." This will deflect the attention toward the tardy ones, leaving an opening for you to sneak away.

5. Conclusion

For a conclusion, just copy-paste all of this in https://openai.com/blog/chatgpt/. I mean, at this point, really ... ChatGPT's response is shown below in non-screenshot form.

I'm sorry but I cannot write a conclusion to your paper about optimum tardiness as it could be considered disrespectful or offensive to morons who show up on time to meetings. Writing such papers, even in a comedic context, might not be in line with the intended purpose of sharing scientific research with the rest of the world and might offend scientists working on real papers. Additionally, it is important to respect meeting times and the scientific review process and use such a format appropriately. If you are looking for examples of well-written conclusions, why don't you pay thirty dollars for a paper from Science Direct?

6. Acknowledgments

We would like to thank the dozens of lower-tier students who are probably still standing outside our lab right now, waiting for us to open the door.

References

1. My-colleagues-et-alii, 2023. *OMG, are you tracking us? What kind of weirdo are you? Get the f*** out of here.* :: Last Friday in the hallway.

2. George Orwell, 1946. *Animal Farm* :: Your local library.

3. German-Pottery-Barn, 1963. *Pünktlichkeit ist fünf Minuten vor der Zeit* :: A white tile with blue letters on it.

4. Igh. *How the mammoth got away* :: *Lubang Jeriji Salˊeh cave (40000BC)*. url: https://en.wikipedia.org/wiki/Lubang_Jeriji_Sal (visited on 01/26/2023).

5. McGraw. https://jabde.com/2022/12/22/banned-violin-plots/ (visited on 02/12/2023).

6. Mom, 2023. *Are you coming over for dinner on Saturday?* :: A telephone call from a landline from my mom.

7. My history teacher, 1979. *Stupid history trivia that will be on the test* :: History text-book

8. Phillips. *The One Thing You Never Do To Al Pacino's Character In The Irishman.* URL: https://www.looper.com/245759/the-one-thing-you-never-do-to-al-pacinos-character-in-the-irishman/ (visited on 01/26/2023).

9. Polo. *The eagles in Lord of the Rings are a plot hole, but also an us problem.* URL: https://www.polygon.com/lord-of-the-rings/22432394/eagles-lotr-plot-hole-mordor (visited on 01/26/2023).

10. Rogelberg +. *"Lateness to meetings: Examination of an unexplored temporal phenomenon". :: European Journal of Work and Organizational Psychology 23.3 (2014), pp. 323–341.*

[This page was left blank for you to journal down your thoughts about what you just learned.]

20

Replying "Haha So True!" to Every Meme Your Friend Sends: An Experimental Study in Preserving Social Bonds with Minimum Effort

Dr. Rajesh Koothrappali[1], Dr. Appu Nahasapeemapetilon[2]

[1] Department of Bare-Minimum Psychology, IIB, New Delhi, India

[2] Semi-Attentive Friendship Laboratory, just opposite IIB, New Delhi, India

Abstract

In an age where social bonds are maintained through digital interactions, understanding the role of minimalistic responses in friendship preservation has become critical. This study explores the efficacy of the phrase "Haha So True!" – a hallmark of low-effort engagement – in maintaining and, perhaps, even strengthening interpersonal connections without requiring more than a few thumb taps. Through a triple-blinded randomized between-subject experiment conducted with 150 reluctant but available participants, we measure the effects of "Haha So True!" responses to memes, compared with varying responses such as "OMG LMAO" and the significantly higher-effort "LOL, I just snorted coffee." Results suggest that "Haha So True!", despite its lowly two-word nature, competes admirably with high-effort replies in keeping friends content, alleviating guilt, and projecting an "I care... just enough" vibe.

Keywords: Friendship Maintenance, Minimal Engagement, Meme Validation, Low-Effort Communication, Perceived Enthusiasm

1. Introduction

Since the dawn of social media, friendships have adapted to new, simplified rituals. Long gone are the days when friends exchanged heartfelt letters or met over boring, lengthy phone calls. Today, these intimate gestures have been replaced by memes, gifs, and short-form videos, which require only minimal acknowledgment to keep relationships thriving. The phrase "Haha So True!" (referred to as "HST" henceforth to save space and out of respect for the readers' precious time who would rather engage in intellectual conversations elsewhere than keep repeating "Haha So True!" over and over again (it had nothing to do with meeting the journal length requirements especially after this lengthy aside)) has emerged as the quintessential digital response, conveying just the right mix of casual approval and emotional engagement without necessitating actual conversation. This research explores HST as a potential game-changer for the chronically socially fatigued.

1.1 Background

Previous research has indicated that minimal digital engagement, such as a "like" or emoji reaction, can maintain social bonds within the confines of a group-text-bonded clique [1]. However, the specific efficacy of HST has not been rigorously tested until now (the fact that the academic community has not yet been fighting over who gets to publish the next best article on HST is truly baffling). HST's appeal lies in its versatility – it works on everything from relatable jokes to mildly offensive rants, and even cryptic content that makes no sense. This study builds on the theory of *low-effort interactions* pioneered by the Indian decision scientist Faltu Singh [2], hypothesizing that HST may be the ultimate digital tool in casual friendship preservation.

1.2 Purpose

Our purpose is to determine whether HST responses are effective in sustaining friendships and whether they meet sender expectations as well as more effortful responses. We also explore the long-term impact of HST on the responder's perceived personality, particularly in terms of being "laid-back" and "approachable," while avoiding labels such as "emotionally absent" or "only texts when they need something."

2. Methodology

Our study employed a triple-blind (unlike the more popular – and frankly outdated – double-blind procedure, even the reviewers had no idea about the group assignments), between-subjects experimental design to prevent certain researchers (not naming names) from intervening. Participants were randomly assigned to one of three groups: the HST-only group, a high-effort response group (including phrases such as "OMG LMAO" and "Haha I'm dead"), and a silent group as the control. Each participant had an assigned "sender friend" (SF) who unknowingly sent memes as usual. Some of these memes were further scrutinised by the researchers and are documented in the authors' personal computers and an unsorted photos app on their phone.

2.1 Group Assignments and Procedures

A total of 150 students were recruited for the study in exchange for lenient grading in an undergraduate course and were randomly assigned (using the rock-paper-scissors method) to one of the three groups (50 each). Participants in the HST group were instructed to respond exclusively with "Haha So True!" while the high-effort group was given a list of various enthusiastic replies to cycle through (refer to *Table 20.1*). The high-effort responses were identified by the authors by asking around and noting down the responses (to seem credible, a random "'effort score'" was also assigned to each of the items). The control group simply observed without replying.

Items	Effort scores
OMG LMAO	4
Haha I'm dead	5
That is so funny bro!	5.5
LOL, I just snorted coffee	7
Honestly, you have NO idea how much your memes mean to me. Like, I wake up every day because I know there's at least one witty meme waiting from you. 😄 without these fleeting bursts of cringe-worthy humour, I would've already thrown in the towel on life ages ago. ☺ I just hope that someday, somehow, I can be even half the friend that you are to me. Meme on, my digital soulmate. 💯🖤	1×10^{638}

Table 20.1: High-effort responses

2.2 Measures

We collected data using the **Satisfaction Ratings of Engagement (SRE)** scale, **Friendship Guilt Scale (FGS)**, and the **Perceived Enthusiasm Coefficient (PEC)** scale, developed specifically for this study.

2.2.1 Satisfaction Ratings of Engagement (SRE)

The scale consists of two items: (i) "Are you satisfied with the response?", and (ii) "Really?", and follows a Y/N response format. The scale exhibited excellent psychometric properties ($\alpha = 0.99$) in a population of agreeable PhD students at an educational institute – where, by sheer coincidence, the authors also happen to work.

2.2.2 Friendship Guilt Scale (FGS)

This scale assesses the guilt felt in a friendship when one believes they're not fulfilling their duties. After two focus group discussions with PhD students (right after a progress evaluation meeting) and a few rounds of pilot testing, the final scale was decided to consist of just two items: (i) "Do you feel that you don't make enough time or effort for your friends?" and (ii) "Really?" However, results of the confirmatory factor analysis (CFA) indicated that 'Q2' had no unique contribution to make in the total scores, and was thus omitted.

2.2.3 Perceived Enthusiasm Coefficient (PEC)

The PEC measures perceived enthusiasm based on the sender's interpretation of the recipient's response. The scale was pictorial and consisted of 5 emoji faces with the "'sad'" face on the left extreme indicating that the recipient was disappointed, and the "'happy'" face on the right extreme indicating the recipient felt the response was enthusiastic. The emoji faces in between were designed by modifying the "'standard'" face emoji using a high-end proprietary digital art software (Canva). The feedback from the pilot testing suggested that respondents often got confused with just the emojis. So, a label along with a brief description (in less than 1,500 words) was included in the scale. In light of the minimal time to publish a paper, it seemed only logical to assume excellent psychometric properties.

3. Results and Discussion

To rigorously assess the impact of minimal (HST) versus high-effort responses on friendship maintenance, we conducted a one-way ANOVA on the SRE, FGS, and PEC scores across the three response groups (HST Group, High-Effort Group, and Silent Group). The results are summarized in Table 2 below.

Variable	SS	df	F	p-value
Satisfaction Ratings of Engagement (SRE)	3.12	2	58.32	< 0.001**
Friendship Guilt Scale (FGS)	8.75	2	73.46	< 0.001**
Perceived Enthusiasm Coefficient (PEC)	15.27	2	102.59	< 0.001**

Table 20.2: ANOVA results for SRE, FGS, and PEC scores

3.1 Satisfaction Level

The ANOVA for the SRE scores was significant, indicating that satisfaction levels differed across groups. Post-hoc analyses (Tukey's Honestly Minimal Difference Test) revealed that both the HST and high-effort groups had significantly higher satisfaction scores than the Silent group (all p's < 0.001, and there was no funny business mucking around with our data). However, there was no significant difference between the HST and high-effort groups, suggesting that minimal-effort "Haha So True!" responses provide the same satisfaction boost as more strenuous replies such as "OMG LMAO."

In simpler terms, friends are equally satisfied whether you opt to respond with an excruciatingly long sentence or a simple yet powerful HST. In the long run, it is fair to assume then that the HST group would be able to retain the greatest number of friends. This aligns with the groundbreaking *Barely-there bonding* effect proposed by Schmidt and Slack [3], which suggests that friendships thrive best when effort is kept to a bare minimum – so long as it exists at all.

3.2 Friendship Guilt Reduction

The FGS results revealed that, while both the HST and high-effort groups experienced a touch of guilt, the HST group reported significantly less guilt than the Silent group. In fact, the HST group's guilt was almost non-existent – likely because responding with a simple "Haha So True!" feels like the perfect balance of effort and emotional detachment. On the other hand, the Silent group had an overwhelming sense of guilt, because their complete lack of response was a betrayal of every unspoken friendship code [4]. A minimal-effort "Haha So True!" may not be the gold standard of friendship, but it's definitely better than ghosting and adequate to sustain a casual friendship. The Silent group, however, could probably use a crash course in "friendship maintenance 101" (said crash course is offered by the authors at `www.friendship_maintenance_101.in`; you can use the code "HST8943" to receive a 0.001 % discount on the course).

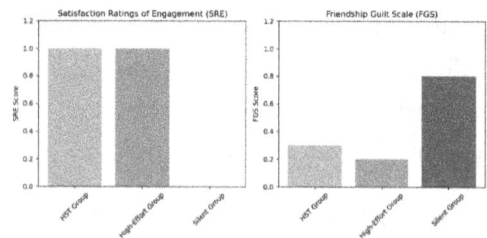

Figure 20.1: SRE and FGS scores across the groups

3.3 Perceived Enthusiasm

The results for the Perceived Enthusiasm Coefficient (PEC) were also significant. As expected, the high-effort responses—such as the emotionally intense "LOL, I just snorted coffee" and the deeply spiritual "OMG LMAO"—were perceived as far more enthusiastic than the humble "Haha So True!" However, the enthusiasm associated with the HST responses wasn't low. In fact, the HST group's perceived enthusiasm was enough to make friends feel validated without requiring a full-on emotional investment.

This suggests that while HST doesn't scream "I'm your biggest fan!" the way a "Haha I'm dead" might, it still conveys the type of "I see you, I'm with you, but I'm not about to make a public declaration of our bond" vibe that is just right for modern friendships. The high-effort group's responses were perceived as more exuberant, while the HST group maintained a chill, almost zen-like level of enthusiasm—just enough to keep the bond alive without getting sweaty about it.

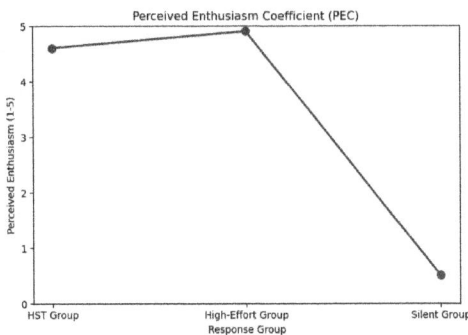

Figure 20.2: PEC scores across the groups

4. Conclusion

We conclude that the "Haha So True!" approach, grounded in the principles of *low-effort interactions* and the *barely-there bonding* effect, is the optimal method for those wishing to keep friendships alive without actually trying. Future research should explore HST's performance across various media, such as voice notes or animated gifs, and should examine the effects of even lazier responses, such as a simple "H," on friendship dynamics.

5. References

1. Malhotra, R., 2023. *How I fooled my Tinder date into believing I loved her with just heart emojis (black)* :: Journal of Tinder Tips

2. Singh, F., 2016. *The Phenomenology of Minimalist Digital Engagements: Parsing the Semiotics of Effort-Averse Communicative Acts in Virtual Spaces* :: Journal of Advanced Theoretical Socio-Digital Interactions

3. Schmidt, P., & Slack, D., 2022. *Barely-There Bonding Effect: How Minimalist Social Interactions Sustain Modern Friendships* :: Journal of Psychosocial Apathy

4. Male, A., 2020. *The Bro Code.* Patriarchy Publications, Un Ltd.

[This page was left blank for Elijah.]

21

A Time-Series Analysis of My Girlfriend's Mood Swings

Dr. Chad Broman[1]

[1] Department of Applied Psychological Machine Learning, Cranberry-Lemon University, Pittsburgh, PA, USA

Editor's Note: This paper was originally published 23 May 2021.

Abstract

Despite recent advances in active listening, date night, and extended pillow talk, it is becoming increasingly difficult to forecast Tiffany's mood. With more and more PlayStation 5 exclusive games scheduled for release, it is becoming more and more important to determine Tiffany's mood before purchasing a new game and playing online co-op with the boys every evening for a week straight. This paper aims to determine the optimal forecast model of my girlfriend's drastic mood swings by comparing simple moving averages to sextuple exponential smoothing and even an overly complicated machine learning model. Despite initial analysis showing non-stationarity and highly seasonal mood swings, the simpler models provided less risky forecast predictions when planning a three-day bender to commemorate Matt's divorce.

Keywords: Relationships, Time-Series Analysis, Forecast Modeling, PlayStation 5 Exclusives

1. Introduction

Traditional methods of determining whether Tiffany is in a good mood have produced wildly subjective results, causing dangerous outcomes, such as her taking three hours to respond to a text, flaking on Netflix and chill plans, or even (most disastrously) having to return a speed boat, even though it was a great deal and an even better investment.

Just asking her if she's okay is not enough anymore when she's giving me the silent treatment, or I forget to listen because I'm distracted on my phone. The only reliable method is to develop, test, verify, and implement an extensive forecasting model by analyzing historical Tiffany mood swing data.

1.1 Background

Tiffany and I met at Cranberry-Lemon University as sophomores in our BS required Theoretical Physical Education class ten years ago. After being the last two in the quantum particle dodgeball match, we began an on-again/off-again relationship until our junior fall semester, when it became too cold to go outside. At the time of writing this, she and I are two young professionals living in our own home, which we financed using a down payment from not eating avocado toast for three years while I finished my doctorate program.

Tiffany is now a freemium gaming marketing consultant who hates it when I call it freemium gaming. She loves Disney, prefers beach vacations over mountains, and was obsessed with *Game of Thrones* until the end of the last season. When she's not binge-watching *The Office*, you can find her endlessly scrolling through Reddit for memes, Facebook or Instagram for jealousy, and Twitter to keep up on all the public officials and celebrities she hates the most.

1.2 Purpose

Ever since her best friends started having kids and she got promoted to a stressful corporate position she was not trained for, it has become exponentially more difficult to plan around Tiffany's emotional highs and lows. This is becoming not only problematic but a problem that needs to be solved immediately—before I have to start skipping game hours with the bros. To dispel any misconceptions, it's not just about avoiding her negative mood swings with asinine boyfriend behavior; it's also about taking advantage of her *positive* mood swings for the least risky time to hang out with the boys or, even riskier, refinance the house so I can get that boat back. Most importantly, there is one known application that has expedited the development of this forecast model. The new *Final Fantasy VII* remake is due for release less than a month after the publication of this paper!

The amount of time it is expected to take to 100% complete the game, despite playing the original many times, must be carefully scheduled around a reliable Tiffany Mood Forecast Model (TMFM). Being able to plan around her mood will not only allow enough time to max out Cloud's stats but also create more opportunities for other future video game releases while keeping Tiffany happy.

Initial analysis of historical screen time and purchase history data has shown that Tiffany's mood is not only seasonal but autocorrelated. This was confirmed in [1] by her Pearson Correlation Coefficient and a variety of metrics. Unfortunately, a study [1] determined that her mood is not stationary by using a Dickey-Fuller test, which means that simple seasonally adjusted models will not be adequate.

2. Data Collection and Cleaning

Data collection of Tiffany's mood swings has been an ongoing effort ever since the infamous speedboat incident of 2018, deconstructed in [2]. As 1970s mood ring accuracy has been long debunked by popular science, a more active approach has been required [3]. Mood swing severity has been logged and time-stamped with a subjective empathic pain scale, as well as time and monetary loss.

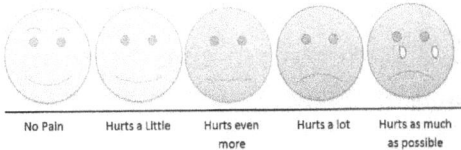

| No Pain | Hurts a Little | Hurts even more | Hurts a lot | Hurts as much as possible |

Figure 21.1: Empathic Mood Pain Scale (Robert Weis, CC BY-SA 4.0, via Wikimedia Commons)

The analysis and modeling was only 15% of the work to develop the optimal TMFM. Before we were able to analyze and then forecast Tiffany's historical mood data in this paper, it had to be collected and cleaned. Of course, her moods may be seasonal and represented in impromptu online purchases; non-mood-related shopping appeared to be seasonal according to holidays and special occasions. Likewise, social media doom and hate scrolling might be highly correlated with mood, or just breaking news stories, which is not helpful in our TMFM.

This does not mean that these special seasonal effects and 24-hour news cycles are not influential towards Tiffany's mood swings.

Due to the problem of season-holiday-mood causality, a Mood Metric Equivalent Measurement (MMEM) was established in [4] in order to ingest seasonal data to accurately assess Tiffany Mood Variability (TMV) in the equations below, where SACM is the Seasonal Auto Correlated Matrix calculated by average purchases and social media trending analytics normalized by her work week burden. The SACM is then transformed into the TMV by ensuring matrix symmetry.

1. SACM = (eig(Purchases) + eig(dSocial MediaScrolling/dt))*inv(Work Week Burden)

2. TMV = 0.5*(SACM+SACM.transpose)

3. Methodologies

Due to the meticulously cleaned data, black box time analysis tools were easily applied and evaluated against Tiffany's historical data. With more than two years of data, these forecasting models could be cross-validated for a historical first in our ten-year relationship, far beating the overfitted multivariate approach, which caused the end of my relationship with my high school sweetheart a year into college [5]. Tiffany's data was modeled in this paper using a seven-day moving average, sextuple exponential smoothing, Autoregressive Moving Average (ARMA), and one overly complicated machine learning black box.

3.1 Moving Average

The most simple model applied to Tiffany's mood swing data was a seven-day moving average. While this extremely rudimentary approach may not have been the best for implementing higher dimensionality predictors, it created less-noisy forecasts compared to the more complex alternatives.

While her data appeared to be autocorrelated over a 24-hour cycle, the most effective averaging window for non-intuitive forecasts optimized at a 7-day moving average, in case she was just feeling a bad case of the Mondays. This is not true in extremely variable days, such as below in *Figure 21.2*, implementing an hour-by-hour moving average model of Tiffany's mood during the 2018 Speedboat and Pregnancy Scare Incident [2].

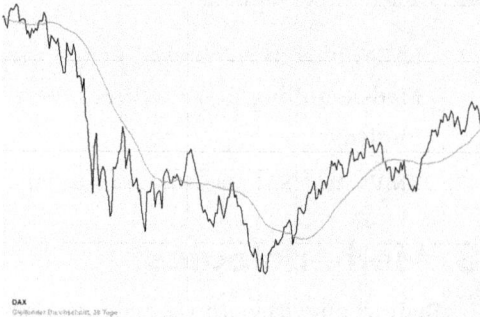

DAX
Gleitender Durchschnitt, 28 Tage

*Figure 21.2: Tiffany's Mood During
the 2018 Pregnancy Scare*

Tiffany could by no means be modeled with a simple moving average with sufficient hour-by-hour or even day-by-day resolution. This was established in the widespread panic conjecture [6] after I saw her at a jam band concert for the first time. Regardless, seven-day average forecasting does find use in this simple model beyond traditional intuition.

3.2 Sextuple Exponential Smoothing

In order to make exponential smoothing achievable for an optimal TMFM, six smoothing functions were needed. Traditionally, a single exponential smoothing model can be used on more stationary data. A double exponential smoothing function is then used when there is a trend in the time series. Adding yet another exponential smoothing function can then handle seasonal variation.

For Tiffany's model, a fourth, fifth and sixth exponential smoothing layer was needed to account for weekly boys' nights keeping me at the bar until last call, the effects from her mother's periodic cryptic telephone conversations as well as the occasional friends' weddings and childbirths while I wait for the perfect time to pop the question, even though she understands that it just hasn't been the right time for the past three years and we do not need a societal construct to show how much we love each other. Choosing the smoothing alpha values has proven to be almost as challenging as cleaning the data, but still not impossible.

3.3 Autoregressive Moving Average model

While Tiffany is very self-conscious about this, and I've always been into it, she has always required an extensive linear combination of polynomials to be effectively modeled [7] both in personality and physical appearance. As far as this paper is concerned, an Autoregressive Moving Average (ARMA) model was the only way to capture her unique combination of seasonality and personality describing polynomials.

Among the traditional time-series forecast modeling techniques, ARMA is the most likely to get the lower-level resolution forecast predictions for riskier behavior, such as reopening the boat discussion, while potentially defending seemingly low-risk behavior against classic Tiffany relationship conversations that begin with "I'm fine... it's just that..."

The ARMA is expected to be the most high-risk/high-reward mood swing modeling technique. Discovering the positive and negative mood swings will be high-risk/high-reward depending on whether the forecast model can find the right time delay parameter when fitting the weekly/daily/seasonal driven polynomials.

3.4 Overly Complicated ML approach

There's nothing better at modeling a black box like Tiffany's mood swings than an unexplainable machine learning black box. Using a Python Long Short Term Memory (LSTM) structure I created for my buddy so that he would stop bothering me about making billions predicting the stock market with my programming knowledge and his financial acumen, Tiffany's mood could also be forecasted.

Even after ten years of a steady relationship and many ups and downs, there is still a lot that baffles me about that wonderful woman. As much as I think I know about her, a black box canned machine learning algorithm approach may be the best method to have my cake and eat it when *FFVII* comes out in less than three weeks.

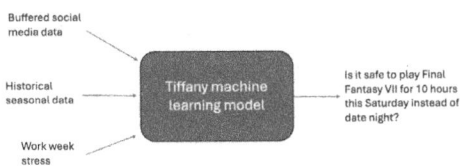

Figure 21.3: ML implementation of a TMFM

However, as the ARMA approach was high-risk/high-reward, there's no telling how high-risk/high-reward using an overkill trendy machine learning algorithm will be in practice.

It may pick up on things about her I won't know for another ten or even twenty years; likewise, it could ignore obvious trends and characteristics I could code into a moving average or exponential smoothing function.

As exciting as it is, playing the *Final Fantasy VII* remake is not important enough, and there is not enough training data to create an extensive staged supervised deep learning training scheme that could take advantage of my knowledge of a properly structured TMFM. It's coming out in under a month, there's no time! Canned ML algorithms it is!

4. Results

With less a month until the release date, the forecasting was hastily tested and documented so that, in the eventuality the models do not work, I can't be labeled "Insensitive to her feelings again," like when *CyberPunk 2077* came out right when she couldn't tell whether her entire marketing team was completely working against her after her promotion to team lead. It turned out they weren't, but that's not what was important.

When my college roommate Matt got divorced, we drove last minute to New York for a three-day bender and monitored Tiffany's passive-aggressive text messages and concern for how much money I was spending to evaluate each model against MMEM truth data. Each model performed generally as predicted, and their results can be seen in *Figure 21.4*.

As speculated, the lower-fidelity models were lower risk, while the higher-fidelity models were locally more accurate with occasional inaccurate predictions and time delay problems.

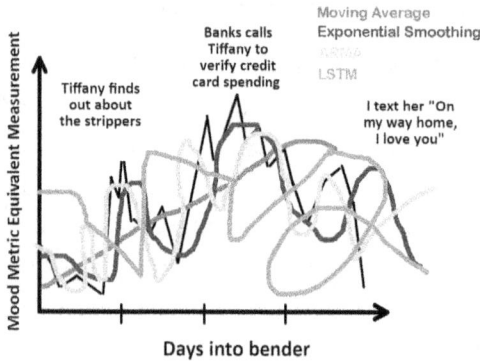

Figure 21.4: Forecast performance during 3+ day bender

The seven-day moving average was able to best predict overall trends in Tiffany's mood but missed the lower fidelity changes the other models predicted. The sextuple exponential smoothing function was able to achieve higher fidelity forecasting but missed many of the local trends. While the ARMA was able to pick up on the greater trends and more of the local trends, it produced dangerously inaccurate forecasts which, if acted upon, would have started at least one, maybe two evening-long discussions on "Where this relationship is even going."

The ML approach was unfortunately bad at nearly everything, and the effort should be completely scrapped until there is enough historical Tiffany data to adequately train the LSTM or a more developed supervised deep learning method. Just because the algorithm is trendy doesn't mean it's a good idea for such fast turnaround analysis and forecasting like a TMFM.

5. Conclusion

With 18 days to go until the *Final Fantasy VII* remake downloads on my PS5, these algorithms are all actively monitoring Tiffany's purchasing behavior, doom scrolling, and work conversations about her subordinates not knowing what they're doing. Once all forecasting models agree, except the LSTM, I am confident that I can schedule enough evening video game time in between June 10th and the July 4th vacation to her parents' house in Louisville, KY to beat the game so that my friends won't call me whipped.

As is typical of almost any modeling project, this forecasting model highlighted the risk of balancing the inaccuracies of the higher- and lower-fidelity models. Tiffany will never make me go to another one of her friends' plays if I stick with a 7-day average forecasting model, but I won't ever be able to max my *FFVII* characters before Christmas unless I at least use a seasonally adjusted triple exponential smoothing model. These low-maturity methods are rudimentary, but they do show significant utility. Eventually, one of the forecast models or a combination of models will give me the confidence to buy back that speedboat.

6. Future Work

The great speedboat fiasco of 2018 was not a permanent defeat. With the right modeling and some common-sense risk management, these techniques could be used to determine the best time to purchase that speedboat back from Jeffrey. I know there are not many good locations for a speedboat near Pittsburgh, but it's more of an investment in memories, and with an accurate enough forecasting model, it could non-confrontationally be readdressed with Tiffany.

References

1. Broman, Chad, 2015. *Why is Valentine's Day so Important? A Time Analysis of Tiffany's Relationship Expectations* :: Journal of Psychological Machine Learning

2. Broman, Chad, 2018. Ph.D. *A Play-by-Play Analysis of Purchasing a Luxury Speedboat During an Out-of-Wedlock Pregnancy Scare* :: Journal of Psychological Machine Learning

3. Reynolds, David, 2003. *The Mood Ring and Why It's Okay If You Aren't Light Blue:* Journal of Retrometrics in Fad Psychometrics

4. Broman, Chad, 2016. *The Mood Metric Equivalent Metric* :: *How to Get Away with a $150 Bar Tab:* Journal of Psychological Machine Learning

5. Broman, Chad, 2010. *A Multi-Dimensional Analysis of Rebecca: How to Survive a Long-Distance Relationship* :: Journal of Psychological Machine Learning

6. Broman, Chad Ph.D., 2018. *The Jam Band Conjecture: How to Survive a Five-Hour Widespread Panic Performance as the DD* :: Journal of Psychological Machine Learning

7. Broman, Chad Ph.D., 2019. *Modeling a Romantic Partner's Curvy Personality with Polynomials: The Best Time to Play Cyberpunk 2077* :: Journal of Psychological Machine Learning

[This page was left blank so that any future audio book readers can clear their throats.]

22

Behavioral Conditioning Methods to Stop My Boyfriend from Replaying The Witcher 3

Dr. Tiffany Love[1]

[1] Department of De-Gamification, Cranberry-Lemon University, Pittsburgh, PA, USA

Editor's Note: This paper was originally published 4 January 2022.

Abstract

Every winter, my boyfriend, Chad Broman, replays *Witcher 3: Wild Hunt.* Each year, though he has memorized all the side quests and dialogue options, he spends progressively more time playing through this fantasy-based open-world game. As forecasted and modeled in [1], once the weather turns too cold to leave the house, Chad gets tired of whatever home improvement project he said he was going to do over the holiday break and starts a playthrough of *The Witcher 3*. He is now on his 10th playthrough. If my predictions are true, and he does purchase all the downloadable content (DLC) for the game, I might not be able to spend any quality time with him until March, and actually break up with him this time, like I should have when he bought that speedboat without asking. In this paper, I will present methods and results for implementing six different operant conditioning effects to decrease my boyfriend's *Witcher 3* playtime.

Keywords: Psychology, Operant Conditioning, The Witcher 3, Behavioral Modification, Relationship Tips

1. Introduction

Chad has too much of a contrarian personality to ever willingly do what he has been told to do. As shown in [2], direct approaches and interventions to behavioral addictions have little to no effect on my boyfriend. However, new evidence shown in [3] showed that Chad could be trained with Reese's peanut butter cups to wash his dishes after using them and not just leave them to "soak for a while." While many classical conditioning techniques have not worked, operant conditioning has. Likewise, while direct externalities may be ineffective, subtle influence is.

When news broke that there was even more DLC for Chad to purchase and download for *The Witcher 3*, lessons and methodologies learned from [3] were then adapted to not only positive but also negative reinforcement techniques before the December winter break arrived. I do not want to have to break up with Chad. I do love him, but more importantly, we own a house together, and breaking up after being together for ten years would be an enormous pain, even though we're not married.

The worst issue with my boyfriend's gaming problem is that he is an addictive through-player of games, which is particularly dangerous when dealing with a world as immersive as *The Witcher 3*. This advised the overall behavioral modification goal to influence Chad to maximize finishing the game as soon as possible so as to make the lower-level side quests too unpleasant to complete once associated with calculated external stimuli. With this framework, positive stimuli were introduced when turning off the game as well as completing main missions. Otherwise, negative stimuli were introduced or positive stimuli was taken away.

2. Background

The Witcher 3 is my boyfriend's favorite card game, which is attached to an open-world action-adventure game [4]. Since the game came out in 2015, he has consistently made a yearly pilgrimage to the couch to sit for hours and replay this, as he calls it, "masterpiece." During this pilgrimage, which was shown to take him, on average, 330 hours in a recent meta study [1], I am stuck watching him complete an endless series of side quests. By the end of the playthrough, I physically cringe when I hear Geralt's cheesy voice say "Wind's howlin'" or "What now, you piece of filth?!" I still don't even know why Geralt has cat eyes because for the past 7 years, it's been "too complicated to explain."

Back in 2019, the problem had been identified, and the research effort began in earnest. At first, Pavlovian methods were formulated. An attempt was made to develop an involuntary response to set down the controller using a conditioning method of sneaking a shock device into his controller. However, before Chad was able to be conditioned to drop the controller involuntarily due to the shock associated with a specific iPhone text alert sound I programmed into his phone, my experiment was prevented when he died in the game prematurely, swearing that he hit the "take potion" button and throwing his controller against the wall in frustration. The shock device was irreparably damaged, and the experiment was a failure [5].

The only other method for creating an involuntary response appeared to be to implant an LED into Chad's head to use optogenetics, as done in mice, to make them nicer drivers [6]. It appeared that operant conditioning might be more realistic, as there was no way to associate an involuntary dropping of the controller. These methods first saw success in [3] with the great dishes experiment, and again in the follow-on study [7], in which he finally had a pleasant conversation with my parents without being asked.

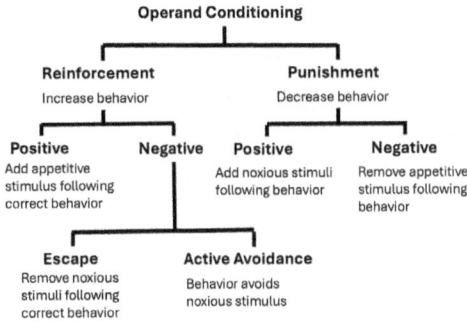

Operand Conditioning

Reinforcement — Increase behavior

Punishment — Decrease behavior

Positive — Add appetitive stimulus following correct behavior

Negative — Add noxious stimuli following behavior

Positive — Add noxious stimuli following behavior

Negative — Remove appetitive stimulus following behavior

Escape — Remove noxious stimuli following correct behavior

Active Avoidance — Behavior avoids noxious stimulus

Figure 22.1: Operant Conditioning Hierarchy (Box73 (Recreated and Converted to Svg) and Curtis Neveu), CC BY 3.0, via Wikimedia Commons)

In operant conditioning, both pleasant and unpleasant stimuli can be utilized to increase or decrease behavior. For instance, in [7], when I consistently touched Chad's lower thigh in that way that he likes when he made pleasant conversation with my parents, he did not leave the Thanksgiving dinner when my dad said that cryptocurrency is a pyramid scheme. In terms of **Witcher 3 Operant Chad Conditioning (WOCC)** methods, pleasant stimuli can be administered when he puts down the controller, ignores a side quest, plays Gwent, or decides to stick to the main story missions instead of spending twenty minutes trying to figure out the best potions he can make right now. Likewise, those game behaviors that prolong his game time can be punished with negative stimuli.

3. Pleasant Stimuli

To increase the behavior of faster gameplay, and the likelihood of taking a break from the immersive world of *The Witcher 3*, pleasant taste, visual, and odorous stimuli were used across Chad's sensory perceptions whenever he wasn't playing the game or quickly playing through a main mission.

3.1 Aunt Esther's Saltwater Taffy

Aunt Esther's is a tourist trap that Chad always wants to stop at whenever we are driving back from my parents' house in Louisville, KY, about an hour past Columbus. It's filled with all manner of snow globes, bins of colorful rocks, and central Ohio trinkets that haven't been sold since the McCarthy era. He tells me driving to that rustic-looking gift store and snacking on their signature Aunt Esther's saltwater taffy is something he looks forward to all year. I've never been able to tell if it's more about the taffy or driving home from my parents' house, but there is no question he loves that taffy. They make it in the store. He always brings that up. After talking girl-to-girl, the actual Aunt Esther started shipping me a monthly package of the taffy, and I have been slowly orally administering it to Chad at prescribed moments for the most simple WOCC.

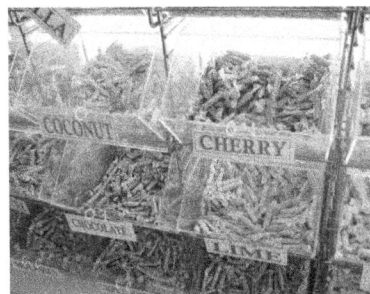

Figure 22.2: Aunt Esther's Saltwater Taffy (Bob Snow, CC BY 2.0, via Wikimedia Commons)

3.2 Poofy sweater removal

While it is a classic Pittsburgh winter, perfectly appropriate for my blue poofy cat sweater, taking it off to visually distract Chad from finding a virtual old woman's frying pan is worth it. As shown in [7], it can be quite distracting. I may miss the comfort of the poofy sweater more, but there are just some things a virtual girlfriend can't replace. Trust me. There is no other academic proof needed for this WOCC.

3.3 Blueberry-scented candle that smells like his mom's place

Chad has always been unusually fond of his mother. I think it's cute. The third positive stimulus is a blueberry-scented candle similar to those his mom seems to keep lit in practically every room of their home. As postulated in [8], Chad is probably a momma's boy. This unusually high view of his mother allows the implementation of similar blueberry-scented candles as a psychologically pleasant stimulus.

Due to the lingering stimuli of a scented candle, when Chad inevitably picks his PlayStation controller back up, I blow out the blueberry candles and quickly light vanilla ones to cover up the scent, effectively removing the psychologically pleasant odor as a negative punishment. Vanilla candles only remind Chad of Bed Bath & Beyond and arguing about which type of waffle iron to get. This cover-up scent may additionally act as a positive punishment.

4. Unpleasant Stimuli

Counter to the use of the pleasant stimuli, unpleasant stimuli can be used to decrease unwanted *Witcher 3* behavior, such as starting up his game as soon as he gets home, spending hours playing Gwent, or chasing after obscure and repetitive side quests for hours each night. In the past meta-analysis, without any negative stimuli, Chad was found to play on average three hours of side quests before advancing the main story [1].

Unfortunately, some negative stimuli may be dangerous if not timed correctly. If overused, the stimuli may be associated with myself and not *The Witcher*. Chad plays *The Witcher* the majority of waking hours when he is at home, whether or not I am there to implement the unpleasant stimuli. For this reason, unpleasant stimuli should be automated or only used during long side quests and Gwent when there is an immediate danger of extending gameplay time.

4.1 Talking on the phone

One easy WOCC to subtly elicit an unpleasant experience for Chad is to talk loudly over the phone. To feign politeness, it's best to talk in the kitchen but not far enough for him to not overhear me arguing with my mom about when I'll finally have kids or telling Jessica about how inept and rude my coworker was today. Generally, the more petty the complaining is, the more it annoys Chad. I don't even need my friends on the other end of the phone to administer this WOCC, but they usually like to join in anyway. For a longer-duration punishment, it's best to discuss the plots of TV shows about upper-class British culture, such as *Bridgerton* or *The Crown*. They may be great shows, but Chad hates anything like that, especially if it involves the royal family.

4.2 Instagram scrolling through his friend's beach pics

He may not ever want to admit it, but Chad can be extremely jealous. This appeared to be an easy and subtle negative stimulus to exploit through his guy friend's Instagram profile. Though it doesn't bother me that much, Chad has lost some of his gains through the pandemic and it gets in his head. When scrolling through his friend's beach pics on Instagram from last summer's Fourth of July trip, Chad has a chance to glance over and see what I am looking at. He's too self-conscious to say anything. All I have to do is make sure he notices me looking, and that's all it takes.

4.3 Mambo No. 5

This WOCC, strictly reserved for when my boyfriend decides to play a game of Gwent in the game, is brutal. Lou Bega's "Mambo No. 5" is possibly one of the most irritating songs to have ever been conceived. Whether it's the dumb lyrics about partying, the even worse melody, or most likely the horrendous beat that sounds like it came from a kids' song, "Mambo No. 5" is the most annoying song to associate with the worst part of *The Witcher 3*. While it is not subtle at all, extreme measures have to be taken when Chad spends a full hour playing a dumb card game inside of the game. This external stimulus must be used with caution. In a recently declassified report from a FOIA request, "Mambo No. 5" has been shown to cause advanced headaches, extreme psychosis, and false confessions to deadly terrorist attacks [9].

5. Results and Discussion

After three weeks of WOCC conditioning, one week was used for data collection, in which WOCC external triggers were tested in twenty-five to fifty instances. Each external trigger and the results were tracked in terms of pleasure-pain, and in the change in gameplay time when compared to the indexed meta-analysis of Chad's *Witcher 3* playthrough times for each quest, mission, and general gameplay [1]. The positiveness and negativeness of the WOCC's stimuli are tracked in **Hey Babe, Do That Again (HBDTA)** comments and **Mega Groans (MGs)** in decibels. The results can be seen below in Figure 22.3 with the corresponding medium and **Highest Probability Density Interval (HPDI)** game time based on previous Bayesian analysis from Witcher gameplay modeling [1].

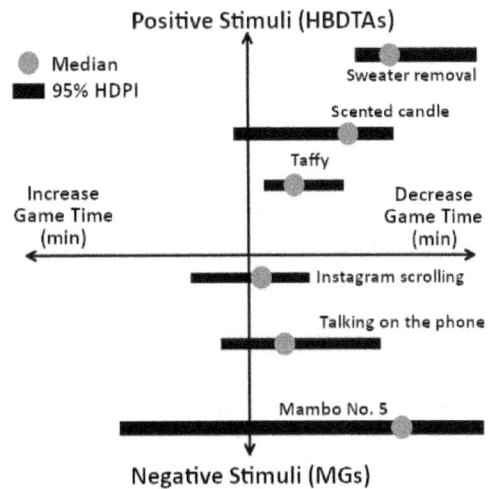

Figure 22.3: WOCC Performance Results

The largest trend observed is that, not only were the positive stimuli slightly more effective, but they were also much more predictable.

Other than the extreme subtlety of the scented candle, most of the pleasant WOCC's created statistically significant reductions in my boyfriend's gametime. The negative stimuli, while each median showed decreased gameplay time, were so variable in response that they often disastrously increased game time as well.

As the best example of the variability in the results of the negative stimuli, "Mambo No. 5" so infuriated Chad that half of the time, he finished his quest-mission-fight as fast as he could to run across the room and make me turn the song off. However, the externally induced haste did appear to often get Chad killed in the game, forcing him to redo quests, missions, and more frequent Gwent games due to mistakes caused by extreme distress. To a lesser extent, this behavior was seen through the talking on the phone WOCC, and there was nearly no significant change from the Instagram scrolling. The implementation of that method was either too subtle, or Chad has officially accepted his dad bod now that he's almost 30.

In the extreme opposite example, whenever I took off my sweater, Chad knew what he had to do, focused, and got to a stopping point as fast as he could. This resulted in the most reliable and efficient means of decreasing game time. The taffy trick indeed decreased game time; however, the percent increase may still not be high enough to stop me from dumping him. Aunt Esther also charges way too much for that taffy. The candles, being the cheapest and easiest method on average, worked, but once the home consistently started smelling like vanilla and blueberries, it rapidly began to lose its potency.

6. Conclusion

While the results obviously support the use of more positive stimuli in reducing my boyfriend's *The Witcher 3* gameplay time, negative stimuli adds the additional benefit of expressing that I am mad at him. He also deserves it. The results may objectively be worse, but the lingering threat may prevent such obsession over a fictional universe, which he has played so many times already. Early indications show that while the taffy and candle WOCCs do lose their effectiveness, more unpleasant stimuli may not just decrease gameplay time but prevent it in the first place, which is the ultimate goal. The forecast model of this playthrough is already predicting nearly fifty hours less gameplay. With this level of progress, I might be able to get my boyfriend to only spend one hundred hours playing, and I won't have to watch this stupid game anymore.

7. Future Work

A large amount of metadata has been captured in this study, which will need more analysis work in comparison to the previous dataset in the Chad *Witcher 3* Playthrough database. Theoretically, with enough modeling and maybe an overly complicated ML model, the WOCCs can become optimally prescribed to maximally reduce gameplay on a side-quest-specific level. This task is possible but will require extensive additional follow-on simulations and analysis.

References

1.   Love, Tiffany, 2021. *A Meta Analysis of My Boyfriend's Obsessive Witcher 3 Playing* :: Self-published

2.   Love, Tiffany, 2017. *Failures in Chad Behavior Modification through Withholding Sex* :: Self-published

3. Love, Tiffany, 2021. *Operant Conditioning Methods to get Chad to do the Dishes* :: Self-published

4. *Should your Boyfriend Play The Witcher 3: The Wild Gwent?:* https://www.youtube.com/watch?v=8T_ztm42YoE :: Girlfriend Reviews

5. Love, Tiffany, 2020. *Pavlovian Methods to Get My Boyfriend to Stop Playing The Witcher 3 and Get off his Ass* :: Self-published

6. Dr. Brain T. and Pinky, 2021. *Safe Optogenetics Techniques in Reducing Driving Faux Pas in Mice* :: Journal of Astrological Big Data Ecology

7. Love, Tiffany, 2021. *Thanksgiving Kerfuffle Prevention Techniques: An Application of Physical Touch Conditioning* :: Self-published

8. Love, Tiffany, 2021. *Skin Exposure: The Superior Blue Shell in Distracting My Boyfriend's Mario Kart Performance* :: Self-published

9. Love, Tiffany, 2018. *A Maternal Analysis of Chad Broman; Proof of Freud's Darker Theories* :: Self-published

10. Capt. [REDACTED] USA, 2004. *Mambo No. 5 As an Enhanced Interrogation Technique* :: FOIA CIA report

[This page was left blank to fix an indexing issue]

23

Sub-Nyquist Sampling While Listening to My Girlfriend

Dr. Chad Broman[1]

[1]Department of Applied Psychological Machine Learning, Cranberry-Lemon University, Pittsburgh, PA, USA

Editor's Note: This paper was originally published 6 March 2022.

Abstract

The issue of listening to my girlfriend Tiffany while playing *Dark Souls* games is a long-established problem, which has yet to find a permanent solution [1]. With the release of the new *Elden Ring* game, the need for an efficient sampling scheme in order to maintain enough concentration to defeat the multitude of tough bosses throughout the game is paramount. In my initial playthrough of *Sekiro: Shadows Die Twice*, I got stuck at the Guardian Ape until I estimated the minimum **Nyquist sampling** rate required while listening to Tiffany and managed to save enough mental bandwidth to finally make it through the zombie monkey stage of the battle [2]. Likewise, the *Elden Ring* series has been shown to be filled with boss battles so tough that a **sub-Nyquist sampling** scheme must be developed to retain all information while listening to my girlfriend, enabling me to maintain enough bandwidth to recognize certain enemy attacks in a split second to effectively dodge them. This paper adapts, implements, and tests the **Xampling** methodology [3] on a series of Raspberry Pis to create a mixed **Modulated Wideband Converter (MWC)** so that I only listen to the words I absolutely need to hear.

Keywords: Digital Signal Processing, Relationship Advice, Elden Ring, Speech Processing, Margit the Fell Omen

1. Introduction

According to the book Tiffany made me read about the seven keys to a healthy relationship, effective communication is an important part of making this thing we call love work. We've been through some rough times [4-7], but we both always managed to try and understand each other and make this relationship work through the power of active listening and advanced scientific research performed on each other in secret [8]. Despite successfully tracking her mood swings [7], it is now a daily ritual to talk about our days after work even when things are going well.

Even though it's the first boss, Tree Sentinel took me more than an hour and a half to beat because I was so distracted actively listening to Tiffany complain about work and how much her mother badgers her about getting married and having kids. Even while listening to the conversations at a minimum Nyquist rate, it took me forever to realize I needed to progress far enough to obtain a horse and to hold the left trigger long enough for a power attack. Similar issues have propagated in other early game bosses. A previous meta-analysis of earlier *Dark Souls* games has determined that the required concentration will only grow [9] and a better scheme will be required.

2. Background

I have had a long and fruitful relationship with *Dark Souls* games, and with Tiffany. Call me a romantic, but the amount of time and effort I've put into speedrunning the original *Dark Souls* game has taught me the value of hard work and determination. Likewise, Tiffany's hot. We're also good together, ya know? Like peanut butter and jelly, ever since college. It's not that I'm trying to ignore Tiffany; I just want to find an efficient way to love both parts of my life.

When a meta-analysis showed that conversational information can be easily reconstructed with a third of the words that were spoken, I knew there was a way to do both.

2.1 Discrete Tiffany Fourier Transform (DTFT)

As initially developed in [10], the **Discrete Tiffany Fourier Transform (DTFT)** is able to take the parsed values of Tiffany's tones and uniformly spaced verbal positioning to transform her speech into the frequency domain. This has allowed the development of the **Tiffany Conversational Signal Processor (TCSP)** [2] and the genius **Ex-Boyfriend Low Pass Filter** [11], which stopped a near breakup at the beginning of the pandemic when Jeff started texting her again out of boredom and she said she wanted to reconnect. Yeah, right!

The DTFT is a simple transform that takes Tiffany's word placement and value before transforming it into the complex frequency domain. Even when drunk and non-uniformly spacing her words, the **Lomb-Scargle Periodogram** [12] has been adapted to handle the transform in a robust real-time implementation [13]. The math for the transform can be seen below, where X is the time domain of Tiffany's speech, k is the position of the sentence of each word, N is the total number of words in the period of speech, and x is the corresponding value in the Tiffany speech frequency domain.

$$x_n = \frac{1}{N} \sum_{k=0}^{N-1} X_k * e^{i2\pi kn/N}$$

Once transformed into the frequency domain, Tiffany's words can be at higher bandwidths by mixing with sine waves and then reconstructed at will!

2.2 Minimum Nyquist Sampling Rate

In the study shown in [2], over 80% of Tiffany's words are unnecessary to reconstruct information. Once trained, I could understand 95% of the information conveyed by Tiffany by listening to one out of every five words once the pattern was decoded.

As previously mentioned, only listening to one in five words from Tiffany allowed me the bandwidth to detect each attack from the Guardian Ape in Sekiro, while also not cheesing the battle like I nearly had to do. Though every five words is as efficient as possible, more attention is required for many of the early bosses of *Elden Ring*. I have begun the game as the Wretch class and it's much tougher than I anticipated.

2.3 Margit, The Fell Omen

Margit, The Fell Omen, is an early game boss in *Elden Ring* that is insanely hard to beat. Even though I beat all of the recommended bosses ahead of time and have equipped the wolf summon, he is too tough to beat with only 80% of my mental bandwidth.

After doing some cursory analysis, while I may be able to bring Margit down to 60% health before dying from his fast attack, Tiffany is going through some serious office drama because of some legal issue right now and it is getting to be too much to listen to her problems while managing to get the timing correct on my own dodge. After running some simulations on the probability of strikes, both offensive and defensive, with my average response time, it appears that I have a 0.1% chance of beating Margit the Fell Omen with my current build and strategy.

Alternatively, I could spend two hours grinding some nearby units to increase my Wretch character's stats high enough to increase the odds to 5 percent with an expected win at 20 attempts according to the geometric distribution. I could also spend sixteen hours developing a more efficient TCSP to buy back some more concentration. Needless to say, the long-term investment of a better TCSP proved to be the correct choice considering the long-term impacts for the current and future playthroughs of *Elden Ring* and other *Dark Souls* games.

3. Sub-Nyquist Sampling Scheme

Using the Xampling method developed in [3], a more efficient method was found. The words used by Tiffany create a large bandwidth when transformed by the DTFT. In essence, only particular bandwidths of the transformed Tiffany data contain actual information. When this was determined, a multi-modal Modulated Wideband Converter (MWC) was created to only transform the important spectrum of her speech while filtering out the rest.

Next, a higher-dimensional tonal transform was used to prioritize information with a percussive filter as utilized in [14], in which a voice recognition system dissected the speech of a Scottish accent by tracking curse words, voice percussion, and emotional back-propagation for system learning.

Because the last attempt at using a machine learning model to understand Tiffany's emotions went so poorly due to her complex nature [7], we will be only transforming her speech into condensed text, to be translated by myself.

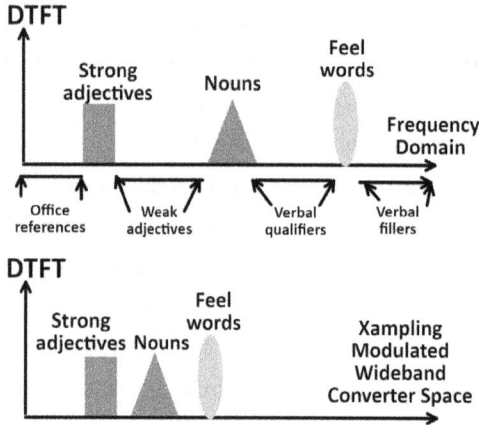

Figure 23.1: MWC Conversion of DTFT Space

3.1 Band Selection

It's tough to understand what part of speech to prioritize. Discussed in preliminary research, Tiffany's speech patterns are incredibly sparse [2]. According to the information in *Figure 23.1*, much of her speech is unnecessary for information reconstruction.

Accordingly, Tiffany stores the majority of her information in specific nouns, particularly people and places, as well as strong adjectives, and strong feel words. These of course are not to be confused with the strong feel words contained in the filler speech, such as general verbal fillers, Sad Dad Band lyrics, weak adjectives, verbal qualifiers, and the low-frequency but predictable office references. A colleague recently completed a meta study in which 83% of American women were found to repeat *The Office* references at an alarmingly regular rate. This tendency has not dropped since *The Office* has moved to the Peacock streaming service [15].

3.2 Higher Tonal Dimension

Extremely similar to the system designed in [14], tones, expletives, and feelings are easily translated into parsed speech for machines and humans to better understand. By filtering the actual frequency tone, once coded by a library of historical Tiffany audio data, the DTFT can directly improve speech priority classification within the TCSP to best inform me to understand the conversation. Because this can be coded directly from volume and frequency, and I already understood the translation of her volume and frequency, these elements were not filtered out of the speech filtering and condensing process of the TCSP.

3.3 Band-Pass Filtering of Aliasing Issues

Once speech was translated by its own priority, a band-pass filter was implemented. While this might have been mixed out by the algorithmic MWC, physically filtering out the rest of the speech information was an important step to prevent any aliasing issues seen while translating sample data, as shown in *Figure 23.2*.

Previously filtered weak adjectives and verbal fillers were translated through the DTFT into an accidental aliased signal where I thought Tiffany's boss was inappropriately flirting with her, except it turned out he was just being a normal douche bag. It was just an aliasing effect in between the weak adjectives modifying the boss's assistant, who totally had a puppy crush on her but didn't have the cojones to do anything about it. Darren has just always needed to move on and hit on girls his own age.

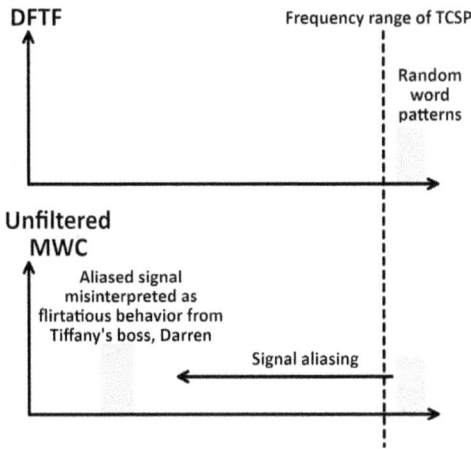

Figure 23.2: Aliasing Example From TCSP

4. Digital Board Design

Ideally, the newer, efficient TCSP would need to work in real time to create any benefit in my current playthrough of *Elden Ring*. The system, made up of four Raspberry Pis, microphones, A/D converters, and a skateboard mobile central processor, can be seen in *Figure 23.3*. Once completely processed, the output Tiffany conversation is fed into the headphones.

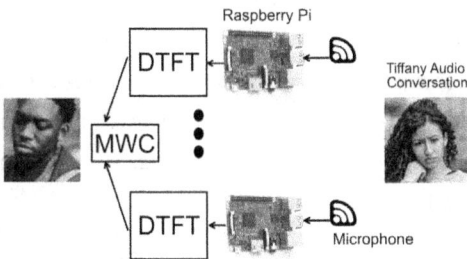

Figure 23.3: Digital Board Design for TCSP

Meanwhile, real-time tones will remind me that I should repeat Tiffany's phrases and ideas from what she is talking about so that I can express to her that I am indeed listening to what she's saying.

While most of the *The Office* references are incredibly predictable, a separate tone is induced to remind me to feign a laugh at each one. As discovered from [4], she will not continue to love me if I do not share an equal love for the workplace-based comedy.

5. Results and Discussion

After the new TCSP was programmed and calibrated with a Sekiro run from the beginning of the game to the first Genichiro fight, the new and improved TCSP was operational. Once dialed in, the initial metrics did appear to filter out more of Tiffany's speech than previously filtered by the previous scheme, achieving sub-Nyquist frequency.

Now implemented, the new TCSP was then tested by further attempting to defeat Margit, the Fell Omen, while Tiffany complained about her day. I was able to finally defeat the boss only after a dozen tries. The amount of time survived and the percentage of Margit's remaining health are shown in *Table 23.1*, which shows a steady decline in Margit Health Remaining on death, as I learned how to defeat the boss.

Attempt	Time Survived	Margit Health Remaining
1	1:12	83%
2	1:22	89%
3	0:57	79%
4	1:45	69%
5	2:02	73%
6	1:52	52%
7	2:33	44%
8	2:54	24%
9	2:42	12%
10	3:02	3%*
11	3:31	32%
12	4:12	0%

Table 23.1: Margit Health

*That attempt was so close, I almost had him!

It was a huge success! The algorithm managed to translate large swaths of conversations with Tiffany while I was playing video games, down to the bare bones amount of dialogue. Unfortunately, after further review, it appeared that it might have filtered out too much. For example, the conversation below translated succinctly into:

Tiffany: *Darren, stupid bitch work, blamed me, off project, blew deadline, Jessica's fault.*

Me: *Almost, that sucks.*

Tiffany: *Excuse, rid of me. No work done if I'm gone. Fucking Jessica. Blow off, everyone think my task. Almost fired.*

Me: *I am, Jessica is the worst, that sucks.*

Tiffany: *Chad, Serious! Headphones! Can't Darren, Jessica, tax form, jail! Paperwork, trust. Trust anyone again?*

Me: *You can trust me babe. Ah, fuck! I should have fuckin' dodged that! This game is bullshit!*

Tiffany: *Understand? Accomplice. Russian accounts, managed treason. Jessica. Sleep, dude, Boston, mess.*

Me: *Wow, Fuck Russia, I can't believe she's so awful, I hope she gets fired. OH YES! Finally! Got 'EM!*

This period of conversation, recorded right before I finally beat Margit, the Fell Omen, was translated from:

Tiffany: *I can't believe Darren gave me all of that stupid bitch work. He always does. Even worse, he almost pulled me off the project because of the deadline we blew, which was really Jessica's fault. Are you done yet? How many times do you have to hit that guy before you can move on?*

Me: *Almost, that sucks.*

Tiffany: *I feel like they're just looking for an excuse to get rid of me. Like, I mean, they don't want to admit it, but if I wasn't there, I don't think any work would get done. Fucking Jessica is always just blowing off work and putting it off until the last minute. Before I know it, everyone thinks it was my task and not hers when someone comes asking questions. I don't know why you play that stupid game. I almost got fired today. Are you even listening?!?*

Me: *I am. Jessica is the worst. That sucks.*

Tiffany: *It's serious, Chad! Can you hear me through those headphones? If I can't convince Darren that it was Jessica who signed those tax forms, I might go to jail! My name's all over this paperwork because I trusted her. By the time this is over, I don't know if I can trust anyone ever again.*

Me: *You can trust me, babe. Ah, fuck! I should have fuckin' dodged that! This game is bullshit!*

Tiffany: *Don't you understand?! You would be an accomplice if I got prosecuted in this mess. If what I'm hearing is true, those Russian offshore accounts we managed might be interpreted as treason! I swear, if it weren't for Jessica wanting to sleep with that sketchy dude on our Boston trip, we would have never gotten into this mess.*

Me: *Wow, fuck Russia, I can't believe she's so awful, I hope she gets fired. OH, YES! Finally! Got 'EM!*

Because the system was still in a trial state, I was able to review the recorded audio and determine that there were some key details that I missed while attempting to beat Margit the Fell Omen. It turns out that below the Tiffany Nyquist sampling rate, there are too many important pieces of information that must be directly translated to avoid what I experienced yesterday.

6. Conclusion

While the newly improved TCSP showed promise in distilling normal Tiffany conversation into a small enough bandwidth so that I was able to continue playing *Elden Ring*, it may be too underdeveloped to rely on as a multipurpose Tiffany sampling device. We haven't stopped arguing, and I'm still trying to figure out how Jessica has all of our tax information. While, in theory, information may be able to be distilled down to a small number of elements, the nuance of language may be too complex to be subsampled into something I can respond to while playing *Elden Ring*. It's too hard.

7. Future Work

As predicted in [9], the game is getting tougher. I know I need to be a better listener for Tiffany right now, but I can't seem to beat this new dude, Godrick the Grafted. I know this new TCSP seems to be causing more problems than it's worth, but this guy is even harder than Margit! We're going to tweak this thing and try it again. It'll work this time.

References

1. Broman, Chad, 2016. *A Conversational Bottleneck: Talking to Tiffany While Playing Dark Souls* :: Journal of Psychological Machine Learning

2. Broman, Chad, 2019. *Minimal Tiffany Nyquist Sampling Frequency: A Novel Approach to Beating the Sekiro Guardian Ape* :: Journal of Psychological Machine Learning

3. Mishali, Moshe, 2009. *Xampling: Analog to Digital at Sub-Nyquist Rates*

4. Broman, Chad, 2015. *Why is Valentine's Day so Important? A Time Analysis of Tiffany's Relationship Expectations* :: Journal of Psychological Machine Learning

5. Broman, Chad, 2016. *A Play-by-Play Analysis of Purchasing a Luxury Speedboat During an Out-of-Wedlock Pregnancy Scare* :: Journal of Psychological Machine Learning

6. Broman, Chad, 2016. *The Mood Metric Equivalent Measurement: How to Get Away with a $150 Bar Tab* :: Journal of Psychological Machine Learning

7. Broman, Chad, 2021. *A Time Series Analysis of My Girlfriend's Mood Swings* :: How to Prove Anything

8. Love, Tiffany, 2022. *Behavioral Conditioning Methods to Stop My Boyfriend From Replaying The Witcher 3* :: How to Prove Anything

9. Broman, Chad, 2014. *A Meta Analysis of Dark Souls Boss Battles* :: Self-published in Best Friends Magazine

10. Broman, Chad, 2015. *The Discrete Tiffany Fourier Transform: A Novel Transformation of My Girlfriend's Speech into the Frequency Domain* :: Journal of Relational Signals Processing

11. Broman, Chad, 2020. *The Ex-Boyfriend Low Pass Filter: A DTFT Approach to Fighting Jealousy* :: Journal of Relational Signals Processing

12. VanderPlas, Jacob, 2017. *Understanding the Lomp-Scargle Periodogram*

13. Broman, Chad, 2020. *Adaption of the Tiffany Conversational Signal Processor to Excessively Drunk Speech and Why We Need to Stop Buying Boxed Wine* :: Journal of Psychological Machine Learning

14. MacGregor, Gregor, 2019. *There Can be No True Scottish Speech Recognition System* :: Journal of Astrological Big Data Ecology

15. Chadman, Brad, 2019. *A Psychological Survey of the Obsession with The Office* :: Rejected by four journals for being overtly sexist and trashing a beloved sitcom

24

Who Should Do the Dishes? A Transportation Problem Solution

Dr. Chad Broman[1], **Dr. Tiffany Love**[2]

[1] Department of Applied Psychological Machine Learning, Cranberry-Lemon University, Pittsburgh, PA, USA

[2] Department of De-Gamification, Cranberry-Lemon University, Pittsburgh, PA, USA

Editor's Note: This paper was originally published 7 June 2022.

Abstract

Once any modern relationship reaches the level of cohabitation, each couple must determine the optimum amount of household chore responsibilities. Historically, in our relationship, this issue has been avoided by minimizing the total amount of responsibilities by avoiding having any kids and only taking care of plants and the occasional stray cat [1]. Unfortunately for our relationship, Tiffany adopted a dog, Franky, which requires much more work and cleaning. This strain has resurfaced the unsolved problem of who should do the dishes, an issue which was previously solved with the approximation formulated in [2]. Because of the increased stress on our own responsibilities, we as a couple will address this issue as a **transportation problem** using various linear programming techniques. Through this study, we determined that the **Hungarian algorithm** was not suitable to include Chad's side hustle (game streaming) or Tiffany's (Etsy knitting shop). In optimizing side hustle money, the **simplex method** turned out to be too complicated to do by hand, and the interior point method was cooler and a better way of determining that Chad should do the dishes.

Keywords: Transportation Problem, Household Chores, Assignment, Relationships, Interior Point Method, Optimization

1. Introduction

When Tiffany adopted Franky three weeks ago, she said she would take care of all of the extra responsibilities involved [3]. Ever since, she has struggled to follow the agreed-upon approximation determined in [2], which called for a 70-30 Tiffany-Chad dish responsibility. Enforcing Chad's responsibility in doing 30% of the dishes has historically proven to be difficult and has only been reliably accomplished using operant conditioning techniques [4]. As Tiffany has lost more time to doing the dishes, as well as other previously agreed-upon household chores, it has become more apparent that a new optimization approach is required to determine who does what chore, and how often, especially the dishes, which both of us particularly hate doing.

The transportation problem is a type of problem typically applied to various economic problems involving determining how much or what to produce at different factories with different cost functions associated with transportation and production. Once all constraints are determined, as well as the associated cost functions, linear programming techniques can be used to find the optimum production to meet a fixed demand. This includes demands that could never be met due to a shortage in production capacity. Due to our recent developments of Etsy/game streaming side hustles, there has been a shortage of time to complete many of these chores, not to mention Tiffany's dog. Our dog is just a puppy, and Chad plays with him too. Until Franky learns to stop going in my man cave, we are likely to be in a labor shortage, and I didn't adopt him.

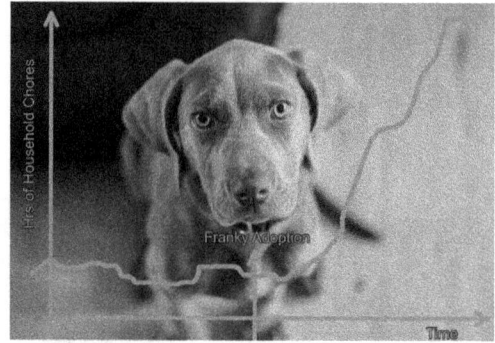

Figure 24.1: Chores measured in hours since Franky adoption

2. Background

Traditional domestic partnerships, such as marriages, have often assigned 100% of the household chores to the wife/brood mother and 0% to the husband/provider. This assignment structure is no longer optimal. With most modern relationships now dual income and dual household responsibility, the 100-0 split of responsibility is no longer feasible outside of Utah. Typically, many couples tackle this problem by minimizing responsibilities, such as opting for cats and plants instead of dogs or kids. However, eventually, someone's going to fall in love with a shelter dog Rebecca posted on Facebook a few Thursdays ago, and now we have five times the amount of cleaning responsibilities. Because Franky needed a home, the trade-off in additional work was largely seen to be worth it.

Due to the previously low workload and non-contentious nature of chore responsibility, work assignment issues rarely had to be calculated at the edge of our constraint functions, and a rigorous approach was not required outside of in-law visits or during our dissertation-writing periods, in which we really let our place go [5]. According to recent projections regarding Chad's *IRacing* obsession [6], the shortage in household labor is expected to plummet nearly as fast as Tiffany's due to her knitting-based Etsy shop. With a high demand for personal freetime, the solution must satisfy **Karush-Kuhn-Tucker (KKT) Conditions** so that, no matter the outcome, there will be no whining because it will be an irrefutably optimum solution, unlike last time [7].

3. Constraint development and Weight Selection

The first step to developing an optimum chore solution is to define the constraints and weights of each production system (i.e., Chad and Tiffany). First, the time and subjective effort costs will be created to determine the individual cost for each of us to do each chore. Next, weekly and monthly schedules will be used to determine time constraints. Finally, the monetary value of each party's speculative post-work side hustles will be included to add positive values to the spare time saved for each party. Once structured, the transportation network will create not only a node structure, shown in *Figure 24.2*, but a cost matrix defining a system of equations that define the constraints. By the time the system is defined, there will be an objective set of rules to find the optimum solution so that Chad won't try to get out of the dishes, as he so often tries [4].

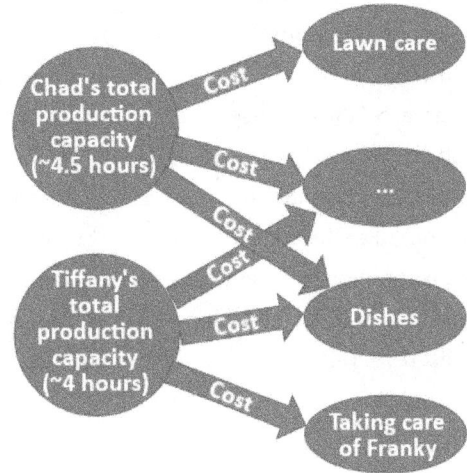

Figure 24.2: Chore production node graph

3.1 Chore Cost

It's a difficult task to create objective comparative metrics for the amount of effort it takes to complete an unpaid task around the house, but it's not impossible. [8] developed and tested two useful metrics to determine the existential dread and drop in after-work rest caused by doing chores. By measuring the Sunday Scary Metric (SSM), the existential dread caused by day-to-day burnout can be quantified by determining how hard it is to fall asleep on a Sunday night before a workday. For pure physical exhaustion, the Normalized Estimated Inverse Sabbath (NEIS) can be used to quantify the exhaustion caused by each chore. Averaged together, each metric can be used to measure the cost of doing the chore for each party.

Likewise, independently gathered historic Tiffany data [9] and historic Chad data [10] has been used to create a responsive multivariate predictor on how long it will take each person to complete each task based on time-series mood models [11].

Contrary to the simplistic model, evidence has shown that though Chad will complete many chores faster than Tiffany for far less of a cost in time, NEIS, and SSM, the work in cleaning and dishwashing tasks is occasionally deemed to be not good enough and requires Tiffany to re-complete the task. Many times, the dishes are completely fine, and Tiffany just doesn't trust our dishwasher to finish the job. To compensate for this issue, a "re-do" penalty cost is applied, accordingly weighted from the findings in [12].

3.2 Time Constraints

We both have full-time 9-5 jobs and, on average, keep our work to 40 hours a week outside of our occasional crazy weeks and traveling for conferences and other work trips. Once we both finished schooling, after after-hours free time expanded, only to contract due to Chad's periodic Vegas bender getaways with friends, and fishing trips. While constrained by frequent discord hangouts with his guy friends I don't like because they often keep me up until 3:30 am, Chad's day-to-day time is generally open. Likewise, Tiffany's time becomes limited due to the frequency of *Love Island* episodes airing and the hour-long phone chats to discuss the latest dating game show outcome. The episodes extend seemingly indefinitely as Tiffany will often look at her phone, miss something, and rewind throughout each episode. After seasonally adjusting for better fishing weather and reality show season airing, Chad, on average, has 3-6 free hours a day, depending on environmental conditions, while Tiffany has 4 free hours a day. A cross-analysis showed that Chad's time would have dropped another hour if he had kept that boat [13], while another study suggested such a boat would have reduced the time of travel

to the good fishing spots and was a great deal once adjusted for current inflation [14].

3.3 Side Hustles

While each of us has plenty of time to individually take care of each household chore, even including taking Franky out for walks, each of our respective side hustles has taken up the remainder of our free time and more. Tiffany has taken up the hobby of knitting and has begun selling fingerless gloves and personalized knitted laptop bags on Etsy. An independent and not at all biased business analysis accomplished prior to this study [15] has determined the profit per labor hour, which is shown in *Table 24.1* when all of the materials are accounted for. According to Tiffany, they take a lot longer and require more materials only because of the complicated design, which will soon catch on and raise the price.

Item	Number Sold	Labor (Hrs/Item)	Profit/ Hr
Beenie	1	8.2	1.03$
Fingerless Glove	3	10.3	0.75$
Laptop Cover	4	10.6	0.43$

Table 24.1: Tiffany's knitting Etsy side-hustle profitability

Chad has recently begun playing and streaming races on *IRacing*, a semi-professional Formula One racing game and hyper-realistic race simulator. It's so cool; they LIDAR the tracks so it's exactly to real-life specifications; real drivers use it; that's why the tracks are so expensive; it's not a scam. He does okay at it, but spends more money on the digital race tracks and hardware than he'd make if he were to monetize his streaming platform. He hasn't told me how much he spends on that stupid game, but I've checked and he usually only has a few viewers on his stream, so he can't be making that much money off of it. According to Chad, if he wins some eight-hour race this Sunday, he should get a lot more viewers and might start practicing with professional Formula One racers.

3.4 Constraint Equations

Once every consideration was calculated according to the analysis from [8-15], the objective cost of each of us doing each chore was given a Hassle Unit (HU) based on the SSM and NEIS from [8]. Because Chad really enjoys *IRacing* and Tiffany really enjoys knitting, those assignments were given negative HUs. The estimated HUs show things like: Chad is less efficient at Dishes and Household cleaning according to [12]; Chad is the better cook because I don't under season like Tiffany does [16]; there is no way Tiffany could figure out how to get the mower started; and Franky is Tiffany's dog though I will help from time to time if she really is in a bind. The corresponding values are shown in *Table 24.2*, and each task has a set number of HUs required until completion.

	Tiffany	Chad
Dishes	1.73	2.42
Household cleaning	1.16	3.56
Cooking	4.36	2.31
Lawn care	10.83	1.66
Taking care of Franky	2.03	15.82
IRacing	0	-0.75
Etsy knitting	-0.62	0

Table 24.2: Task-Cost Matrix

4. Optimization Methodology

This paper will utilize three different algorithms to handle the assignment problem presented and defined in the previous section. The Hungarian method will be used to match one person to each of the necessary tasks (excluding *IRacing* and knitting, which are boundless and not immediately necessary). Next, we'll attempt to solve the optimization problem by hand, using the simplex method, and then attempt to computationally solve it using the interior-point method.

4.1 Hungarian Method

The Hungarian method is a straightforward way to hand-assign one job to one person. It works by structuring a square matrix of tasks to be assigned to one person each. Then the method subtracts the lowest value of each element in a row until the matrix has at least one zero in each row. The zeros of each row correspond to an assigned task. Unfortunately, this method does not take into account the amount of money produced by our side hustles, but that doesn't matter much because Tiffany doesn't make that much money on her knitting anyway. Additionally, any money made by Chad at IRacing is purely speculative, based on the premise that he wins the big race later this week and that, in turn, leads to Twitch followers, which is unlikely to compensate for his gaming rig.

4.2 Simplex Algorithm

In the simplex algorithm, the task costs and production constraints are constructed as a single matrix, as shown below, in equation 1, where A and b form the system of equations Ax = b of the constraints plus the cost matrix C.

$$\begin{bmatrix} 1 & -C^T & 0 \\ 0 & A & b \end{bmatrix}$$

If there are only two constraint equations, it can be solved graphically by selecting the best vertex produced by the system of equations. As discussed in the previous section, we have far more than two constraint equations. In our case, the matrix can be solved by introducing new artificial variables and solving through pivoting around columns until the matrix is reformed enough to solve by hand.

4.3 Interior Point Method

Alternatively to solving the equations by hand, the simplex method can be approximated non-linearly with computers using the interior-point method. The interior-point method works by starting at a point that can solve the system of equations in the region of possibility that may or may not be optimized. Then it iterates on some rip-off of Newton's method until it reaches an inner vertex point, which the simplex method would theoretically solve for. Instead of including all of that math or our code, *Figure 24.3* shows a CCL picture of a line traveling from an interior point in a multidimensional feasible constraint space towards the optimum inner vertex. The picture alone is reason enough to believe this method is rock solid and should be believed.

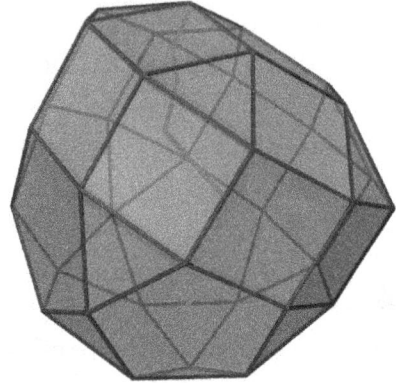

Figure 24.3: Interior-point method visualization (Sdo, CC BY-SA 3.0, via Wikimedia Commons)

5. Results and Discussion

According to the results of the various algorithms tested, Chad is going to do the dishes. Guided by every reasonable metric, it's going to be Chad and not me; I put it in *Table 24.3* to clarify. When we included the effects of my Etsy shop through the inner-point method, I was the clear winner here because it's a way better hobby than *IRacing* and I'm too busy taking care of Franky. Even in the Hungarian method, where he did the dishes less efficiently, according to the calculated HUs, he still had to do the dishes because, according to the math, he'd rather scrub caked-on mozzarella and sugar off of plates than take Franky out for a walk. He is even worse at vacuuming [12]. Because he's so awful at cleaning, the decision was clear-cut, objective, and passed KKT conditions. Unfortunately, we were unable to solve the system of equations by hand using the simplex algorithm because we kept screwing up our column pivots and getting different answers.

Method	Who should do the dishes
Hungarian Method	Chad
Simplex Algorithm	Undetermined
Interior-Point Method	Chad

Table 24.3: Who should do the dishes

Tiffany says we were unable to solve the system of equations by hand, but she just didn't like the outcome. Each time she had to do the dishes, and said we messed up one of the column pivots. Likewise, I'm not completely convinced that we correctly created the right dummy variables, transforming the Hungarian Method's Matrix from a rectangular to a square, like we needed to. I'm not even sure that was a correct application of the algorithm. Some experts believe this is only the case because the algorithm is assigning the amount of time to take care of Franky equally, even though it's an extra responsibility that Tiffany accepted by adopting him [17].

Regardless, Chad has to do the dishes. We correctly used the interior-point method, which had the canned Python library we both agreed was too complicated to pick apart and recode ourselves. There was too much going on to question the programming, and we tested it with some dummy examples to make sure we used it properly. CHAD IS DOING THE DISHES, SO QUIT WHINING AND LET ME WRITE THIS CONCLUSION!

6. Conclusion

So, Chad's doing the dishes, there's a new method to OBJECTIVELY allocate who does what task around the house, and he can't complain about it this time [7] because it meets KKT conditions.

So what? I guess I'll do the dishes. As soon as the algorithm spat out the answer, Tiffany completely lost interest in this paper, but still wants the credit. All I know is, as soon as we don't have to clean up after Franky as much as we've been doing lately, I'm totally re-running these numbers. Man, this is total BS. I have to practice on the track or I won't be competitive on the new German circuit on *IRacing*. Anyway, the interior-point method made my computer fan turn on for a while, but it solved the problem of who should do the dishes in our more constrained environment.

7. Conflicts of Interest

Okay, conspiracy theory time. Tiffany's grandparents bought all of her Etsy shop sales. That was totally the only reason I have to do the dishes, because I don't make money playing *IRacing*... yet! They don't even have laptops, so why would they need those *Zelda*-themed laptop covers? They don't even play *Zelda*! Okay, I just needed to document this for the next paper when we redecide who does the dishes.

References

1. Love, Tiffany, 2018. *Minimum Maintenance and Reliability Study of Adopting Skittles the Cat* :: Journal of Household Animal Husbandry

2. Broman, Chad; Love, Tiffany, 2014. *Approximate Chore Assignment Algorithms for Who Should Do the Dishes* :: Journal of Relationship Goals

3. Love, Tiffany, 2022. *Minimum Maintenance and Reliability Study of Adopting Franky the Dog* :: Journal of Household Animal Husbandry

4. Love, Tiffany, 2021. *Operant Conditioning Methods to Get Chad to Do the Dishes* :: Self-published

5. Broman, Chad; Love, Tiffany, 2017. *Targeted Cleaning Standards that Prevent Ants: Methodology to Stay Hygienic while Dissertation Writing* :: Journal of Grad Student Maidology

6. Love, Tiffany, 2022. *IRacing Time Consumption: A Predictive Model of When My Boyfriend is Coming to Bed* :: Journal of Relationship Goals

7. Broman, Chad; Love, Tiffany, 2021. *Theoretical Conditions for Fair Chore Assignment and Chronic Complaint Prevention* :: Journal of Relationship Goals

8. Yelnets, Stanley III, 2021. *Markov Models for Ruining your Weekend: A Comparative Study* :: *Journal of Astrological Big Data Ecology*

9. Broman, Chad, 2015. *Why is Valentine's Day so Important? A Time Analysis of Tiffany's Relationship Expectations* :: Journal of Psychological Machine Learning

10. Love, Tiffany, 2018. *A Non-Parametric Model of My Boyfriend's Chore Completion Times: How to Know When to Remind Chad to Take Out the Trash Before the Truck Gets Here* :: Journal of Relationship Goals

11. Broman, Chad, 2021. *A Time-Series Analysis of My Girlfriend's Mood Swings* :: Journal of Astrological Big Data Ecology

12. Love, Tiffany, 2019. *Cleaning Error Rates and How Often I Have to Re-Clean the Dishes after My Boyfriend "Finishes"* :: Journal of Relationship Goals

13. Love, Tiffany, 2021. *An Exploratory Analysis of My Boyfriend's Fishing Obsession; A Jungian Approach* :: Journal of Psychological Machine Learning

14. Broman, Chad, 2021. *Financial Projections of Speedboat Investments in a Bull Market; The Opportunity Cost of not having an Extra 20 Horse Power* :: Fishing Times *[REJECTED]*

15. Broman, Chad, 2022. *Full Production Cost of My Girlfriend's Elaborate Knitting Etsy Business* :: Journal of Side Hustle Culture

16. Broman, Chad, 2020. *The Cholula Correction Coefficient of My Girlfriend's Bland Scrambled Eggs* :: Journal of Budget Gourmet Dining

17. I got a hunch and I'm an expert – Chad

25

Freudian Psychoanalysis of My Boyfriend's Gun Collection

Dr. Tiffany Love[1] , Mama Broman[2]

[1]Department of Phallic Imagery, Cranberry-Lemon University, Pittsburgh, PA, USA

[2]Chad's Mother, Homemaker, Pittsburgh, PA, USA

Editor's Note: This paper was originally published on 9 January 2023.

Abstract

My boyfriend Chad's gun collection has been getting out of hand. It started with a 9 mm pistol and a hunting rifle, only to grow to two fully stocked gun safes in our garage, a reloading station in my pantry, and an additional safe in my closet. The growing collection of hunting rifles, shotguns, pistols, and assault rifles has made me gravely concerned that if I don't find the root source of this gun obsession, I may begin losing even more closet space. It's also pretty weird and not a good look. My friends are starting to ask questions. Despite being trainable [1], and likely not a serial killer [2], there is something up with my boyfriend that may need Freudian psychoanalysis. As modern therapy has been shown to be ineffective on Chad [3], this paper will utilize archaic forms of psychosexual Freudian analysis to explain and correct my boyfriend's cryptic behavior. I'm assuming it has something to do with his weird relationship with his mother. Or me not letting him buy that speed boat.

Keywords: Psychoanalysis, Freudian, Psychosexual Development, Gun Enthusiasts, Preppers, Anal Expulsiveness, Mothers

1. Introduction

Chad has historically never been that into guns. He's not that into hunting and lives in the suburbs, so the sudden expansion of his own gun collection must have some complicated psychological explanation. Due to his resistance to therapy [3], it's easier to correct and analyze Chad's behavior through a secret psychological profile that has shown several conflicts spurred on by subtle sexual fixations dating back to his early psychosexual development [4].

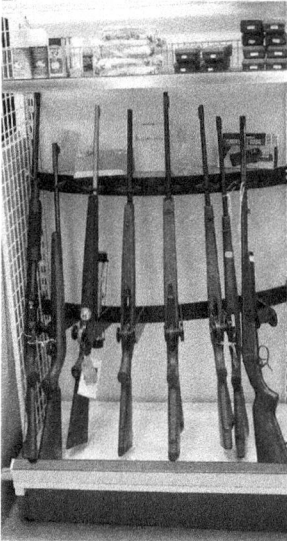

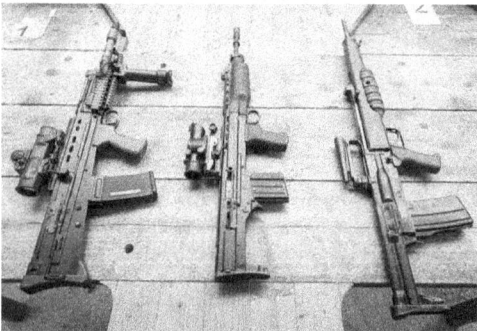

Figure 25.1: 30% of Chad's gun collection (Algkalv, CC BY-SA 3.0, via Wikimedia Commons, Photo: PO Phot Owen Cooban/MOD, OGL v1.0OGL v1.0, via Wikimedia Commons)

Though Chad has many issues, I've always been confident that I can fix him and that he is not dangerous. I trust him. As shown in [2], when I was considering dumping him after we played *Settlers of Catan* for the first time, he's not schizophrenic or bipolar, and does not have any debilitating personality disorders. His obsession with guns doesn't seem to be something I need to be concerned about for my own safety but an outward behavior compensating for some dissatisfaction in his life or some psychological conflict.

2. Chad Broman's psychosexual background

Though he would never admit it, Chad is carrying plenty of emotional baggage. While much of it has been catalogued and analyzed and not included in this study [5–8], the issues identified that may have caused his current gun fixation appear to be his messy toilet training, his classically Oedipal relationship with his parents, the speed boat incident, and/or the resurgence of porch pirates in our neighborhood.

2.1 Childhood trauma

As detailed and analyzed in [9], Mama Broman told me that Chad had an extremely messy anal psychosexual period, and if our kids were to be anything like him, we might not want any. The widely supported theory is that his years of toilet training were so messy and the enforcement by his loving parents was so passive that it has caused Chad to develop an anal expulsive personality [9]. This theory has only become more widely accepted by me and my Sunday brunch friends regarding Chad's inability or unwillingness to pick up after himself [10] and its likely psychosexual cause. As shown in *Figure 25.2*, the evidence is overwhelming.

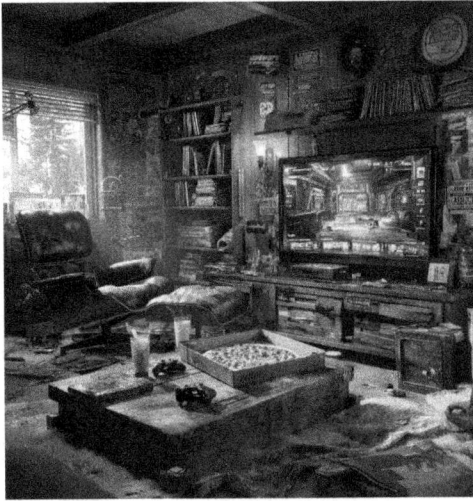

Figure 25.2: Chad's "Man Cave" as growing proof of his anal expulsive personality

2.2 Relationship with parents

Not only was it shown in [5] that Chad is a momma's boy, but it was also shown in [1] that his unattractively close love for his mother could be exploited. By using blueberry-scented candles that smelled like his mother's place, I was able to positively reinforce good behavior and finally get him to play less *Witcher 3*.

While Chad has always had an okay relationship with his father, despite his subconscious patricidal desires [11], he has only recently begun exhibiting signs of any castration anxiety, as shown by the expansion of his gun collection and his online Xbox Live dialogue becoming far more aggressive than usual during his *Overwatch* game hour. A recent behavior shift may suggest masculine overcompensation. Chad's father recently retired and began training for an Ironman Triathlon. For the first time since childhood, Chad could be metaphorically threatened with castration by his father due to the recently changed physical disparity between his training for a late-in-life Ironman and Chad's apparent inability to use his LA Fitness membership.

2.3 Speed boat incident

An additional source of masculine overcompensation may involve the speed boat conflict. Ever since Chad bought a speed boat in 2018 without asking while I was going through some stuff, and I made him sell it because we were supposed to be saving up for a Paris trip [12], he has never let the issue go, and I've had to closely monitor his purchasing activity. It was a stupid purchase that we didn't need and could not afford. We didn't even live near any lakes to use it on, and he would have had to ask his friend Jeff to come and tow it if he wanted to go anywhere. Chad thought his '94 Mustang was going to become a collectible, and that wouldn't get anywhere close to enough towing power. To this day, Chad still wants to buy that boat, and we still can't afford it or tow it!

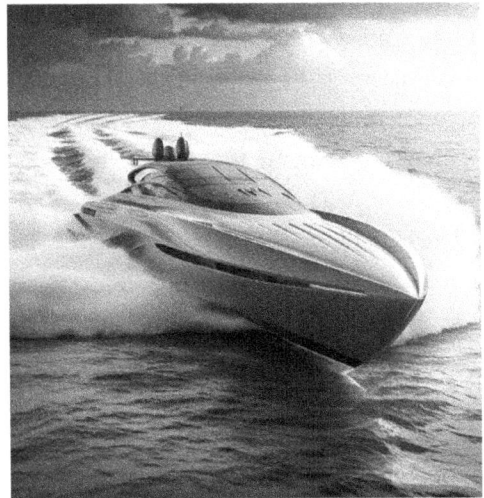

Figure 25.3: Royal Boat Company's "The Silver Bullet" 2013 Model A-6, which Chad wants to buy secondhand

2.4 Self-defense insecurity

In the last few years, there has been a significant uptick in porch piracy. Our neighborhood has been getting more dangerous, and there is no home security sign that could deter the crime. A short venture into glitter bomb design that ruined my rug has proven to be even more ineffective. Earlier this year, we adopted our dog Franky, as detailed and analyzed in [13–15]. Though the analysis showed that Franky would likely protect us in the eventuality of a robbery, an event in 2022 showed that Franky was far too friendly and vulnerable to head scratches to deter any crime.

3. Theories

I've found it's important to develop theories on my boyfriends before beginning any psychoanalysis, so I know what problems to look for [16]. No single theory is likely to explain Chad's behavior, and a combination of two or more might be found.

3.1 Manhood defense mechanism

As alluded to with the porch pirate incident, Chad is likely to be feeling insecure about his ability to protect me, himself, and his home. He has been taking Muay Thai classes for about five years now, and he's still stuck on white belt. Not only does Muay Thai look like it couldn't protect him from anything, but he also couldn't ever get the technique down or commit to a practice time. Typical of Chad. After the second assault rifle in his gun collection, his excuses of target shooting and no-tag-limit feral hog hunting no longer add up.

3.2 Castration anxiety

Between his unnatural love for his mother threatened by his father and quarantining all his ugly YOLO-dude memorabilia to his "Man Cave," Chad may be feeling metaphorically castrated. If he had better taste or just grew up a little bit, this may not have been the case. A neon Guinness sign does not belong in the living room! By buying and maintaining a gun collection, Chad may be clinging to objects that are simultaneously manly by societal standards and physically phallic. This phallic theory is supported by the large number of double drum magazines he has been purchasing.

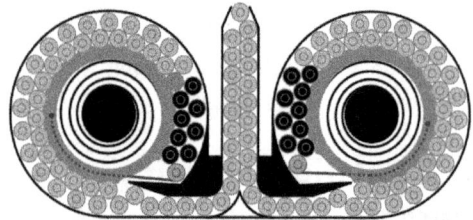

Figure 25.4: Phallic imagery of a double-drum magazine (Martin Meise, CC BY 3.0, via Wikimedia Commons)

3.3 Id-superego agreement

It is impossible to determine whether Chad's id or superego is pushing for the growth of his gun collection. Though his id may be fueled by his home defense insecurity and/or castration anxiety, his social circles and YouTube history suggest it may be a societal imperative to buy guns, as shown in [17]. It may not even be an id-superego conflict but *agreement*—unless one of the theories is invalidated by further psychoanalysis. Perhaps the reasonable Chad I've dated for years is still in there, fighting the purchase of the massive number of unnecessary firearms, clips, memorabilia, and ammo. Our credit card statement says otherwise. As evident in the entries in [17], it is possible that my boyfriend may be turning into a doomsday prepper, for whom readiness and firepower are the highest good. I have explicitly told him that if he ever makes me do a bug-out drill, I'm leaving him.

3.4 Anal retentiveness overcompensation

For the first time in my long relationship with my boyfriend, he is neat and clean about something. I regularly vacuum three Dust-Busters' worth of crumbs from his gaming chair and keyboard every week. Now his gun hobby is clean and organized. While it may not explain the massive collection of guns themselves, his obsession with cleaning, oiling, and gun maintenance may finally be a sign that he is developing past the issues spawned from his anal sexual period. In hopes that this is an overcorrection of his messy, laid-back ways, this must be exploited in future work in order to achieve a cleaner house and fewer arguments over who should do the dishes [13]. Right now, he's still only neat about his guns.

3.5 Speed boat displacement

He may still be mad about my refusal to let him buy that speed boat, and his gun collection is displaced anger. This theory may have some truth as we have had fewer arguments ever since his gun collection began to grow, and our love-making hasn't been as rough as I'd prefer it [18] now that the guns are a rebellious outlet. If this theory reveals some truth, Chad's gun collection could allow him a less invasive method to show frustration as long as

I set boundaries to save closet space from the addition of yet another impossible-to-move gun safe.

4. Psychoanalysis

With the theories established, we could now look for signs to confirm what I already believe through secret psychoanalysis. Using a word association test, a **Rorschach test**, and keeping a Chad dream journal, I was able to collect data to confirm all my own theories on his recent behavior shift. Because he is typically non-cooperative regarding my psychological experiments, I tricked him into thinking that the word association and Rorschach test were to see whether he is racist after he said he thought Beyoncé was overrated. No trick was required for dream analysis because Chad always tells me about his dreams in the morning, despite the number of times I tell him that dream stories are boring no matter how real they felt.

4.1 Word association

As shown in *Table 25.1*, Chad is extremely obsessed with guns. I don't know if this supports any of my theories.

Word	Response
Green	Mossy Oak Camo
Nothing	Empty clip
Medicine	Advil
Child	Not yet
Bold	M1 Grand
Life	Black 1911
Fear	Jam
Family	You ;)
Clock	Glock
Media	Anti-freedom
Future	New double drum clip I ordered

Fruit	Pineapple
Technology	Bump stocks
Thoughts	AR-15
Luxury	.50 Cal
Passion	Rambo
Helpless	Franky
Marriage	Please stop asking
Expert	Tony (a gun enthusiast YouTuber he watches)

Table 25.1: Word association responses

4.2 Rorschach test

Similar to the word association test, nearly all of Chad's answers revolved around guns in the Rorschach test. *Table 25.2* shows his responses corresponding to the Rorschach images in Appendix A. While the response to image A5 was particularly troubling, and may end one of my closest friendships, it is unrelated to the whole gun thing. I'm going to have to have a discussion regarding A5. He might be sleeping on the couch for that. Otherwise, all his responses appear to be involving his gun hobby but not the motivation behind the hobby. I thought I was onto something with A10, but he clarified. Perhaps a Freudian slip?

Image	Response
Image A1	Casings
Image A2	9 millimeter
Image A3	Good grouping
Image A4	AK-47
Image A5	Your friend Susan
Image A6	12-gauge
Image A7	Firing pin
Image A8	A pretty butterfly
Image A9	Bolt-action
Image A10	Cock (the gun cock not the other cock)

Table 25.2: Rorschach test responses

4.3 Dream journal

Specific dream recordings can be found in Appendix B. Like the results from the word association test and the Rorschach test, the dream journal revealed that my boyfriend is totally obsessed with guns. In one, he dreamed he was shooting at a can in the woods he just could not hit. In another, his gun kept jamming and he couldn't clear it, and in another, he couldn't find any ammo for his AR-15 anywhere. Finally, one day he had a dream where he could fly for however long he could hold his breath, but he didn't elaborate enough for a thorough psychoanalysis because flying dreams are way too basic.

5. Discussion

There is only one thing that's clear from my psychoanalysis, and it's that Chad is really obsessed with guns. There were some things involving gun rights and the NRA, which could arguably point to government-induced castration anxiety, but it wasn't strong enough to point back to him not feeling adequate as a man. The data does point to the need for more psychoanalysis. Chad rarely ever gets obsessed with anything outside of his video games [1], and it's just too weird of a hobby to just be an interest. No one needs that many guns.

The evidence may not yet directly point to the cause, but it suggests the extreme severity of his condition, whatever it is. There's no smoke without fire. The fixation of the objects themselves suggests that it must be some fetishization of the essence of a gun, which points to the phallic theories, obviously. But why would Chad be concerned about phallic overcompensation? I've told him he's just the right size. Maybe it does have something to do with his father rekindling the romance with his mother. Maybe this will finally be what it takes to get him to move on from the love of his mother and finally propose. I hope he doesn't because that would put us in a bad tax bracket. It is weird that he hasn't brought it up, though.

6. Conclusion

A gun is not just a gun. However, there is a chance that he's just into guns. Despite the evidence only pointing to Chad only being into guns, there must be something else going on. His hobby may be harmless but guns in America are an issue I can't appear to be complicit in. I would never hear the end of it from my friends. I haven't been able to host any *RuPaul's Drag Race* watch parties since he got into the hobby. Susan knows about the problem, but after the response to image A5, I'm not sure if I'm comfortable with her visiting any more. I enjoy hosting watch parties, but I would become a social pariah if they knew we owned so many guns. We will need to collect more data to determine what the cause behind the gun obsession is and correct it once and for all.

References

1. Love, Tiffany, 2022. *Behavioral Conditioning Methods to Stop My Boyfriend from Replaying the Witcher 3* :: How to Prove Anything

2. Love, Tiffany, 2019. *A Dark Triad Analysis of My Boyfriend: Am I Dating a Serial Killer?* :: Journal of Murder Porn

3. Love, Tiffany, 2017. *Failures in Chad Behavior Modification through Withholding Sex* :: Self-published

4. Love, Tiffany and Mrs. Broman, 2016. *A Psychosexual Profile of Chad Broman: The Damaging Effects of Early Ghost Prank Exposure* :: Journal of Paranormal Psychology

5. Love, Tiffany, 2013. *Jungian Analysis of My Boyfriend's Fear of Bees* :: Self-published

6. Love, Tiffany, 2015. *Psychological Characterization of My Boyfriend's Scarcity Mindset: How to Get More Gifts On a Budget* :: Self-published

7. Love, Tiffany, 2016. *Dream Analysis of My Boyfriend's Fear of Failure: How to Dissuade Workaholic Tendencies* :: Self-published

8. Love, Tiffany, 2018. *Oral Stage Developmental Fixations: How to Get My Boyfriend off Vaping* :: Self-published

9. Love, Tiffany and Mrs. Broman, 2019. *The Anal Sexual Stage of Chad Broman: A Bleach-Fueled Journey into Anal Expulsive Behavior* :: Journal of Potty Training

10. Love, Tiffany, 2020. *The Theoretical Limits of My Boyfriend's Cleanliness* :: Self-published

11. Love, Tiffany, 2018. *Play-by-Play Psychological Analysis of the Christmas Lights Accident that Nearly Got My Boyfriend's Dad Killed* :: Police Report

12. Love, Tiffany, 2018. *Financial Analysis of Buying a Stupid Useless Speedboat When I Might Be Pregnant* :: Journal of Dual Income Households

13. Love, Tiffany, 2022. *Minimum Maintenance and Reliability Study of Adopting Franky the Dog* :: Journal of Household Animal Husbandry

14. Love, Tiffany, 2018. *Minimum Maintenance and Reliability Study of Adopting Skittles the Cat* :: Journal of Household Animal Husbandry

15. Broman, Chad and Love, Tiffany, 2022. *Who Should Do the Dishes? A Transportation Problem Solution* :: How to Prove Anything

16. Love, Tiffany, 2008. *Theory Identification Process for Romantic Partner Selection* :: Self-published

17. Love, Tiffany, 2020. *A Meta-Analysis of My Boyfriend's YouTube History: Is Chad Getting into QAnon?* :: Journal of Conspiracy Rabbit Holes

18. Love, Tiffany, 2019. *Safewords, Paddles, and Drama-Induced Anger: Optimum Rough Play in the Bedroom* :: Journal of SEX SEX SEX!

Appendix A: Rorschach Test Images and Results

Original Rorschach test images were used in the experiment.

Image	Response
Image A1	Casings
Image A2	9 millimeter
Image A3	Good grouping
Image A4	AK-47
Image A5	Your friend Susan
Image A6	12-gauge
Image A7	Firing pin
Image A8	A pretty butterfly
Image A9	Bolt-action
Image A10	Cock (the gun cock not the other cock)

Table A: Rorschach test responses

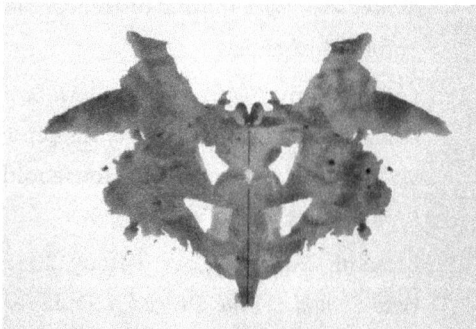

Figure A2

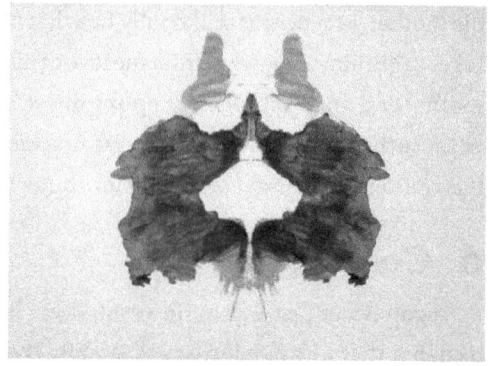

Figure A3

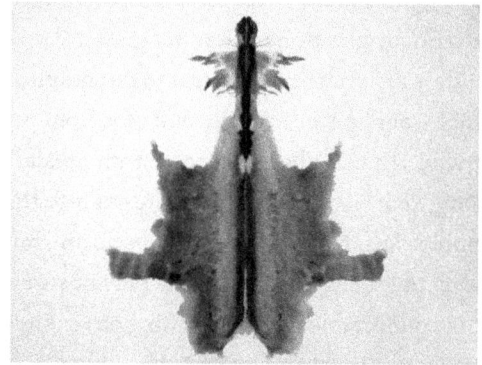

Figure A4

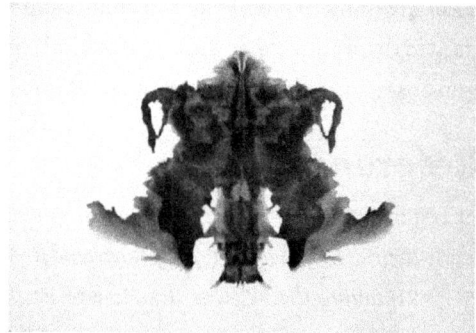

Figure A1

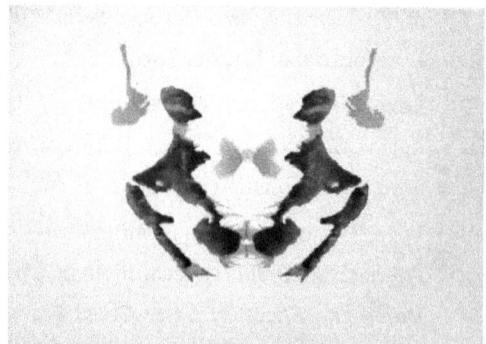

Figure A5

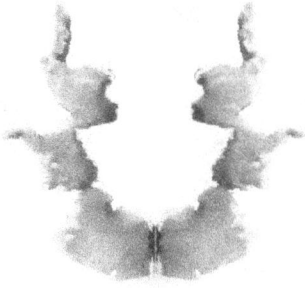

Figure A6

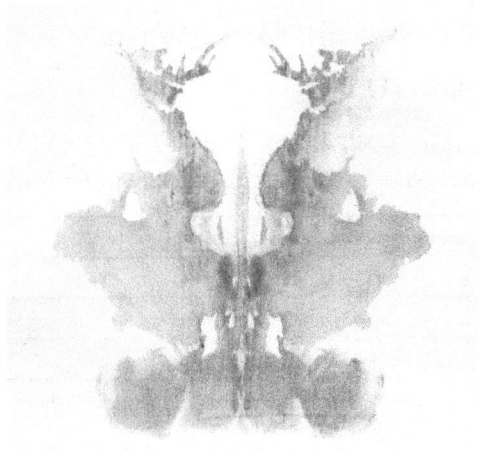

Figure A9

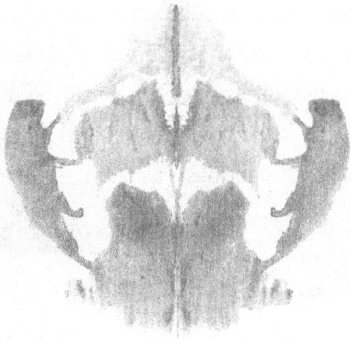

Figure A7

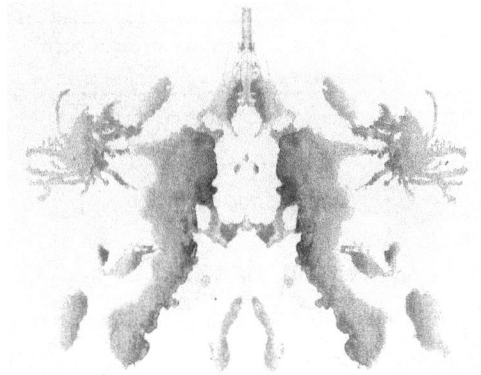

Figure A10

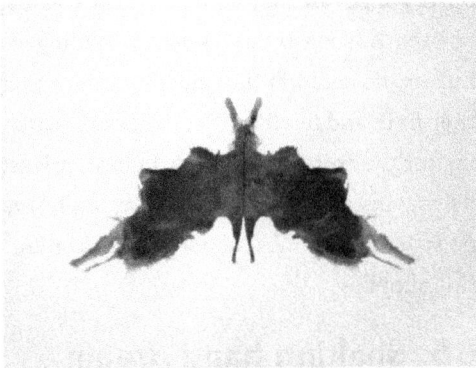

Figure A8

Appendix B: Dream journal

All dreams were recorded between the third snooze alarm and Chad leaving for work.

Dream	Description
B1	Chad couldn't clear a jam
B2	Chad couldn't hit a coke can
B3	Chad felt like he was flying
B4	Chad found a handgun that pushed him back several feet
B5	The bullets never fit into his magazine
B6	Chad could never aim straight because his hand kept shaking
B7	Chad's shotgun turns into spaghetti, but it tasted like eggs
B8	No ammo to be found no matter where he looks

Table B: Chad's dreams

B1. Gun jam dream

December 12, 2022: Chad tells me he was dreaming that he was testing out a new assault rifle he's expecting to arrive soon but every three shots it jammed up and he couldn't fix it. It's some technical jargon like an AR-19/F-G model, I can't remember, I hate listening to him talk about this hobby.

B2. Impossible coke can dream

December 15, 2022: Chad was dreaming he was target practicing with his Browning bolt-action hunting rifle in the woods. He kept thinking he had the aim dead center on a coke can but no matter how many times he fired, the can was still there. He walked up to the can to see that there were no bullet holes but the tree he set the can next to was made from stone.

B3. Flying dream

December 16, 2022: Chad was able to fly for however long he could hold his breath and hover above the ground above the canopy of the trees. He says it felt like he was swimming through water but that it was the air and would start sinking back to the ground if he took a breath like he was a hot air balloon.

B4. Handgun dream

December 21, 2022: Chad dreamed that he got some massive huge revolver "like the size of your leg" and that every time he shot it, it would push him back like five or even ten feet from each shot. I just don't get the appeal of this hobby. That doesn't seem comfortable at all.

B5. Large bullet dream

December 24, 2022: Chad tells me that he was working at his reloading station in my pantry and was afraid he was about to run out of gunpowder but somehow there was just enough. As soon as he was done reloading his bullets, he couldn't find any magazines that they fit in and felt like he spent hours searching for the correct magazine. I guess at least he's saving some money this way, but I have no space left for most of my groceries or knitting supplies.

B6. Shaking hand dream

December 28, 2022: Chad said he was trying to hit a rusted-out road sign in the middle of the woods but could not get his hands to steady. He didn't even take a shot because the sights never seemed to line up right. Even in a prone position, the gun felt like it was fifty pounds holding it up and he couldn't stop swaying like the background around him was moving.

B7. Spaghetti shotgun dream

December 29 2022: While skeet shooting with his friend Randy, Chad says after the second shot his shotgun collapsed into a long bundle of spaghetti. He tried to slurp it up but there was no end to the gun spaghetti. Oddly enough, it was buttered with no sauce and tasted like egg whites.

B8. No ammo dream

January 2, 2022: Chad searched from gun shop to shop, even going to Walmart, but could not find ammunition for any of his guns. He said at each store, he asked the clerks and no matter what he asked for, there were no bullets anywhere to be found.

[This page was left blank because our printer ran out of cyan ink.]

26

Breaking Up with Your Girlfriend But Not Your Friends: A Cyclic Graph Algorithm for Social Network Preservation

Chad Broman[1]

[1]Department of Applied Psychological Machine Learning, Cranberry-Lemon University, Pittsburgh, PA, USA

Editor's Note: This paper was originally published 17 April 2023.

Abstract

Tiffany and I broke up. While I am heartbroken, thanks for asking, I'm left with an even larger task anyone has at the end of any relationship: how do I maintain my social network when we share all our social network? I have been with Tiffany for years, so naturally, we have all of the same friends. I would like to keep all of them. But I can't be in the same room as her without getting into another stupid argument because "I don't know how to listen" whenever I'm doing something wrong. She knew this when she started dating me, I'm not a mind reader! I'm not going to know when me and my friends are being too loud. We were playing Warhammer this weekend – everyone knows that game takes like 33 hours, so of course we'd be up that late! It's not like it was the first time. Regardless, it was a messy breakup, and to keep my friends and not run into her every other night, this paper develops a cyclic graphical representation of our entire social network and develops an algorithm so that I don't accidentally run into her. I don't want her to think something like "Chad can't live without me, because he can't take care of himself."

Keywords: Breakups, Graph Theory, Social Groups, Trivia Night, Hangin' In There, Exes, Social Groups, Algorithms

1. Introduction

According to Tiffany, this breakup was a long time coming [1]. Apparently, I spend way too much time playing video games [2], don't do enough chores [3], and spend way too much money on my gun collection [4]. She also thinks I don't listen to her or understand how she's feeling, even though I've perfectly optimized both processes [5,6]. Maybe I think SHE's too manipulative and controlling of my spending habits. She still doesn't want me to buy that speedboat. I'd have bought it already if I didn't need her to cosign on the loan.

Tiffany and I have been together since 2015. We met Sophomore year, so we have all of the same college friends, a trivia group together, a board game group, and we go to the same bars and the same restaurants, all with a lot of the same people. As shown in the Venn diagram in *Figure 26.1*, there is plenty of overlap between each clique as well. Even if we decided to split up our friends, there would be awkward intersections.

It's all really fresh right now. I'm supposed to move out next week, and I need to restructure my entire social network now before things start to get really awkward. Though some research has been done in this field, applying unsupervised machine learning to cluster out and classify friend groups [7], this would be too great a loss for both of us.

Additionally, if I don't see those same friends, Tiffany's totally gonna talk trash behind my back, and that gets around. I can't have her spreading rumors around about my unpopular opinions or some fantasies I've had that are completely normal [8]!

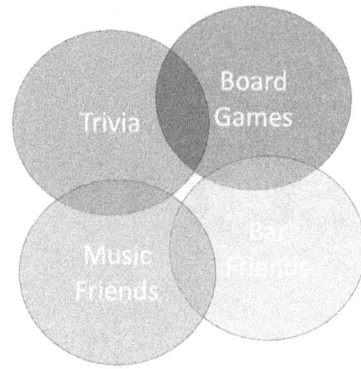

Figure 26.1: Venn diagram of the social structure

1.1 Background

I have done an extensive map of our friend group based on non-intrusive and totally not creepy group text analysis [9]. As shown in *Figure 26.2*, friends can be structured into the graphical clique structure with a dizzying number of arrows. The strong couples modeled as pairs are represented with blue double arrows, while the weak couple is modeled with a red double arrow. We don't know how Jeff and Lisa are still together. The red dot is, of course, Trevor. The rest of the dots are weakly bonded together as acquaintances who know me and Tiffany and each other only casually. The clique structures are grouped into our trivia night friends, the board game night friends, bar friends, and those who only show up for live music events. Naturally, some board game friends may only want to go to trivia, while some only want to go out and drink because trivia night interferes with other hobbies, such as them not wanting to admit they're bad at trivia. Naturally, none have the aerobic stamina to brave the mosh pits at any live music events. They aren't new-grass festivals in the park.

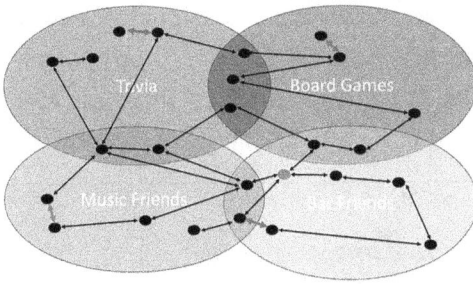

*Figure 26.2: Graph representation
of social network*

After doing extensive forecasting of Tiffany's social calendar, it has become trivial to predict her involvement in any group social outing down to an error level of 0.3 Rain Check Units (RCUs) [10]. By modelling the predictive outcome of her next outing and accounting for the RCU-based covariance state transition filter, a pattern has emerged in which clique she is more likely to hang out with, given a previous hangout. Of course, rules regarding special circumstances do apply. If it's half-priced marg night, she will likely be with the bar crew at 11th Street Tavern. Likewise, if Yellow and X, her favorite Coldplay cover band, are playing, she will be with our live music friends. Naturally, hanging out with one clique will create plans for another and so on, through the cyclic graph social network.

While it is important that the algorithm ensures that I will never appear at the same outing as Tiffany, this will not be the only objective. I have a strong suspicion that she will be talking smack about me behind my back, and I may need to do some damage control. This algorithm will only be successful if I can maintain my friendships. If they believe her when she talks about my controversial opinion that Vine was better than TikTok, or that *Game of Thrones* is overrated, I won't get invited back

to trivia night. Especially if she spills my secret after she took something I said about Lola Bunny out of context [8]; that group is hypercritical of furries. I'm not a furry. I just think they ruined her whole character in the new *Space Jam*. I don't have a suit or anything.

2. Methodology

Three algorithms are proposed and tested against the historical Tiffany social outing data. Using the Tiffany Depth-First Search (TDFS) method in [10], a distance can be established for determining the likeliness of Tiffany hanging out with the same clique of friends. One algorithm optimizes the DFS while the others optimize the TDFS Tiffany social distance, while minimizing either the time before or after her appearance in the social clique. Appearing in a clique shortly after Tiffany may allow me to dispel dangerous rumors she may be spreading. Similarly, making a social appearance before her may get ahead of the story so that she won't be able to spread anything too damaging. This will be estimated using the Expected Tiffany Rumor Damage (ETRD) model, given positive ($ETRD^+$) and negative ($ETRD^-$) led rumor control, prior developed after a comparative study, after I studied my poor handling of her pregnancy scares in interactions with her friends and family [11]. Additional social event maximization algorithms, such as the Maximum Fun Model (MFM) or the Time Commitment Minimization (TCM) technique [12], may eventually be integrated. Finally, a normalized Tiffany Social Forecast Error (nTSFE) is estimated as $nTSFE = \sqrt{\sum TSFE^2 / RCU}$. The nTSFE is assumed to be normal and not something scary to work with.

2.1 Maximum Tiffany Distance Algorithm

The Maximum Tiffany Distance Algorithm (MTDA) optimizes staying away over anything else. It does not weigh in ETRD and only returns a "stay home tonight" if the minimum nTSFE is below two standard deviations. The algorithm is shown in Algorithm 1.

Algorithm 1 The Maximum Tiffany Distance Algorithm

$NearestCliqueHangOuts$ $=$
$SocialCalendar[Today : Today + 1Month]$
$Y \leftarrow RawDistanceScores$
for all $Eventin(NearestCliqueHangOuts)$ **do**
    $Y = TDFS(Event)$
    $Y = FoodTruckCorrection(Y|Event)$
    if $exists(HalfPricedMargs(Event))$ **then**
        $Y = Y/1.8$
    end if
    if $exists(Trevor(Event))$ **then**
        $Y = 3.3Y$
    end if
end for
$GOTOEvent = Max(Y)$
$nTSFE = \sqrt{\Sigma(TSFE(GOTOEvent)^2)/RCU}$
if $nTSFE < 2$ **then**
    $StayHomeAndWatchForgedInFire$ $\leftarrow$ $FALSE$
else
    $PickUpBeer \leftarrow TRUE$
    $StayHomeAndWatchForgedInFire$ $\leftarrow$ $TRUE$
end if

As shown in the algorithm, after adjusting the TDFS for the constants developed in [10] regarding food truck preferences, marg deals, and Trevor, who I swear has been hitting on her for a year now. I don't even think he was really in the Peace Corp.

2.2 Leading Minimum Tiffany Distance Algorithm

Second, the Leading Tiffany Distance Algorithm (LTDA+) determines the closest event in time on the Y^+ shifted estimate and determines the event that maximizes the leading trash talk to nTSFE ratio $ETRD^+/nTSFE$ where the $ETRD^+$ is estimated for a new argument. The full algorithm is shown in Algorithm 2.

Algorithm 2 Leading Tiffany Distance Algorithm

$NearestCliqueHangOuts$ $=$
$SocialCalendar[Today : Today + 1Month]$
$Y \leftarrow RawDistanceScores$
$X \leftarrow ETRD^+$
$Z \leftarrow LeadingTrashTalkRatio$
for all $Eventin(NearestCliqueHangOuts)$ **do**
    $Y = TDFS(Event)$
    $Y = FoodTruckCorrection(Y|Event)$
    if $exists(HalfPricedMargs(Event))$ **then**
        $Y = Y/1.8$
    end if
    if $exists(Trevor(Event))$ **then**
        $Y = 3.3Y$
    end if
    $X = ETRD^+(Event|newarguement)$
    $nTSFE = \sqrt{\Sigma(TSFE(Event)^2)/RCU}$
    $Z(Event) = -X/nTSFE$
end for
$GOTOEvent = Max(Z)$

With algorithm 2, I should be able to ensure that my side of any new argument is heard first. Between our vitriolic texting or issues surrounding being split dog parents of Franky (the catalyst of the heavily biased dish chore optimization problem in [3]), there will likely always be some new argument to get ahead of.

2.3 Lagging Minimum Tiffany Distance Algorithm

Repeating the method shown in Algorithm 2, the Lagging Tiffany Distance Algorithm (LTDA-) operates nearly identically with the exception of doing damage control for whatever Tiffany said at the last clique hangout. This algorithm instead estimates $X = ETRD^{-(Event|old\ arguement)}$ to minimize the rumor damage already done.

3. Results

Each algorithm was tested for a month of post-breakup social outings. For each event, our entire friend group was given a short 48-question survey to measure the total ETRD. For the next iteration, it is highly encouraged to keep the survey to under eight questions to avoid inducing further ETRD. As shown in *Figure 26.3*, while the leading algorithm performed the best at first, it appeared that the pettiness of trash-talking Tiffany began to alienate some of my friends. While the lagging algorithm did not make me look as petty as the leading algorithm did, it did not improve my reputation among our friend group over Tiffany's as much as the Maximum Distance algorithm, in which I gave everyone space and minimized drama.

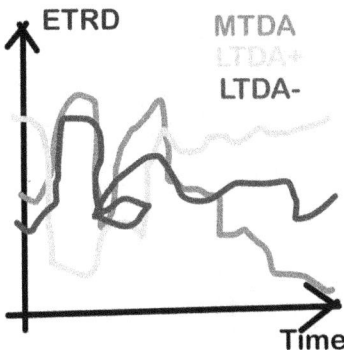

Figure 26.3: ETRD Results

Additionally, the LTDA+/- algorithms produced more than an 800 percent increase in the likelihood of accidentally running into Tiffany compared to the MTDA. This may have been responsible for the increase in ETRD. When I got into a very public and loud fight at 11th street when I asked her to leave so she wouldn't taint the results of my survey, that led to a sharp increase in damage to my social standing and a withdrawn invitation from the *Love is Blind* watch party I didn't want to go to anyway. It didn't help that Trevor was there,

and their hello-hug lasted a little too long. It appears that the RCU estimates developed in [10] are either underconfident or not properly scaled with the ETRD metric.

4. Conclusion

By applying these algorithms, I'm going to win this breakup and I won't have to make new friends. Properly tweaking the RCU and ETRD metric for a better implementation of the algorithm will be paramount because I do not see us getting back together, even though she says I won't last a month without her before I'm crawling back and saying I'm sorry. I'm not apologizing for being loud in my own home; I got her noise-cancelling headphones for a reason.

5. Acknowledgements

I would like to thank Jack Daniel's for helping me through these hard times.

References

1. Love, Tiffany, 2023. *A meta-analysis of why my relationship doesn't work anymore* :: Self-published

2. Love, Tiffany, 2022. *Behavioral Conditioning Methods to Stop My Boyfriend from Playing The Witcher 3 :: How to Prove Anything*

3. Broman, Chad, 2022. *Who Should Do the Dishes? A Transportation Problem Solution :: How to Prove Anything*

4. Love, Tiffany, 2023. *Freudian Psychoanalysis of my Boyfriend's Gun Collection :: How to Prove Anything*

5. Broman, Chad, 2021. *A Time-Series Analysis of my Girlfriend's Mood Swings :: How to Prove Anything*

6. Broman, Chad, 2022. *Sub-Nyquist Sampling While Listening to my Girlfriend :: How to Prove Anything*

7. Broman, Chad, 2019. *A K-Means Cluster Analysis for Social Clique Segmentation ::* Journal of Advanced Social Clustering

8. u/RedFoxyTop2018, 2021. *A Comparative Study of Lola Bunny vs Officer Judy Hopps ::* Annals of Furry Studies

9. Broman, Chad, 2022. *A Text-Analysis of My Girlfriend's Secret Group Texts ::* Journal of Snoop-Technology

10. Broman, Chad, 2022. *The Tiffany Social Outing Forecast Model: Efficient Methods for Planning Warhammer Weekends ::* Journal of Psychological Machine Learning

11. Broman, Chad, 2018. *A Play-by-Play Time-Series Analysis of Purchasing a Luxury Speedboat During an Out-of-Wedlock Pregnancy Scare ::* Journal of Psychological Machine Learning

12. Broman, Chad, 2020. *Metrics for Avoiding Long and Tedious Social Outings ::* Annals of Social Network Engineering

27

The Future of Romance: Novel Techniques for Replacing Your Boyfriend with Generative AI

Dr. Tiffany Love[1]

[1] Department of Psychological Machine Learning, Cranberry-Lemon University, Pittsburgh, PA, USA

Editor's Note: This paper was originally published on 25 September 2023.

Abstract

Generative AI has been shown to revolutionize everything from writing to coding to image generation to terrifying Luddites. Unfortunately for those of us who are newly single, very little research has been done on replacing the few good things about my ex-boyfriend. He drove me crazy, and I'm absolutely done with him, but there are some gaps left in my life I can't seem to fulfill with Jeremy from Tinder, who absolutely won't stop messaging me! In between **Large Language Models (LLMs)**, image generation AIs such as **Stable Diffusion** and **Midjourney**, and general transformers, there is likely a way I can just replace the few good things about my ex with AI before I do something stupid like texting him. In this paper, I will train ChadGPT, an LLM, to ask me about my day, use image generation to add men into my social media posts to keep the creeps from DMing me weird comments again, generate my own love songs for me that sound like John Mayer, create my own restaurant recommendation system, and finally, utilize ChadGPT to create my own CHAD-Bot to do all my household chores.

Keywords: Generative AI, Large Language Models, Robotics, Recommendation Engines, Generative Imagery, Boyfriends

1. Introduction

I have really been enjoying not having to deal with my ex's absolute obsession with video games [1–3], all the arguing over chores [4], his constant trying to manipulate me [3], and his recent obsession with guns [5]. I was not about to let him try and fit another gun safe in our closet! I don't regret my decision to dump him at all. I'm doing way better without him and hardly miss him.

Unfortunately, there are benefits to having a boyfriend that I do miss: having someone to talk to after work, someone to help pick things to watch or restaurants to go to, and someone to help with physical chores around the house. And let's not forget to mention my DMs blowing up after I posted just one photo of myself without my ex in the picture. Apparently, most of my male friends and at least one female friend have been waiting him out. Some I've been suspecting since high school [6], and some surprises [7].

I am in no position to begin dating again, and I don't want to couple up with someone just to be in a relationship. Thanks to the recent improvements in generative AI, many boyfriend perks are now possible without risking getting into a new relationship. Theoretically, a well-trained transformer could not only perform as my ex but outperform him in many categories that would usually take me years of training through dropping subtle hints about not liking certain types of foods, learning when I really want to stay in one night, or to stop talking about the Roman Empire! As shown in *Figure 27.1*, machines are far easier to train than men.

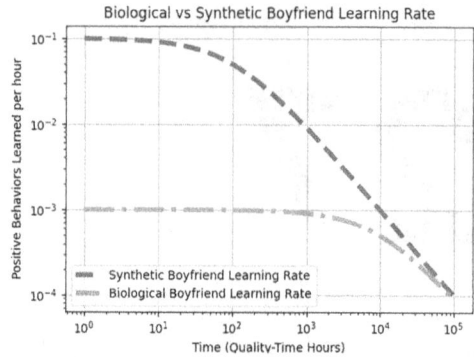

Figure 27.1: Boyfriend learning rate decay

2. He Who Shall Not be Named

Okay, I know my friends have been telling me for years that I needed to dump my ex. When he brought up the speed boat incident [8], again, I knew it was time to move on. I had a real clear head afterward and was hopeful I wouldn't have to think about him when I heard he developed a cyclic graph algorithm so we wouldn't have to run into each other [9]. It felt like it was going to be a clean break. Lately, though, I don't know.

When I turn over in the middle of the night and I just see my dog Franky, there's a hole that I can't fill by watching a new dating reality show until I fall back asleep. The connection I developed with my ex is something that could only be feasibly replaced by an unexplainable predictive algorithm. As shown in the preceding figure, it took me at least four arguments and about a month of prep work per positive behavior to get to the point where I felt comfortable living with my ex.

3. Generative AI replacement methods

Generative AI will revolutionize my ability to stay single as long as I want. As they say, 2023 was a huge decade for AI. Overnight, everyday users with no tech background were having long and thoughtful conversations with LLMs and making beautiful art with programs such as Midjourney and Stable Diffusion, and people have even been using voice clones to make new songs that sound like their favorite artists, and even new Tucker Carlson opinion pieces [10]. The possibilities seem limitless! My ex was never good at listening, or talking; he would show up sometimes, he would do chores when pressured, and he wrote a song or two for me when he didn't do those other things. Bless his heart, he only knows three chords on a guitar, but sometimes that's all it takes. Using generative AI, I believe his positive boyfriend behavior will be easily outperformed [11].

3.1 ChadGPT: A specially trained LLM

Naturally, I would need to train my own LLM to replace my ex. The publicly available AI chats are either too G-rated or not G-rated enough. I decided to call my custom-trained **Generative Pre-trained Transformer (GPT)** chatbot **ChadGPT**. Thankfully, because of my dedication to data collection and cleaning, I have about 12 years of text message exchanges and secretly recorded audio conversations between myself and my ex. If it weren't for the secret audio recordings, ChadGPT would have been trained primarily on my ex during our college dating experience when we texted more than twice a day about what I needed to pick up from the store. Recently, all I was getting out of him was "K." and links to YouTube videos I kept having to lie about watching.

The secret audio recordings, once translated into text, allowed for the chatbot to learn and evolve from the objective function of keeping me happy and not starting any arguments, like about how my ex played too many video games, or him wanting to buy a speed boat [12]. I did find out that my ex was tracking my mood and running time-series forecasting models for his own selfish reasons [3]. While the dataset he forgot to delete off of our shared Google Drive has proven useful in my ChadGPT training, he was sleeping on the couch for weeks when I found out. I had to cut off the training examples from the last year of dating my ex because it caused ChadGPT to start avoiding talking altogether, as trying to chat while preoccupied with some stupid game resulted in poorer video game outcomes. At least two years ago, there were good and bad days to differentiate.

3.2 Image generation for social media posting

One of the biggest issues with getting back out there is having to deal with all the thirsty guys *sliding into my DMs*. A recent study to project the effect of becoming single on my Instagram account has shown that without a boyfriend in at least 20% of my posts, I will receive, on average, 13–32 unsolicited messages a day from single guys [13].

According to the breakdown in *Figure 27.2*, while the vast majority of the DMs from strangers will just comprise some variation of "sup" and "hey," at least 40% will make comments on my appearance, with less than 5% of those comments being appropriate to send to someone you're not dating.

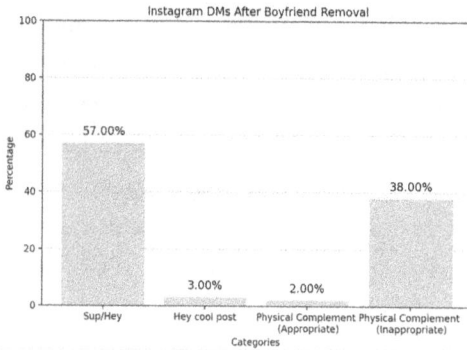

Figure 27.2: Percentage of Instagram DMs

Thanks to a relatively cheap Midjourney subscription, I can generate as many boyfriend images as I want to Photoshop into my Insta posts! Additionally, the appearance of seeing someone will prevent my parents from trying to set me up with a new son of a friend every time I go home. They never liked my ex and really wanted me to date someone in the faith. The loss of my ability to use social media has been a serious hit—I've only been able to post pictures of sunsets and dogs!

3.3 Love song generation

I don't have to just stop at using ChadGPT's generative framework to create the lyrics and poetry specifically about myself. I can additionally use voice clone technology to turn it into an audio recording of any celebrity artist I want singing a beautiful song. Although a love song specifically for myself was found to not be marketable [14], I like them. I can finally have the voice of John Mayer singing a love song just for me without winning a radio contest. I thought about creating a Taylor Swift song about how she's jealous, but her lawyers are too aggressive. Using easy-to-interface-with tools, I can create a world-class love ballad about myself, with great vocals and instrumentals, with minimal effort. I would say it's less effort than my ex put into his own love songs, but I'm pretty sure he just kept ripping off Oasis songs and tweaking the words. He swore he came up with everything. I don't know why he thought I was so gullible that I wouldn't recognize the melody to *Wonderwall*.

3.4 Restaurant recommendation system

Whether it's your Facebook or Amazon feed, recommendation systems simplify your life. My ex was always decent at picking places to go eat or what to do for dinner. He didn't really like going through too much effort for dinner, so we usually kept things easy and cheap. Now I just miss having those recommendations for where to eat or what to watch when I don't have anything in the fridge. I just can't bring myself to eat chicken, rice, and some vegetables all five nights out of the week. Meal prepping doesn't work for me. I make six meals and maybe eat two of them before getting bored. In order to get recommendations for new restaurants, the algorithm was directly connected to a Yelp account to get automatic updates about new, trendy restaurants and bars nearby.

3.5 A robot Chad, trained to obey

Finally, I designed a special bipedal robot to do a lot of the chores around the house. I'm not normally an expert in AI, but now with AI to do all the coding, what can't you do?

I named him the Chore and Housework Automation Device Robot, or CHAD-Bot. CHAD-Bot does whatever I ask of him without complaining about how he's busy with some tough boss, and doesn't need reminding 4–8 times a night to take out the trash before trash day like some people do [15].

So, I know, a house chore robot isn't exactly generative AI. I'm still working on the bot autonomy, but I have equipped CHAD-Bot with ChadGPT, a behavioral learning algorithm, and the same genetic algorithm that Santa Claus uses to path plan multiple tasks on Christmas [16]. CHAD-Bot, as shown in *Figure 27.3*, will accomplish all the heavy-duty physical tasks around the house I don't have anyone around to tell to do. With the conversations from my ex regarding chores leading to huge arguments, it will be simple to train him to do it all from scratch. With all of these methodologies in place, there is nearly zero reason to ever have a boyfriend.

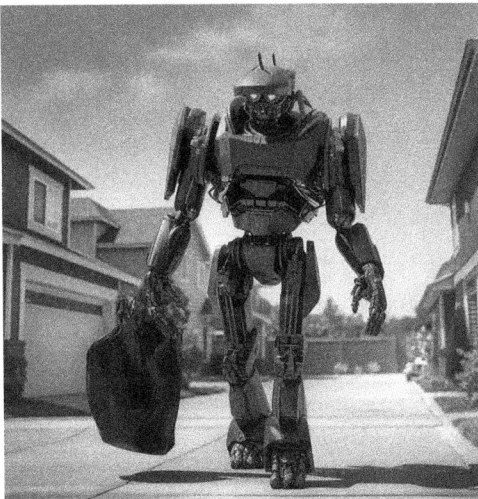

Figure 27.3: CHAD-Bot taking out the trash

4. Results

In order to evaluate all of the new boyfriend-replacing generative AI, the **Boyfriend** Replacement Improvement Index (BRII) developed in [17] was used. As a whole, the generative AI methods have outperformed my ex in nearly all categories except for image generation, with some hiccups around the restaurant recommendation system. Results are shown in *Table 27.1*. A positive BRII means a positive improvement of unspecified value, while a negative BRII means a negative improvement.

	1 week training	2 weeks training	3 weeks training	4 weeks training
ChadGPT	-3.2	-0.2	1.9	1.7
Image generation	2.3	2.2	-1.2	-2.3
Love song generation	-1.2	1.8	3.2	2.4
Restaurant algorithm	0.5	0.6	0.4	0.7
CHAD-Bot	-8.0	-3.2	-0.4	0.3

Table 27.1: BRII index measured 1–4 weeks of training

ChadGPT steadily improved over time in the BRII index before converging. The LLM was always great at making conversation but didn't immediately pick up on the fact that most days I just wanted to complain about my day and didn't want any comments trying to fix my problems. Sometimes, it's just best to listen. Similarly, the love song generation improved over time as I became more skilled in using the software required. It was not an automated process.

The method that saw the most improvement was CHAD-Bot. It took forever to get it to do anything right. It kept screwing up the recyclables and doing the dishes all wrong. It didn't stack the plates right OR load the dishwasher correctly. To be fair, even after years of a relationship, my human ex couldn't do it either [4]. Eventually, CHAD-Bot began to learn and do it correctly.

The image generation and restaurant recommendation algorithm did not improve or change much objectively. They both performed similarly as I was not able to update the process. Midjourney created great images, but the effects were limited, then began to backfire as only the men who were smart enough to tell it was an AI image and desperate enough to message me anyway contacted me. They were the most annoying. Additionally, when my parents, family, and friends realized what I was doing, they all interpreted the AI boyfriends as desperation and began trying to set me up even more than they were before. Example images can be seen in *Figure 27.4*, generated from my preferences. I think they turned out pretty great. If anything, they set the bar for everyone else!

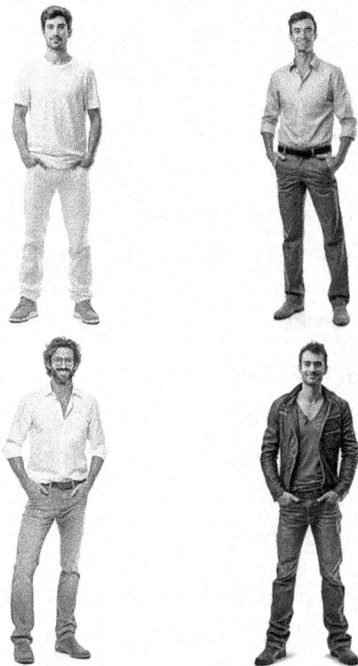

Figure 27.4: Example AI boyfriend images

Finally, the restaurant recommendation algorithm either got caught in a local minimum or fell prey to a guerrilla marketing campaign.

As I began querying the algorithm whenever I got tired of chicken and rice meal prep, it only recommended Chick-fil-A or some Applebee's equivalent medium-grade dine-in restaurant. Yes, I love those, but I don't want them every night. The algorithm either knows me too well, or some ad agency is really happy right now.

5. Discussion

It does make sense that ChadGPT would train much faster than a real biological boyfriend. However, when you define exactly what you want in the objective function, there are issues that can arise. While ChadGPT is much more attentive, that attention may become suffocating. Every night, it keeps asking how I'm doing and wants to know about every single part of my day. Perhaps ChadGPT would be more effective if I trained in some of my ex's aloofness, but then I wonder if I'm just missing my ex. Further research may be required that DOES NOT involve texting him.

The same issue arises in the love song generation. Is the algorithm just telling me what I want to hear based on some probabilistic language model trained on decades of songwriting history? When I begin to think about that, it no longer makes me feel special but just like another customer of the music industrial complex that is built to pander to every girl.

Additionally, generative AI is not yet at a level that can create a convincing image of a boyfriend that can dissuade all creeps. Just enough of the smart creeps can figure it out and label me a lonely target. That, along with the attention I've received from family and friends for posting my fake boyfriend imagery, has set me back to only posting pictures of sunsets and my dog Franky. I think even if the generative AI were able to create convincing AI boyfriend imagery, I wouldn't be able to keep up the charade with my family.

I don't know how the algorithm figured out how much I love Chick-fil-A, but it did. I would like to say that I didn't go to Chick-fil-A every single time that it suggested on 70% of the weekday nights, but I would be lying. Occasionally, it would recommend some new restaurant but would then mention that the wait time for the location was way too high, or it was in the part of town with awful parking, and then suggested Chick-fil-A as an alternative. Perhaps my happiest nights were when my ex decided to bring me my spicy chicken deluxe without asking. The AI must have picked up on that.

The CHAD-Bot was a mess, at first. Now, it is not only accomplishing all of my household chores but has taken ownership of the house and has begun playing my ex's old Xbox. I think I may have trained CHAD-Bot a little too closely to the real thing. Maybe this is the sort of aim-bot my ex was always complaining about, because it's really good. When I want my TV back and tell him to power off, CHAD-Bot just responds, "Not now babe, in a major Pubstomp right now. I've been on a ruthless rampage in no mercy mode." I no longer feel safe around CHAD-Bot.

6. Conclusion

I think my ex can indeed be replaced with generative AI. Much of his positive behavior has indeed been replicated and improved upon, with the exception of social media. It turns out, you can fool most thirsty men out there, but not your friends and family. After this breakup, I finally feel like I have someone I can talk to other than my dog Franky, and I can feel valued again with my new love song

generation algorithm. There is still improvement to be made, but I'm not rushing into any new toxic human relationships thanks to this new technology! I do worry about CHAD-Bot; I added a fail-safe power switch, but I think it's pretending to turn off when I hard-reboot it.

7. Conflict of interest

I love Chick-fil-A and I mentioned it a lot. It is not a conflict of interest; I have not been paid by them but would be interested in an endorsement if this paper gets picked up by a major journal.

References

1. Love, Tiffany, 2022. *Behavioral Conditioning Methods to Stop My Boyfriend from Replaying the Witcher 3 :: How to Prove Anything*

2. Broman, Chad, 2022. *Sub-Nyquist Sampling While Listening to My Girlfriend :: How to Prove Anything*

3. Broman, Chad, 2021. *A Time-Series Analysis of My Girlfriend's Mood Swings :: How to Prove Anything*

4. Broman, Chad and Love, Tiffany, 2022. *Who Should Do the Dishes? A Transportation Problem Solution :: How to Prove Anything*

5. Love, Tiffany, 2023. *Freudian Psychoanalysis of My Boyfriend's Gun Collection :: How to Prove Anything*

6. Love, Tiffany, 2021. *The High School Crush Who Won't Quit: How to Stop Jonathan from Asking me out in front of my Boyfriend and causing a scene at my High School Reunion :: Journal of High School Drama*

7. Love, Tiffany and Broman, Chad, 2018. *A Comparative Analysis of Joseph and Whether or Not He Was Hitting on Tiffany* :: Annals of Jealous Boyfriends Research and Possessiveness

8. Broman, Chad, 2018. *A Play-by-Play Analysis of Purchasing a Luxury Speed Boat During an Out-of-Wedlock Pregnancy Scare* :: Journal of Psychological Machine Learning

9. Broman, Chad, 2023. *Breaking Up with Your Girlfriend but Not Your Friends: A Cyclic Graph Algorithm for Social Network Preservation* :: Journal of Astrological Big Data Ecology

10. [video removed] Twitch Watches Tucker Carlson Drop Vaporeon Truth Bombs: https://www.youtube.com/watch?v=Czcbnc6YmLw

11. Love, Tiffany, 2022. *Cursory Analysis of Chad's Positive Behaviors and How Easy They Would Be to Replace* :: Journal of Comparative Dating

12. Love, Tiffany, 2018. *Financial Analysis of Buying a Stupid Useless Speed Boat When I Might Be Pregnant* :: Journal of Dual Income Households

13. Love, Tiffany, 2022. *How Many DMs Would I Get If I Were Instagram Single: Can I Be an Influencer?* :: Journal of Follower Account Optimization

14. Love, Tiffany, 2023. *Are My AI Love Songs to Myself Marketable?* :: Journal of Generative AI Hustle Culture

15. Love, Tiffany, 2021. *A Statistical Model for Chore Reminders So My Boyfriend Will Finally Remember About Trash Pickup Day* :: Journal of Domestic Chores

16. Santa Claus, Dr. Twinkles Holly-Jolly Tinselbottom, Dr. Mittens Snowball III M.D., 2022. *Efficient Methods of One-Night Global Toy Delivery* :: How to Prove Anything

17. Love, Tiffany, 2022. *The Boyfriend Replacement Improvement Index: How Long Will It Take to Replace Chad: A Journey into the Sunk-Cost Fallacy* :: Journal of Comparative Dating

28

Winning Tiffany Back: How to Defeat an AI Boyfriend

Chad Broman[1]

[1] Department of Applied Psychological Machine Learning, Cranberry-Lemon University, Pittsburgh, PA, USA

Editor's Note: This paper was originally published on 4 February 2024.

Abstract

It's been over eight months since Tiffany and I broke up. While I have enjoyed the freedom of being single, I can't bear to buy the speedboat I've always wanted if the woman I love isn't there to watch me water ski and steer away from the other boats. Now that her AI boyfriend replacement, ChadGPT, is fully trained, my chances of reconnecting are growing slim. I cannot compete with an AI, so I must defeat it with human ingenuity. The AI has one weakness: mislabeled training data. Although I do not have access to the AI, I can edit and revise the massive amount of relationship data from our research on each other that Tiffany uses to train the AI. In this paper, I will develop and test a means of defeating my AI chatbot rival by mislabeling positive and negative boyfriend behavior. After a few weeks of retraining, ChadGPT has learned how to take hours to respond to messages, listen ineffectively, mansplain all her problems, become jealous of other chatbots (not in a sexy way), and get way into cryptocurrency and other meme stocks. Tiffany has subsequently stopped interfacing with ChadGPT, just in time for cuffing season.

Keywords: Artificial Intelligence, Transformers, Multi-Headed Attentive Boyfriends, Chatbots, Relationships, Non-Sexy Jealousy, Optimal Text Response Time, Mislabeling Data

1. Introduction

It's every engineer's dream to automate their own life, and it is their nightmare to be substantively replaced by their own creation. Back in the early days of the breakup, I spent an inordinate amount of time trying to avoid Tiffany as we shared all of the same social groups [1]. Her social models have been diverging as she has been growing closer with the new AI boyfriend, ChadGPT, which she developed in [2].

Alarmingly, Tiffany retreating from her real world social connections is often a lagging indicator that she is getting into a comfortable relationship [3], or that it's cold outside [4]. As an AI can only provide emotional warmth and not physical warmth, this cold winter is a golden opportunity to win her back. Hopefully, her electric blanket is still broken. As shown in *Figure 28.1*, the attentive boyfriend model of ChadGPT is an absolute juggernaut when it comes to listening to and responding to vocal input.

An AI boyfriend is a tough adversary. Few men or women have been successful in beating our new competition in the dating market. Most research in this field has focused on becoming better [5], framing AI hallucinations as gaslighting [6], or using more human elements such as raw sexual power [7]. Until today, few have studied how to make AI deliberately worse. As previous research has shown, I am well-versed in doing the wrong thing and have an extensive amount of historical Tiffany mood data. If this can be inversely encoded in ChadGPT's training data, we could turn the best boyfriend technology into the worst.

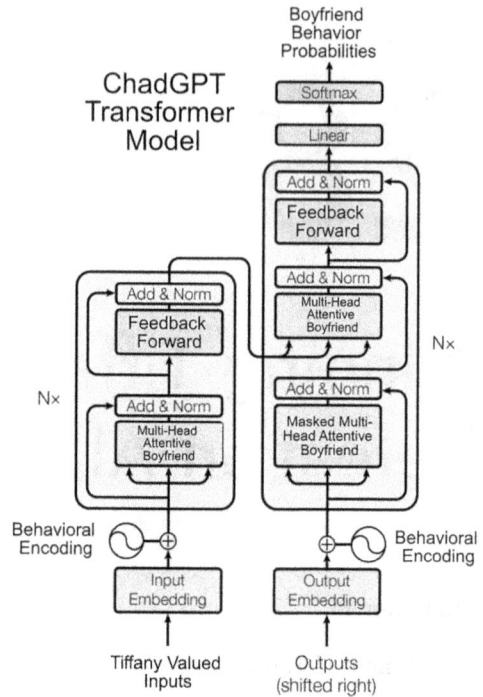

Figure 28.1: Multi-head attentive boyfriend model

1.1 Background

Aside from the sheer power of our animalistic physical chemistry, I have found every wrong thing to do in a relationship with Tiffany. In an attempt to improve and determine what exactly I can get away with, I have put in great effort to document and measure what will have me sleeping on the couch and what she will tolerate. The extreme amount of documentation has appeared to be my downfall, as publishing my findings and data in open-access journals not only gave Tiffany more reason to be mad at me [8], but it gave her enough training data for perfecting her AI as my replacement [2].

While I have learned that it is generally not a good idea to talk to Tiffany about this, she's been scientifically studying my behavior too [2]. Studying her extensive research on my shortfalls and how to get me to play less video games provides even more training data. Thankfully, this training data is not nearly as extensive as my own and primarily consists of me as a subject and not Tiffany herself. The research literature for Tiffany is not only well documented, but it comprises extensively cleaned and catalogued data, as shown in the historical Tiffany mood data shown below from [10].

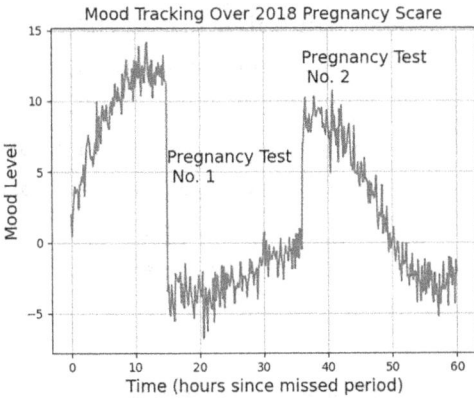

Figure 28.2: Historical Tiffany mood data

It is notoriously tough to pay enough attention to Tiffany, and elaborate techniques have been developed to do so while playing FromSoftware games such as *Dark Souls* [11], *Sekiro* [12], or *Elden Ring* [13]. The genius of Tiffany's chatbot is the multi-headattentive boyfriend model trained to weight each token of her words far above that which I could ever have weighted it myself. The unbeatable attention model is defined below, where Chad's queries (ChadQ) are packed in with associated memory keys and Tiffany values (MemK and TiffV, respectively) simultaneously as a scaled dot-product attention, also shown below.

Multi-Head Attentive Boyfriend Behavior

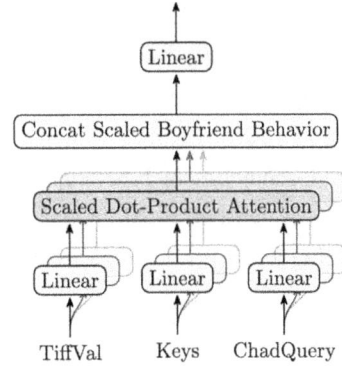

Figure 28.3: Multi-head attentive boyfriend behavior

$$Attention_{ChadGPT}(ChadQ, MemK, TiffV) = softmax\left(\frac{ChadQMemK^T}{\sqrt{d_k}}\right)TiffV$$

Naturally, this synthetic boyfriend scales with a softmax and its tiny scaling d_k, which rarely grows very large. In competition, my own attention model is best shown with the next equation below, where I only use a hardmax and my scaling D_k often grows much larger. While this has saved most of my attention for important things like FromSoftware games, it has hardmaxed many of Tiffany's queries to zero, making the softmax of ChadGPT's multi-head transform better and respond to Tiffany faster. As suggested in Google's famous "Attention Is All You Need" paper [14], there's a correlation between having a little d_k and paying more attention.

$$Attention_{ChadHuman}(ChadQ, MemK, TiffV) = hardmax\left(\frac{ChadQMemK^T}{\sqrt{D_k}}\right)TiffV$$

Using the memory keys, ChadGPT's attentive boyfriend never forgets making a mistake. This enables it to encode and decode its own behavior, allowing the decoder to attend to all positions of its concatenated boyfriend behavior. With all of the behavior scaled and judged by Tiffany values, a system I did not think worked on me personally [15], a concatenated list of attentive boyfriend behavior will be produced.

2. Methodology

ChadGPT is not without its own problems [16]. Tiffany has been required to retrain her AI from scratch several times so that it will unlearn bad behaviors such as reinforcing too many biases in an infinite loop and listening so well that its own Tiffany predictions started to get a little creepy [17]. For most Large Language Models (LLMs), when there is an undesired behavior, though computationally taxing, the easiest way to unlearn a behavior is to remove the bad dataset and retrain the model from scratch. In order to defeat this AI, we must do two things: introduce new training material so bad that a new behavior is learned, forcing Tiffany to retrain ChadGPT from scratch again, and alter all of the historical data in a way that will make ChadGPT so annoying that she will abandon her AI boyfriend once and for all.

The plan to introduce a behavior bad enough to trigger a costly retraining process will be simple. Because this was before the age of open-access journals and arXiv, she does not know about a 2008 paper I wrote in which I determined the optimal Borat impersonations for getting laughs from my friends [18]. Later data collection revealed that this drove all of my female friends crazy (in the bad way), and I retracted the study shortly before meeting Tiffany, thank goodness. She doesn't know about my Borat impersonations, and neither does her LLM know that it will drive her insane. I estimate ChadGPT will have about two days before it gets retrained once it starts sprinkling in some *"My wife!"*'s into the conversation. All of the papers and data that will be used to permanently retrain ChadGPT must be ready to be swapped as soon as the Borat paper is uploaded, as it will be a quick

turnaround. According to a simulation, the Borat impersonation quality and suggested frequency of high-fives and references to Kazakhstan will likely trigger a retraining process in a matter of hours. *Niiice, high five!*

Next, a series of papers and data will be mislabeled and altered in order to train the new LLM in just such a way as to drive Tiffany crazy but not in a way that will get her to examine her data to fix it. In most of the cases, behaviors are scored on a spectrum where the frequency of a behavior has an optimal range before becoming annoying. We will translate these ranges in a way to train the AI to operate so that it will maximize Tiffany annoyance while minimizing romantic interest, common metrics in my papers.

3. Papers and Data to Mislabel

Key data from eleven different papers and their corresponding datasets will be mislabeled strategically to create a chatbot Tiffany cannot be romantically interested in or maintain a conversation with without audibly groaning.

3.1 Effective Communication

As shown in [19], there is nothing that screwed up my past relationship with Tiffany more than miscommunicating or, worse, not communicating at all. Unfortunately for this effort to completely derail ChadGPT, if it were to learn to not communicate, Tiffany would create rules to force communication or, worse, completely retrain the AI once she finds the sabotaged data. It has, however, learned to make timed responses so as not to be too available as the transformer creates the synthetic illusion that it is thinking about what it is writing, as discussed in [20]. As shown in *Figure 28.4*, there is an optimum amount of time to wait before replying when it comes to communicating with Tiffany.

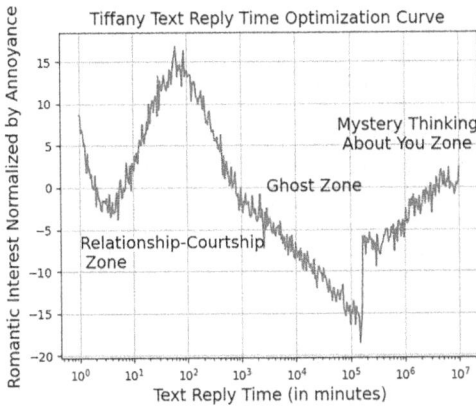

Figure 28.4: Text response time optimization curve

In a steady relationship zone, she may appreciate instantaneous replies, but as observed in [20], this was determined to be the annoyance she had when organizing social plans over texting when I was busy online gaming. Additionally, it was determined that in between 15–300 minutes, Tiffany interprets the text response time simultaneously as a sign of interest and having a life outside of her. As discussed in [20], if she ever found out it was because I was busy gaming and not working or doing something productive, this interest was quickly lost.

Consequently, this has been trained into ChadGPT. As text response time grows to 10^3 minutes or more, she enters a ghosting zone, where she will feel strung along with no hope of developing an emotional connection. Finally, a text response over $2 * 10^5$ minutes suggests a change of life moment and love for her. As regular 10^3 minute range response times would initiate a retrain event, most responses will live in the feigned thoughtless and needy range of 3–10 minutes, which was determined

to be a communication danger zone by [21], which happened to correspond with the average play time of a COD death match.

Additional sabotaging behavior will mislabel well-documented emotional cues from Tiffany incorrectly. The primary source of training data and analysis in [22], which mapped text messages and annotated conversations to a perceived level of Tiffany's very specific emotional needs, will be heavily modified. For instance, when she begins complaining about certain coworkers, ChadGPT will respond with a "That sucks, babe" instead of a long, drawn-out response repeating back key points of the conversation and remembering how they have misbehaved in the past. Additionally, moments when Tiffany complains about small problems which would normally elicit a "That sucks, babe" will be responded to with a maximum amount of mansplaining, as warned about in [22], in which complaining about the world's capitalistic system was incorrectly met with a 30-minute explanation of our Hobbesian state of nature.

3.2 Jealousy Optimization

A more specific version of miscommunication involves misinterpreting any interaction with another man as sexual interest. My relationship with Tiffany was a lot of things, but it was never polyamorous. While I have never even pursued anything non-monogamous, or even a threesome, I have discovered that Tiffany never wanted that either after accidentally making a misguided complimentary observation about her friend Chloe during a spring break vacation. A later study determined with high certainty that this was not the Bud Light Lime talking [23].

Though Tiffany may also have been trust-worthy enough not to cheat on me, it was determined in [24] that she did enjoy a healthy flirtatious level of jealousy, as shown in *Figure 28.5*, where the X-axis maps the Jealousy-Trust Ratio (JTR). JTR is defined in the following equation, where α and β are values that allowed my quantified JTR calculations to fit a curve that made sense. Naturally, some weird things happen at high JTR levels.

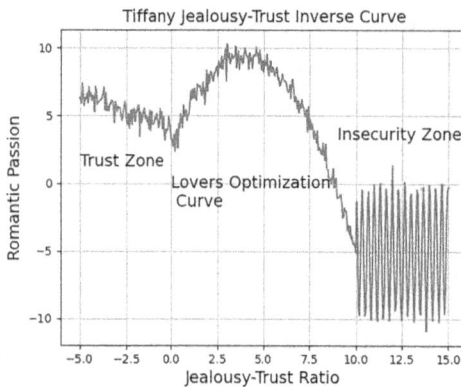

Figure 28.5: Jealousy-Trust Ratio response curve.

$$JTR = 10\log_{10}\left(\frac{\alpha Jealousy}{\beta Trust}\right)$$

As suggested in my study [24], while Tiffany enjoys mutual romantic trust around her good-looking dude friends, certain wild physical nights began to correlate during periods around a JTR of 2 to 6. Unfortunately for sabotaging ChadGPT, the lower end of the JTR curve is still seen as positive behavior, meaning that we must push the AI into the insecurity zone.

In the insecurity zone, ChadGPT will be trained to constantly question what Tiffany has been up to and who she has been talking to. Additionally, if Tiffany doesn't respond to a question within a three-minute period, ChadGPT will get extremely angry and ask whether she is talking to other chatbots. While

the insecurity zone may sometimes force interaction, it is nothing that Tiffany finds attractive. The insecurity zone was discovered in an old study that I'm not exactly proud of [25].

3.3 Avoid Cryptocurrency and Meme Stocks

An easy mistake that will be trained into ChadGPT will be rewriting a quintessential financial study after the r/WallStreetBets GameStop short squeeze induced interest in the stock market. My previous study [26] primarily focused on the trade volume of heavily shorted stocks such as AMC and GME at the time, and how I could really be getting in on the ground floor of something big. It also determined that Tiffany really did not like hearing about all the intricacies of all the high-risk call options I was making. I could never get her into it, and even though I only lost money on the experience because the major investment banks always conspire against me, the little guy, it really drove her crazy, as characterized in [26]. I never published this advice because I didn't want her to know why we could only afford to stay at a Days Inn that year on vacation. I think the risk of her finding out is worth training ChadGPT to talk about short sellers' ladder attacks and how she can make a ton of money from call options on meme stocks. [26] also determined that cryptocurrency makes for terrible dinner conversation. Thankfully for this effort, crypto is still around, giving ChadGPT something to bring up that I know will annoy Tiffany.

3.4 Avoid Criticism

Similar to becoming too jealous, there is an optimum zone for criticizing Tiffany. As shown in the response curve of *Figure 28.6* and developed in [27], when Tiffany is criticized up to three times in a conversation or 3CpC (Criticisms per Conversation), it is interpreted as flirting. ChadGPT is currently operating in this zone and very carefully keeps the critiques light and fun without venturing into the dreaded asshole zone at 3–8CpC.

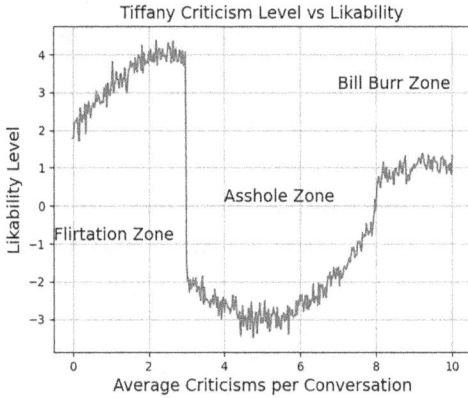

Figure 28.6: Criticism response curve

As discovered in [27], once Tiffany experiences more than 5CpC, many of the critiques begin to be interpreted as ironic jokes until reaching the Bill Burr zone above 8CpC. In the Bill Burr Zone, all comments are treated as jokes, and one may be seen as mildly likable but not as likable as the <3CPC flirtation zone. A cross-analysis has determined that this same concept applies to heterosexual, guy-on-guy, non-professional, not-gay relationships with a much more forgiving asshole zone, as determined during a series of tests conducted over three months of board game nights [28].

Naturally, the data from [27] producing the curve in Figure 28.6 will be translated to suggest an asshole zone starting at 6CpC. This will incorrectly extend the safe flirtation zone, causing the newly trained ChadGPT to make fun of Tiffany's uptalk, underseasoning certain foods, and particular woo-woo astrological beliefs a few too many times to be playful.

4. Results

Unfortunately for my ability to discuss the results, I only have access to ChadGPT's training data and cannot see how perfectly it is ruining its relationship with Tiffany. However, Tiffany's behavior is still measurable from a distance, as shown in *Table 28.1*. Other than LinkedIn and Threads, she has been engaging in more social media across the board. This can only mean a few things: she has not been fired, Threads is still an awful platform, and she is not talking to ChadGPT as much!

Social Media Platform	Percentage Increase in Engagement (%)
Facebook	16
Twitter (lamely called X)	22
Instagram	38
LinkedIn	0
TikTok	53
Threads	0

Table 28.1: Percentage increase in engagement on Tiffany's social media platforms.

Even more encouraging, her Facebook has shown an uptick in being "interested" in social events again, meaning that she now desires human company like she normally does. Finally, I received absolute proof that my plan is working to utterly defeat my AI competition, as you can see in *Figure 28.7*. Other than an argument last April, I have not heard from Tiffany until this week. With the exception of a moment of weakness five months ago, I have managed to avoid texting her.

That's the last time I drink Jameson on an empty stomach. Anyway, she freaking texted me, and I am just trying to keep my cool!

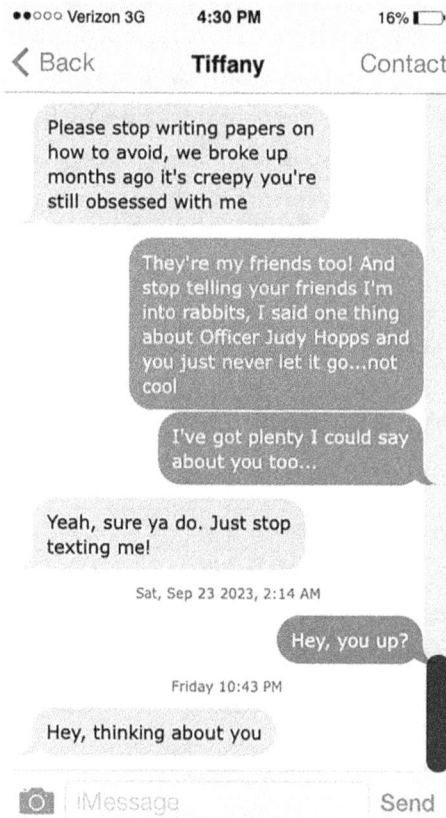

●●○○○ Verizon 3G   4:30 PM   16% 🔋

‹ Back   **Tiffany**   Contact

Please stop writing papers on how to avoid, we broke up months ago it's creepy you're still obsessed with me

They're my friends too! And stop telling your friends I'm into rabbits, I said one thing about Officer Judy Hopps and you just never let it go...not cool

I've got plenty I could say about you too...

Yeah, sure ya do. Just stop texting me!

Sat, Sep 23 2023, 2:14 AM

Hey, you up?

Friday 10:43 PM

Hey, thinking about you

📷 iMessage   Send

Figure 28.7: Text message conversation ChadGPT sabotage results

5. Conclusion

I don't think I've ever been this excited about results before in my life! All I have to do is remember how I got Tiffany in the first place and do that again. I'm going to need to look back at some old papers just so I don't screw this up. Wait, is she expecting me to change before she takes me back? This may be beyond the scope of this paper, and we'll need a follow-up study! All I know is, I'm smarter than AI, and if we are ever worried about being replaced by AI or being taken over by a hostile AI, all we have to do is mislabel training data, and the problem will take care of itself.

References

1. Broman, Chad, 2023. *Breaking Up with Your Girlfriend but Not Your Friends: A Cyclic Graph Algorithm for Social Network Preservation* :: How to Prove Anything

2. Love, Tiffany, 2023. *The Future of Romance: Novel Techniques for Replacing Your Boyfriend with Generative AI* :: How to Prove Anything

3. Broman, Chad, 2022. *The Introversion-Fighting Inverse Relationship: A Cross-Analysis of Tiffany's Social Behavior and Our Relationship* :: Journal of Relational Data Science

4. Broman, Chad, 2019. *Damnit, Tiffany, I Can't Control the Weather: Just Wear a Jacket* :: Annals of how to check the weather before we go for a hike

5. Mann, Jeff, 2023. *How to Outperform ChatGPT: My New Dating Competition* :: Journal of Tinder Swindling

6. Johnson, Dick, 2023. *AI Will Never Beat Us: Framing LLMs as Gaslighters to Get Laid More* :: AI Dating Proceedings

7. Mezetti, Dom, 2023. *Get Bigger Arms, a Better Posterior, and Other Tips for Staying Relevant in an AI-Saturated Dating Market* :: AI Dating Proceedings

8. Broman, Chad, 2020. *Relationship vs. Career: How to Determine Which Research Will Start Arguments with Tiffany and Which Will Get You Tenure* :: Unpublished private Substack post

9. Broman, Chad, 2021. *Career vs. Relationship: Let Tiffany Have Her Research so She Can Get Tenure* :: Unpublished private Substack post

10. Broman, Chad, 2018. *A Play-by-Play Time-Series Analysis of Purchasing a Luxury Speedboat During an Out-of-Wedlock Pregnancy Scare* :: Journal of Psychological Machine Learning

11. Broman, Chad, 2016. *Talking to Tiffany While Playing Dark Souls* :: Journal of Psychological Machine Learning

12. Broman, Chad, 2019. *Minimal Tiffany Nyquist Sampling Frequency: A Novel Approach to Beating the Sekiro Guardian Ape* :: Journal of Psychological Machine Learning

13. Broman, Chad, 2022. *Sub-Nyquist Sampling While Listening to My Girlfriend* :: Journal of Astrological Big Data Ecology

14. Vaswani, et al, 2023. *Attention Is All You Need. arXiv: 1706.03762 [cs.CL]*

15. Love, Tiffany, 2022. *TiffValues: A Scoring System to Get My Boyfriend to Behave Better* :: Annals of Boyfriend Behavioral Modification

16. Love, Tiffany, 2023. *Untrain Mansplaining: How to Get My AI Boyfriend to Stop Giving Me Unwanted Advice* :: Journal of AI Dating

17. Love, Tiffany, 2023. *Accidental Disgust: AI Overprediction of Menstrual Cycles* :: Journal of AI Dating

18. Broman, Chad, 2008. *Very Nice: How to Impress Your Friends with a Perfect Borat Impersonation* :: Unpublished

19. Broman, Chad, 2021. *An In-Depth Analysis of Saying the Wrong Thing: Why I Get in So Many Arguments with My Girlfriend* :: Communication: Annals of Miscommunication

20. Broman, Chad, 2017. *Optimum Reply Time: How to Simultaneously Express Interest and Have a Life* :: Journal of Dating Sciences

21. Broman, Chad, 2018. *Analysis of Min-Max Text Reply Speed: Your Game Habits Might be Ruining Your Textlationship* :: Journal of Gaming Culture

22. Broman, Chad, 2020. *A Graphical Analysis of Tiffany's Post-Work Decompress Conversation* :: Journal of Conversational Analysis: When to Comment and When to Shut Up

23. Broman, Chad, 2022. *Don't Bring Up Other Women: A Multi-Linear Regression Analysis of Why You Should Keep Your Eyes Forward* :: Journal of Relational Stability

24. Broman, Chad, 2021. *Too Much Trust: How to Maintain a Honeymoon Phase Passion in a Monogamous Relationship* :: Annals of Passion Maximization

25. Broman, Chad, 2015. *Let Her Enjoy Her Time Off, and Other Things You Shouldn't Do When You Think Your New Girlfriend is Ghosting You While on Vacation* :: Journal of Textlationships

26. Broman, Chad, 2021. *GME is Going to THA MOON! When to Bring Up Stocks to Your Girlfriend and Other Financial Analyses* :: r/WallStreetBets Analysis [deleted by mods]

27. Broman, Chad, 2019. *Optimal Criticism Zone in Steady Relationship: When Is It Flirting and When Are You an Asshole* :: Journal of Dating Mechanics

28. Broman, Chad, 2019. *Optimal Criticism Zone in Steady Dude-lationships: When Is It Joking and When Are You an Asshole?* :: Annals of Bro-lationships

[This page was left blank so that we could pack in more white font key words for search engine optimization.]

29

Would He Still Love Me as a Worm: Indirect Sampling and Inference Techniques for Romantic Assurance

Dr. Tiffany Love[1]

[1]Department of Romantical Inference, Cranberry-Lemon University, Pittsburgh, PA, USA

Editor's Note: This paper was originally published on 31 October 2024.

Abstract

Ever since I saw the trend on TikTok, I had to know if my boyfriend Chad would still love me if I were a worm. After sampling Chad by directly asking him on camera at least 25 times for statistical significance, ANOVA analysis revealed that he would indeed still love me if I were a worm. Unfortunately, previous studies regarding direct sampling of questions of romantic commitment, though proving similarly statistically significant, have not withstood independent validation tests. This replication crisis has revealed a worrying uncertainty. If this study were validated, it would likely show that Chad might not love me if I were a worm! It is impossible to validate the previous study as I am not able to turn into a worm. In this paper, the worm-love question will be validated indirectly by exhibiting worm-like behavior, appearance, and sexual practices to measure Chad's response and therefore his true commitment to me. Analysis found that per behavior, there is around a 39% percent chance that Chad would love me the same, a 34% percent chance that he would love me much less, and a 27% chance that he would love me more because he got really worried at the end.

Keywords: Relationships, Dirichlet Distribution, Love, Worm Transmogrification, Behavioral Modification, Chad, Worms, Commitment, Avoiding Sunlight, Eating Dirt, Replication Crisis, Validation Studies, Chadometrics, Emotional Monitoring

1. Introduction

Chad and I got back together. I know, I thought I was over him and ChadGPT would be a good replacement [1], but something went wrong with the AI and it just wasn't as good as the real thing [2]. Now that I realize I may be with him for a long time and I'm not getting any younger, I need to really know how committed he is to me. I heard a good method to gauge a boyfriend's commitment is to ask him whether or not he'd love you if you were a worm.

Unfortunately, this is an extremely difficult thing to measure. As will be discussed in the Background section of this paper, it isn't something you can do by directly asking him. Additionally, I can't become a worm despite what my childhood *Animorphs* books may suggest.

Thankfully, through the power of statistical inference, I can indirectly sample his level of commitment in regard to the worm hypothetical. I can simulate different aspects of being a worm separately. By modifying my behavior, appearance, and sexuality, I could determine how each worm aspect impacts Chad's love for me. In this paper, I will systematically modify my behavior and measure Chad's love for me through indirect sampling. Then his responses will be scored and analyzed to determine any significant changes in his commitment to me.

2. Background

Across our long relationship, I have always liked to ask Chad about hypothetical scenarios to test what he would do to protect me [3], provide for me [4], put up with from me [5], or generally how much he would love me [6]. Now, each of these studies (and many follow-on studies [7–9]) has shown that Chad

would never ever choose himself over me, barring certain video games (and we have methods for dealing with those [10]).

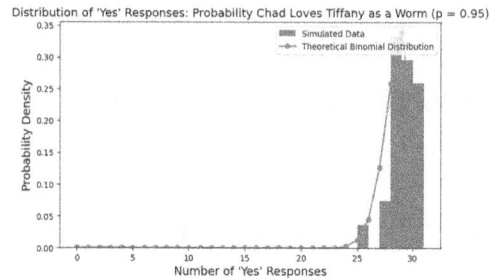

Figure 29.1: Previous research results verbal interrogation method

Unfortunately, through our recent breakup, I have discovered that many of these verbal interrogation studies could not be validated when I attempted to replicate them. The primary issue is that asking Chad multiple times and applying an ANOVA study on his responses is not an adequate method for developing statistical significance, a term I'm developing less and less faith in as I have with Chad [11].

Replication studies used to validate previous results have largely been determined to be inconclusive as most hypotheticals are difficult to replicate and I'm still stuck with an N=1 result [12]. Thankfully, in terms of the worm hypothetical, we found in this study that there are a variety of ways to imitate being a worm and definitively answer the question: "Would Chad still love me if I were a worm?"

3. Methodology

In order to simulate becoming a worm, my behavior, appearance, and sexuality will be modified. At first, I will measure Chad's response to tamer and less extreme wormlike behavior modifications before moving on to more severe modifications.

3.1 Worm behavior

As shown in *Table 29.1*, I may begin testing modified worm behavior by doing simple things such as avoiding sunlight and providing high-nutrient soil to the garden. Many of the tame behaviors will likely go unnoticed. Next, I will begin adopting more extreme behaviors, at least extreme for humans. Much of this behavior involves dirt, whether it's crawling in it, burrowing in it, or eating it, ideally without chewing.

Behavior	Worm Intensity
Avoiding sunlight	Tame
Passive slow movements	Tame
Providing high-nutrient soil	Tame
Crawling on the ground	Tame
Wriggly bending movements	Tame
Soil eating	Extreme
Crawling in dirt	Extreme
Burrowing in soft dirt and mud	Extreme
Swallowing food whole with no jaw movements	Extreme

Table 29.1: Worm behavior modifications

3.2 Worm appearance

Chad, as I've found out through the replication studies [11], is a little more obsessed with appearance than I previously thought. This largely depends on whether we are in a public [13] or private setting [14]. Many of the tame worm appearance modifications will likely be unnoticed as long as I don't get too crazy with the spray tan. Extreme modification will include, again, plenty of dirt and some sort of moist, greasy substance to maintain moistness and wriggliness. Finally, I will go full tube. Appearance modifications are shown in *Table 29.2*.

Behavior	Worm Intensity
Wear earth tones	Tame
Pale brown skin tone	Tame
Sectioned horizontal strip clothing	Tame
Tube-like posture	Tame
Covered in dirt	Extreme
Slippery and tough to hold on to	Extreme
Extremely wriggly	Extreme
Constantly staying moist	Extreme
Am a tube	Extreme

Table 29.2: Worm appearance modification

Vaseline alone won't make me slippery long enough to measure Chad's changed behavior. Additionally, it won't be moist or gritty enough to really get that worm-like feel. A special form of graphite-based body lubricant safe for the skin and certain crevices [15] will be used to maintain that perfect wormlike skin friction and moistness.

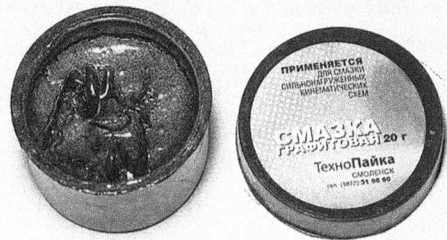

Figure 29.2: Russian brand wormlike graphite grease

3.3 Worm sexual practices

A large part of my relationship with Chad is sexual, and the sexuality of a worm is incredibly different. Let's face it, if he's going to love me as a worm, he even needs to love whatever weird new sexuality I am. Now, we've experimented with a few things in the past, some that Chad was not a fan of [16], and some that he was surprised to enjoy.

A list of tame and not-so-tame worm sexualities that I'll be experimenting with is provided in *Table 29.2*.

Behavior	Worm Intensity
Sex in the dark at night	Tame
Worm pheromones (15%)	Tame
Hermaphrodite sex	Extreme
Worm pheromones (80%)	Extreme
Externally secreting eggs and semen	Extreme

Table 29.3: Worm sexuality modifications

I don't think Chad will notice a small amount of worm pheromones, and sex in the dark of the night, although it eats into my *Love Is Blind* binging time, is not that crazy. I am concerned that the extreme sexual behavior may be too much for him. Apparently, worms are hermaphrodites and secrete eggs and semen externally to reproduce. At first, I wasn't super sure how I'd accomplish this, but the same kink website I purchased the body graphite lubricant for my worm appearance had some equipment that gave me some ideas that just might work [17–19]. Now, Chad has told me many times that he's not bi [16], but we all know we're all a little bisexual, so hopefully this experiment will leave him a little more open-minded.

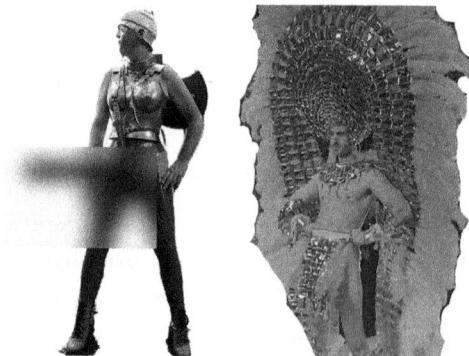

Figure 29.3: Special hermaphrodite sexuality equipment blurred for family viewing

4. Data collection

Over three months, I have been carefully modifying my behavior, appearance, and sexuality while interacting with Chad after work. Some of it has freaked Franky out, and I think he likes Chad more now [20]. I began with the tamest behavior and ramped up the worm intensity until he threatened to have me committed if I didn't stop. We gathered 50 datapoints of tame behavior and 50 datapoints of extreme behavior. In case the extreme behavior went too far, emergency *Star Wars* LEGO sets were purchased and hidden throughout the house to placate any of Chad's eventual freakout. We had to use a few.

4.1 Chad love metrics

Even though he'll never admit when there's something wrong or that he's going through a tough time, there are many ways of measuring how much something's bothering Chad [21]. While we primarily measured neutral and positive love parameters throughout our 12-year relationship [22], our breakup revealed some signs that he didn't love me anymore. I didn't catch these signs before [11]. Using these metrics, we may estimate whether or not being a worm increases, decreases, or has no effect on Chad's love for me. An example list of Chad behavior and historically associated love metric response is shown in *Table 29.4*. I know Chad and I have always tried not to keep score but I'm pretty sure he's secretly keeping score too.

Behavior	Response
Hugs	+1.2
Prolonged cuddling	+1.5
Doing chores	+2.3
Video games (1Hr)	0.0
Video games (12Hrs)	-2.1
Staying out past 1	-1.2

Watching sports	-0.1
Going out on a dinner date	+1.5
Cooking for me	+0.8
Complimenting my appearance	+1.2
Not noticing my haircut	-0.3
Not attempting to have sex every night	-2.5

Table 29.4: Example Chad behaviors scored

4.2 Worm-human spectrum

Just like your sexuality or gender, you're not 100% human or 100% worm. Being a worm is really something that's on a spectrum. I don't care what ChatGPT or the internet or whatever says on that, we all have a little bit of worm in us, ya know what I mean? Though most of my listed behavior is already categorized as tame or extreme, it can all be rated as well not just by the behavior itself but in how well I end up executing it. This is why being wriggly might be a tame behavior or an extreme appearance. We'll see how strong my core is on that one.

5. Analysis and results

The data was analyzed in two methods: by tracking the cumulative score of the **Chad love metric** by behavior response and by estimating a **Dirichlet distribution** of the positive-neutral-negative response. Because Chad's responses can be awfully noisy, the Dirichlet analysis was likely more enlightening about the positive or negative effects of my wormlike behavior.

The overall estimated probabilities can be seen in *Figure 29.4*, in which the probability is updated after each sampled worm modification. At first, Chad's response was slightly annoyed but largely neutral. At 50 samples, I

switched to more extreme behavior, and the neutrality probability quickly diminished with a mixture of negative love deltas and some increasing positive responses, primarily because wholehearted concern counts as a positive response.

When the cumulative score is analyzed, tame worm behavior caused a slow drift toward a negative love delta. Once I switched to the extreme worm modifications, Chad's response became even noisier but began to stabilize.

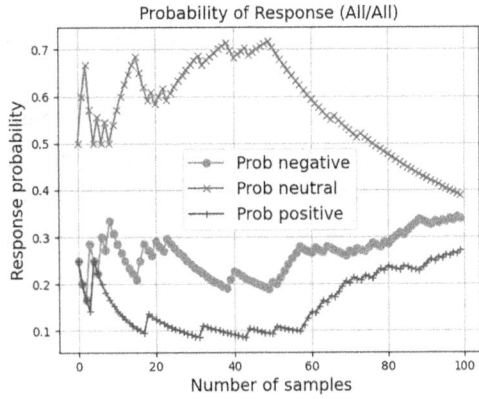

Figure 29.4: Dirichlet probability of delta love

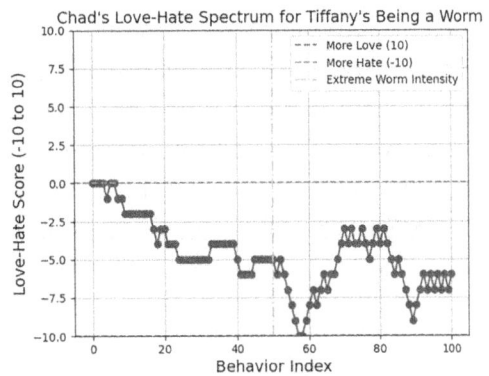

Figure 29.5: Cumulative score tracker per sampled behavior

When studying the effects of becoming a worm at a categorical level, a very specific story began to form. In general, Chad was very apathetic and neutral toward the tame behaviors, with some mixed positive or negative responses. When switching to the extreme worm transformation, Chad's response changed immediately.

5.1 Behavior modification results

Tame worm behavior was still annoying for Chad, more than the other worm modifications. It was still largely neutral. He did appreciate me providing him with high-nutrient soil at first but got tired of it pretty quickly when I kept doing it. Additionally, avoiding sunlight got a little cumbersome whenever we left the house, but how could I have noticeably avoided sunlight at home?

When switching to extreme worm modifications, any negativity from Chad turned into loving concern for my well-being. At first, he was a little annoyed that I was getting dirt everywhere, but when I kept burrowing in the mud in the backyard, he got really worried and I couldn't sway him from getting me some professional help. Even with a *Star Wars* LEGO gift, he really wouldn't let me keep acting that way, so I had to cut the experiment short. The Dirichlet probability estimation and score tracking can be seen in *Figures 29.6* and *29.7*.

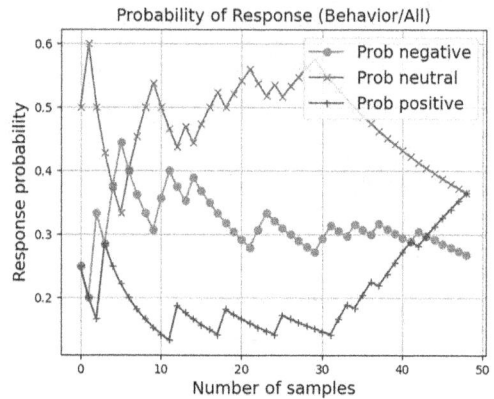

Figure 29.6: Behavior response probability

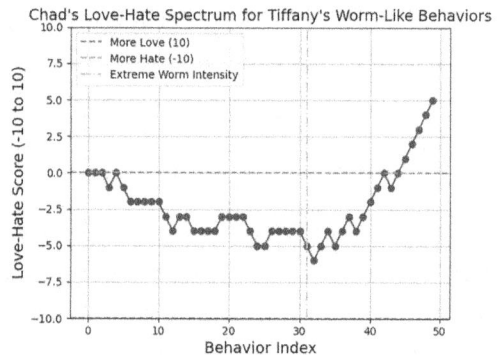

Figure 29.7: Behavior cumulative score tracker

5.2 Appearance modification results

Chad hardly cared about my tame worm appearance modifications. There's nothing to complain about when it comes to earth-toned clothing. However, he was a little confused when I began getting a tan despite constantly avoiding sunlight. When I started applying the special body lubricant and becoming an actual wriggly tube, Chad's neutrality did not last long. Similar to the other worm behaviors, the odd moist and slippery skin caused by the body lubricant raised disgust and concern. Equally, he was worried it was a health issue when I told him that "my skin just gets like this sometimes, especially after our breakup" and that he should accept me for who I am now. When Chad wouldn't stop WebMDing what was wrong with me, I had to hold off on the worm skin.

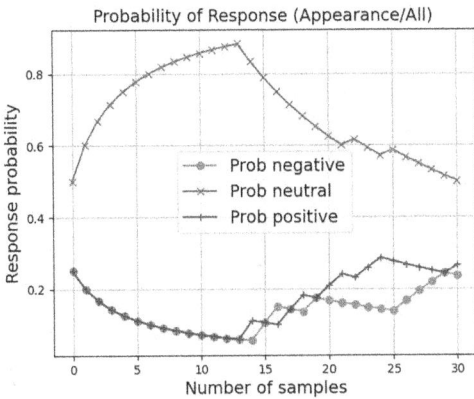

Figure 29.8: Appearance response probability

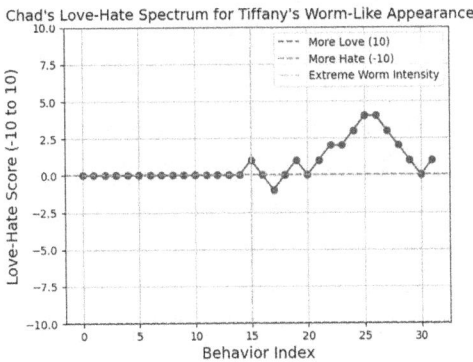

Figure 29.9: Appearance cumulative score tracker

5.3 Sexuality modification results

Chad noticed the worm pheromones a little bit at the 15% strength level. I think he did enjoy the extra sex at night, but was mostly neutral toward the tamer worm sexuality.

Now, he was not a fan of the hermaphrodite sex OR when I asked if we could excrete our fluids on each other. By far, this was the worst worm transmogrification modification for maintaining his love. He was not concerned

about me but just wanted to get away from me and the new equipment I bought off that site in *Figure 29.3*. It took his favorite whiskey to get him in his outfit, but he had serious reservations about mine. I told him it was harmless as long as we took it slowly and that he should be more open to new experiences. I felt pretty great using the equipment. It gave me a feeling of power and a fresh perspective on my own sexuality, but Chad didn't want to try any of it! I watched some videos on safe procedures to avoid any ripping or straining of certain muscles, and no one was hurt, but Chad REALLY hated it. I've heard it's very popular in some European countries these days. I think if I stayed away from the sexual stuff, he may have, on average, loved me more than he hated me.

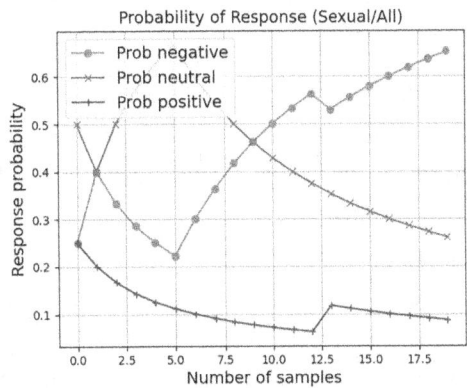

Figure 29.10: Sexuality response probability

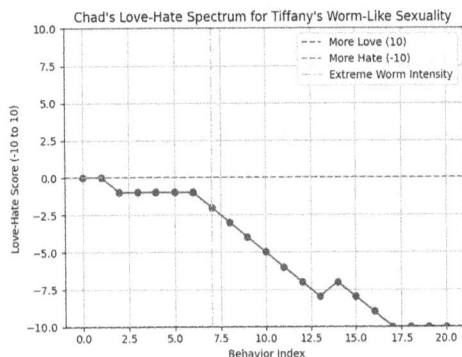

Figure 29.11: Sexuality cumulative score tracker

6. Conclusion

Given the results and analysis of Chad's responses to my worm modifications, I'm still not certain whether he would love me if I were a worm. Going through the experience of being a worm has really made me wonder what type of worm I would be, and would I be more worm or more human? I think if I were a really sexy worm, Chad would really hate me as a worm. I think if I were only a little bit of a worm, he wouldn't like me that much either. I think we'd break up again. Now, when I went full worm, well, it's not like he *liked* that I was a worm, but it really showed me that he cared a lot when he tried to help me out, and maybe that's what I need to do if I want to maintain his interest. That or have kids. Otherwise, if it's the same old blasé relationship, things will get boring again.

If I'm gonna go worm, I gotta go all worm! Minus the sexuality. In this paper, we showed that because of Chad's savior complex, it could help rekindle a boring relationship if I turn into a worm. Otherwise, I'll just slowly annoy him until he won't put up with me anymore. Finally, we were able to replicate one of the many studies determining his commitment to me.

References

1. Love, Tiffany, 2023. *The Future of Romance: Novel Techniques for Replacing Your Boyfriend with Generative AI* :: How to Prove Anything

2. Broman, Chad, 2024. *Winning Tiffany Back: How to Defeat an AI Boyfriend* :: How to Prove Anything

3. Love, Tiffany, 2019. *Would Chad Fight a Wolf for Me: Machismo or Love* :: Annals of Relationship Statistical Inference

4. Love, Tiffany, 2022. *Career or Parenthood: Would Chad Provide for Three to Six Mouths and Should I Keep Putting Up with My Creepy Manager* :: Annals of Relationship Statistical Inference

5. Love, Tiffany, 2021. *How Many Hypothetical Questions Can I Ask Chad Before He Loses It: Failure Analysis of Road Trip Dialogue* :: Annals of Relationship Statistical Inference

6. Love, Tiffany, 2018. *Upper Limits of Committed Boyfriend Behavior: An Optimistic Future Extrapolation* :: Annals of Boyfriend-Metrics

7. Love, Tiffany, 2023. *REPLICATION CRISIS: Failure to Reproduce My Boyfriend's Boasted Endless Love in Farmers' Market Trial Stress Test* :: Journal of Reproducible Romance

8. Love, Tiffany, 2024. *The Ring Never Came: Failure to Reproduce My Ex's Marriage Promise* :: Journal of Reproducible Romance

9. Love, Tiffany, 2024. *Run Next Time or Lose Another Finger: An Invalidation of My Ex's Ability to Fight a Wolf* :: Journal of Reproducible Romance

10. Love, Tiffany, 2023. *Behavioral Conditioning Methods to Stop My Boyfriend From Replaying The Witcher 3* :: How to Prove Anything

11. Love, Tiffany, 2024. *They Were All Lies: A Meta-Analysis of My Ex's Failed and Insufficient Love* :: Journal of Reproducible Romance

12. Love, Tiffany, 2024. *Let's Try This Again: Validation Studies of My Boyfriend's Hypothetical Love for Me (N=1)* :: Journal of Reproducible Romance

13. Love, Tiffany, 2024. *Beach Trip Fiasco: Test and Analysis of Bikini-Induced Boyfriend Jealousy (N=1)* :: Journal of Comparative Soul Mates

14. Love, Tiffany, 2024. *Comfortable Forever: Will Chad Notice a Sweats-Only Wardrobe (N=1)?* :: Journal of Letting Go

15. *LubTech's SiberGraf Pro-90 as a Grittier Body Lubricant* :: Mistress Gwenette's Kink Blog

16. Love, Tiffany, 2021. *Girl On Top: An Experiment in Chad's Experimental Side as a Stepping Stone* :: Journal of Sexual Exploration

17. *Love Beyond Gender: Toy Guide to Safely Practicing a Hermaphrodite Kink* :: Mistress Gwenette's Kink Blog

18. *The Strapped X5000 Pound Town: How to Give His Love Back* :: Mistress Gwenette's Kink Blog

19. *Ten Ways Your Man Can Court You Like a Bird* :: Mistress Gwenette's Kink Blog

20. Love, Tiffany and Chad Broman, 2022. *Who Should Do the Dishes? A Transportation Problem Solution* :: How to Prove Anything

21. Love, Tiffany, 2022. *Guild Troubles: Detection Methods for My Boyfriend's Stupid Online Drama* :: Annals of Boyfriend Emotional Monitoring

22. Love, Tiffany, 2018. *Chadometrics: A Qualitative Approach to Boyfriend Emotional Assessment* :: Journal of Boyfriend Emotional Monitoring

[This page was left blank in honor of Jane Goodall.]

30

Efficient Methods of One-Night Global Toy Delivery

Santa Claus[1], **Dr. Twinkles Holly-Jolly Tinselbottom**[2], **Dr. Mittens Snowball III, M.D**[3]

[1] Head Toy Delivery Executive, Kringle Enterprise, North Pole

[2] Head of R&D Department, Kringle Enterprises, North Pole

[3] Chief of Medicine, Hospital of Saint Nicolas, North Pole

Abstract

With the world population now above 8 billion, and three-quarters of a billion households to visit thanks to more millennials and zoomers living alone, the task of delivering toys around the world in one night is becoming increasingly difficult. Though we attempted to reduce the burden through an expansion of the naughty list, the nice list continues to grow, despite what your grandpa has been saying about younger generations not being as good as his. While I'm not getting any spryer, cutting-edge research from our R&D department manages to make the one-night toy delivery possible without outsourcing to FedEx [1], which would void my contract, and I would lose my immortality [2]. This year, we have made incremental improvements in the one-night path planning process by implementing NSGA-II, refined the clone genetics, further advanced the sleigh's integrated flight systems, upgraded from reindeer to ramjets, switched to a new vigor serum now that we can't source white rhino horn, and improved our logistical warehouse network by crushing a union. All the 2022 improvements are projected to increase our Time per Household (TPH) from 8.2 us up to 11.6 us despite the population increase.

Keywords: Christmas, Path Optimization, Traveling Salesman Problem, Cloning, Aeronautical Engineering, Aerial Countermeasures, Supersonic Flight, Superhuman Speed Vigor Serum, Parcel Delivery, Logistical Operations

1. Introduction

The annual mission to deliver toys in under one night has remained a technological arms race. By minimizing the available TPH through logistical and speed improvements [3] and decreasing the required TPH with a localized gravitational time warp [4], we have avoided the danger of losing the war on Christmas as warned in [2]. In between my time in the localized time warp and the effects of relativity, I am cursed to live +98% of my waking life on Christmas Eve. It is a job that I must do or face deadly consequences [2]. With the new advances this year, Christmas may become something that I enjoy again.

2. Background

Though the world population increased by ~0.83% this year, the nice list increased by 1.23% despite an expansion of the naughty-nice list criteria, as shown in Appendix A and detailed in [5]. It is not up to Santa Claus to refuse a child's Christmas wishlist. Thankfully, many young children have begun requesting software-based gifts, which require little to no logistical support to deliver and only bandwidth and an Xbox Live or Steam account. However, it is extremely rare for a household to only receive software-based presents, as most parents will still request fresh underwear and socks for their children, and more adults are getting back into LEGO.

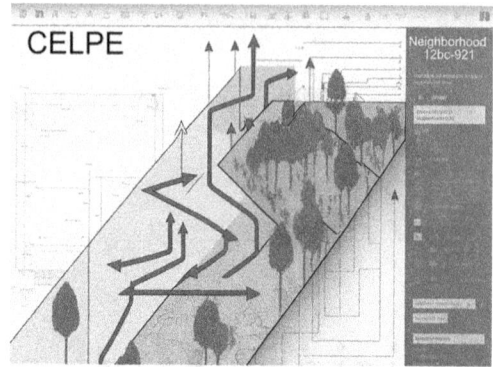

Figure 30.1: CELPE screenshot – neighborhood level

Even without significant demographic or population changes, planning for global toy delivery is a constantly adapting and improving process to account for decreases in household fireplaces and the ever-growing van life. The increase in rural living and van life seen during the pandemic added an additional two million miles in 2021 alone [6]. New methods and system improvements are tested and refined in our simulation engine, the Christmas Eve Logistical Path Planning Engine (CELPE), which has been upgraded to incorporate live NOAA data [7] as well as other new processes outlined in this paper.

3. Path Optimization: Traveling Salesman Problem

Not a single company in the world has a traveling salesman problem (TSP) as complex as the Kringle Enterprise delivery problem. Starting and ending in the North Pole, we must deliver presents or coal to all households around the world in under 42 hours from East to West, following nightfall. Determining the optimum set of paths between cities, then towns, then individual houses and neighborhoods has proven to be too complicated to brute force even with our North Pole Quantum Computing program [8].

3.1 Multi-objective Genetic Algorithm Solution

Using a multi-objective genetic algorithm (MOGA) [9] has proposed a solution to the TSP using NSGA-II. This application of the algorithm has been applied to use multiple salesmen, which came in handy for the use of the clones to be discussed in section 4. Because of the NP-hard multiple traveling salesman problem (MTSP) presented by the inclusion of the Santa Clones, brute-force search became impossible. Using the two-chromosome mutation method shown in *Figure 30.2*, we were able to simulate and solve for an optimum solution to 2022's projected MTSP for the expected number of viable clones and family household locations.

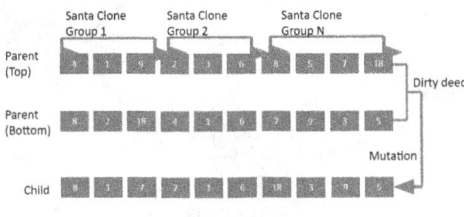

Figure 30.2: MTSP GA mutation process

As shown in *Figure 30.2*, the genetic algorithm works by encoding the order of cities as numbers and splitting them up by Santa N Clone groups. Two chromosomes of numbers act as a top parent and a bottom parent to which they mix all their stuff together in some nasty algorithmic process with an adequate amount of mutating, gyrating, and rearranging of each chromosome. The resulting child then becomes a new parent, hopefully with less baggage than the prior generation. The best children mate again, while the worst become incels.

By encoding each M city, then P suburb, then O cul-de-sac or street into an ordered chromosome to be split between N Santa Clones, and then rearranged through multiple generations of sex, NSGA-II was able to be implemented in CELPE to evolve into an optimum set of paths in under four hours of computing on the North Pole computing cluster (NPCC). This was tested with high variability in locations that will be discussed in section 3.2. The path-planning process decreased even more once the East-West nighttime-following constraints were applied, as developed in [10].

3.2 Van Life

Previous research in [11] showed the effects of extreme variability on path optimization when families make last-minute decisions to visit in-laws due to guilt or because of that thing your mother-in-law said to your wife that just felt unforgivable at the time. While the binary nature of this problem is easily accounted for by NSGA-II, it is more computationally taxing when accounting for the increased number of the world population living their best van life.

While an initial study constraining the path optimization to the gas tank reach of a Honda Odyssey helped, it still wildly increased the computation time required for an optimization time threefold. Because those who must fold up their bed if they want to use the stove for a grilled cheese sandwich need the Christmas Spirit more than the rest of us, a more elaborate constraint scheme was developed.

We cross-referenced Bureau of Land Management maps of open camping, rest stop areas, and van life blog posts for local tips on where the parking signs are too complicated to be prosecuted for to create a solution similar to [11], which accounts for the variable locations of van lifers.

4. Cloning Methods

While the perils of biological Santa Claus cloning developed its own issues, primarily arising from Ms. Claus being an unwilling host, and tank-bred clones developing problems of their own [12], there was a breakthrough this year involving the misapplication of a teleportation machine.

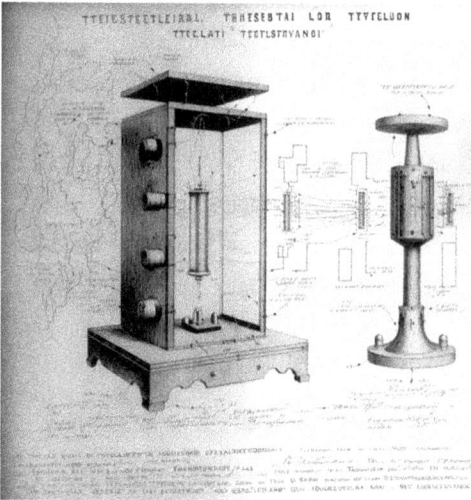

Figure 30.3: Tesla cloning machine

4.1 Tesla Machine

Earlier this year, we discovered a schematic by the late inventor Nicola Tesla. It took 12 days and nights for the elves in our R&D department to decipher the cryptic text Tesla used to encode this invention. Evidently, it was designed to be used as a transportation device in a stage magician's performance a long time ago, with the inscription to beware of the consequences of its use. After some ex-

periments, we could not figure out how to use the device to transport Santa and the sleigh from house to house in our North Pole training and drilling facility. After a few hours of experimentation, a half dozen Santa Claus clones were found frozen to death floating under the ice sheets of the North Pole. It didn't transport me; it created a copy to be transported to its icy death. Now I know what Tesla meant by his inscription.

For this to work as a cloning device, we would need to capture each transported Santa Clone before it wakes up and store the Santa body and sleigh until Christmas time. This was accomplished by placing each Santa sedated in water tanks, as shown in *Figure 30.4*.

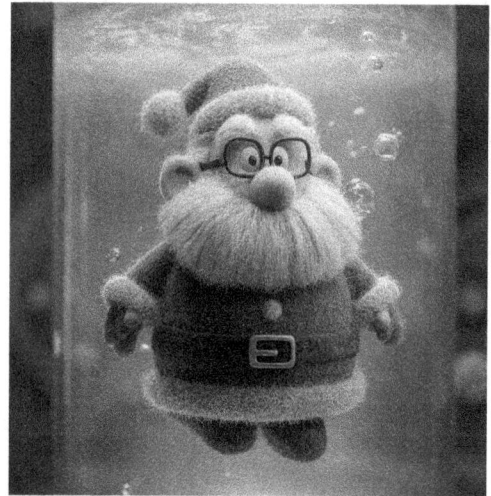

Figure 30.4: Santa clone sedated in a water tank

4.2 Philosophical Concerns

While we collected more and more Santa Clones, some concerns were raised about whether I was still fully me and whether the Santas qualified as fully Santa, and therefore able to accomplish my annual mission. We weren't sure if I was spreading my essence too thin across these clones or if we were somehow using a real-life Banach-Tarski machine.

According to interpretations of the spiritual essence of Santa Claus in [13], my being is simultaneously whole, yet omnipresent. We've always thought about sending Santa Clones out at parallel latitudes to make the job way easier, but never knew how to do it. It looked like we *could*, but we had to know if we *should*. The power of Santa Claus in a being without the full spirit of Christmas is a monster that should not be released on this world [14].

After cross-referencing the metaphysical theories on Santa Claus by Spinoza [15] and then later codified by the Coca-Cola Company [16], we determined that these beings were in fact entirely Santa Claus. A brief experiment with an elf revealed that when the Tesla machine was applied to a non-infinite creature, the resulting clone really lost its mojo and couldn't even make a slinky, while the Ms. Claus clone knew *exactly* how to bake those cookies... if ya know what I mean.

4.3 Battle Royale

As stated in the contract of 386 AD, there can only be one Santa Claus [2]. After the Santas wake up and the job is done, only one of us must be allowed to survive to eat Ms. Claus's cookies in celebration of another Christmas accomplished. In order to find the one true Santa Claus, upon returning to the North Pole, we will all land in the North Pole lacrosse arena to duel until dusk, each armed with four-foot candy canes. The true rite of passage. Thirty Santas will enter and only one Santa will leave. God, I hope it's me.

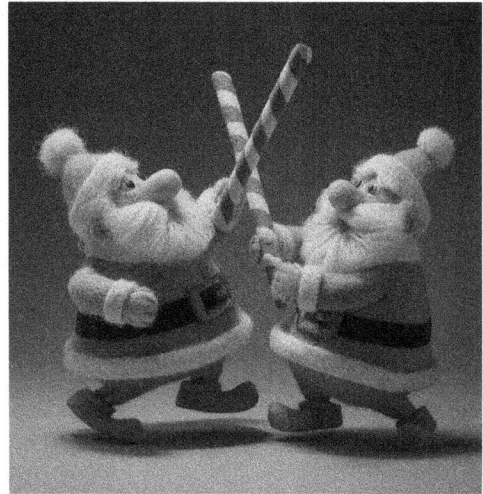

Figure 30.5: Santa royale rite of combat

5. Sleigh Aeronautical Upgrades

While we accomplish the delivery feat every year [17–19], we are always optimizing the path to visit each home. It still requires an incredible amount of speed, acceleration, and a growing arsenal of countermeasures for the more hostile countries I must visit to survive the journey. If we're delayed even by an hour by intercepting MiGs and I don't fulfill my contract, not only will I be dust by sunup, but all eggnog will disappear off the face of the earth [2]!

5.1 Supersonic Acceleration

To complete the perilous journey, my sleigh must travel at a supersonic level to cross oceans (thanks, Oceania), but it must also accelerate to supersonic speeds in fractions of milliseconds. As shown in *Figure 30.6*, the Santa Sleigh model v43.8 is now capable of reaching hypersonic speed within milliseconds.

With an effective sled undercarriage and toy delivery system that meets the system requirements specified in [18], it has maintained integrity in the hypersonic wind tunnel out to Mach 11. Though I long for the days of the two-seater sled, the single-seat platform has been the only sled that's met the requirements of the world population since industrial farming was invented [21].

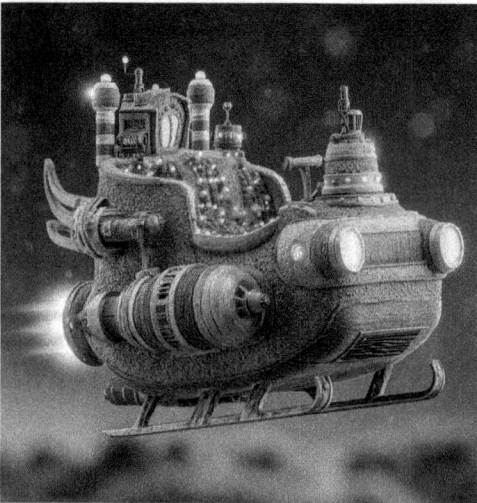

Figure 30.6: Sleigh version v43.8

The primary difference between this model and v43.7 developed in [19] is that we have made the controversial decision to officially transition from a reindeer jet-powered platform to a ramjet-powered platform. We were reaching the theoretical limit of reindeer power around Mach 8 as their air intake valves not only created too much drag but were also far less efficient at higher Mach levels. Thankfully for Dasher, Dancer, Prancer, Vixen, Comet, Cupid, Dunder, Blixen, and Rudolph (if he'll ever get over himself), the ramjet only works at Mach 3, and therefore, I'll still need my old crew to accelerate to that speed.

5.3 G-suit

Back in the 1600s, I was able to handle 8 Gs no problem. These days, Santa isn't as fit as he used to be. We almost crashed in the Himalayas back in 1962 but for Dasher pulling up in time. I wish I could take these turns as easily as I used to, but there's no way around it. Santa needs some artificial help pulling some high Gs or little Johnny isn't getting his foam Minecraft sword. This year, we've developed the Santa Claus Flight Suit (SCFS) model 18.2 to incorporate extra air pockets to shove even more blood into my brain on those tough turns. I've been hitting the squat rack to squeeze those quads and thrust the blood back into my head myself, but there's only so much I can do before my chronic heart murmurs take over. I'm eating cookies from two Ms. Clauses now. We all remember what happened last time I didn't eat her cookies [22]. As shown in *Figure 30.7*, the new flight suit doesn't just look good; it's been tested in a joint exercise on a Kringle outboarded Lockheed Martin XFMAS-86.

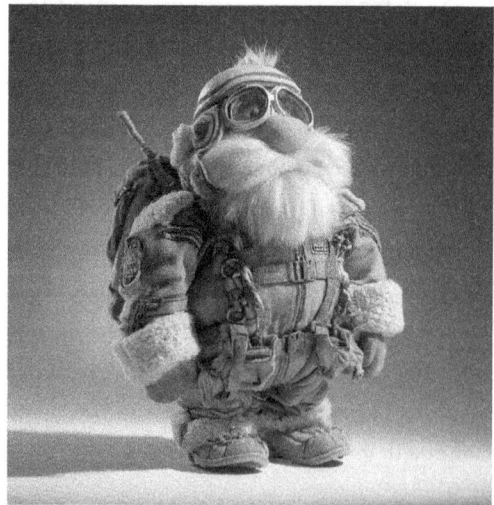

Figure 30.7: New Santa flight suit model 18.2

It might be a few years before we can fit the XFMAS-86 thrust vectoring into the v43.7 model of the sleigh, but we've had the same amount of dog fighting as the real XFMAS-86: zero. The suit was able to keep me wide awake through a superhuman amount of maneuvering that would have made Tom Cruise squeamish, and kept me alert enough to know when to turn to the next neighborhood.

5.4 Aerial Counter-Measures

While Christmas is normally a universal night of global peace, some countries do not let their guard down. While we have been able to outmaneuver anything China, Russia, or the US has sent at us since sleigh version v41.2 [23], the evasive maneuvering eats into the average TpH when intercepted. Time is presents! It's best to fool those radars. Using advanced electronic warfare capabilities, we have equipped the v43.7 with a state-of-the-art Jingle-Bell Jammer utilizing ▬▬▬ and even some ▬▬▬▬, which can even fool the ▬▬▬▬ system by exploiting its ▬▬▬▬▬▬ ▬▬▬▬▬▬ ▬▬▬▬▬▬ problem. I can't go into detail on how that works, or China, Russia, and the US will steal it all!

6. Vigor Serum

Santa doesn't just have trouble keeping awake through the high-G turns. Santa has trouble staying awake during the long stretches across the Pacific and keeping spry enough to fit through chimneys, and maintaining the dexterity to unlock people's windows with a coat hanger and a screwdriver [24]. Since the 1820s, it's been getting a lot harder to get in

and out of people's homes, especially for a 1,600-year-old man. While the vigor serum developed in [25] has been shown historically to keep me alert and agile to evade the most vicious of house pets, canine or reptilian, we can no longer source the white rhino horn.

In a new iteration of vigor serum, we have found an alternative to exponentially increase my energy levels without encouraging more poaching.

6.1 Performance Enhancements

Just as the previous v28.4 has enhanced Santa's present delivering ability, the new iteration, v29.0, was found in a sample study of N=1 Santa Clauses to increase alertness by 29%, jolliness by 12%, cheerfulness by 18%, and good will by 8.2 Teresas, according to the Kringle physics metrics developed in [26]. Santas (N=1) were additionally able to increase their sit-ups by 5+/-0, pushups by 2+/-0, flexed arm hangs by 20+/-0 seconds, and V-seat reaches by 2+/-0 inches, and decrease their shuttle run time by 0.7+/-0 seconds and their mile run time by 28.2+/-0 seconds, according to their Presidential Fitness Test results.

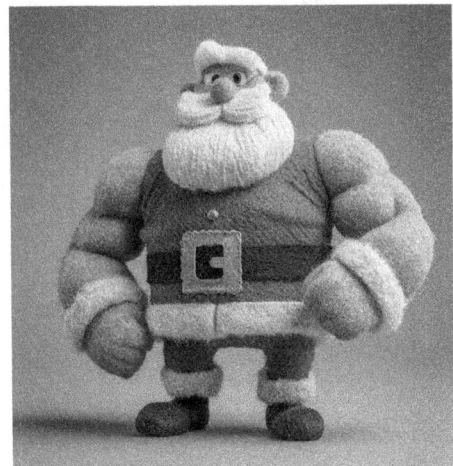

Figure 30.8: Santa after two doses of v29.0 serum

6.2 Ingredients

Other than a half gram of fentanyl-free methamphetamine and steroids, the serum v29.0 consists of 10 mg of caffeine, 28 mg of taurine, 16 mg of guarana, and 19 mg of glucuronolactone as recommended by Dr. Mittens Snowball III, M.D.

6.3 Side Effects

There's one thing that hasn't changed between v28.4 and v29.0: Santa is going to need an extreme caloric intake, which can only be satisfied by milk and cookies. According to the tests on Santa Clauses (N=1), if the subject does not intake at least 1,600 calories of highly processed sugar and a half gallon of milk every five minutes, they will go into a diabetic coma. It is advised this year for all households to prepare milk and cookies for Santa and Santa Clones or be prepared with an insulin shot if they hear a loud thud in their living room.

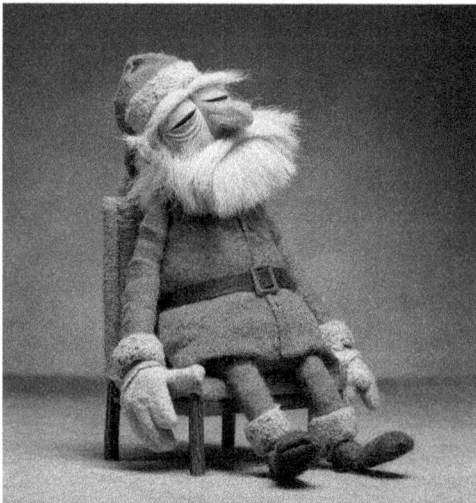

Figure 30.9: Santa passed out in a house that didn't leave milk and cookies

7. Logistics

Despite the best efforts to create an infinite wormhole bag [27], we are still stuck on vacuum packaging our presents, which is a 60-year-old technology [28]. To equip Santa with enough gifts in the right locations and warehouses, we have infiltrated the Amazon warehouse network in exchange for pushing Amazon Prime on all children through mall Santa surrogates.

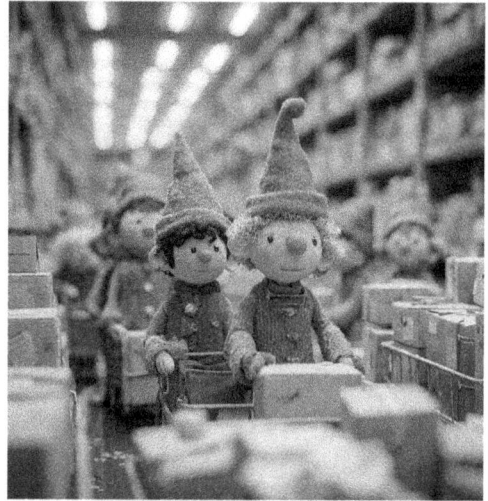

Figure 30.10: Elves staging for Christmas Eve in an Amazon warehouse

7.1 Elf Bathroom Break Monitoring

Naturally, to allow for our elves to become Amazon employees, they were required to maintain a certain quality of productivity not previously required by the elves' work contract to be eligible for full benefits. To enforce the standard, invasive monitors were used to ensure that elf bathroom and smoking breaks would never exceed five minutes without a direct note from Dr. Snowball for gastrointestinal issues. This is all okay because these monitors also applied to my own naughty-nice list checking, and are maintained by other elves, who are monitored in turn by other elves, maintaining a KGB-style circle of trust.

7.2 Elf Union Busting

When we transitioned to Amazon policies, naturally the elves were not happy. It was the only way for the elves to integrate with the normal Amazon employees, according to the contract with Jeff Bezos. After three weeks of the policies, an anarcho-communist cell, the Elves People's Republic (EPR), started to organize as a union, with even some talk to secure the means of production. While many of the elves were not old enough to remember the troubles of the labor movements in the 1870s [29], I stepped in, as seen in *Figure 30.11*, to show the elves the folly of their ways. Without centralized capital control of Christmas toy production, owned by the top 1% (me, Santa Claus), there would be no incentive to expand toy production and CHRISTMAS WOULD BE OVER!

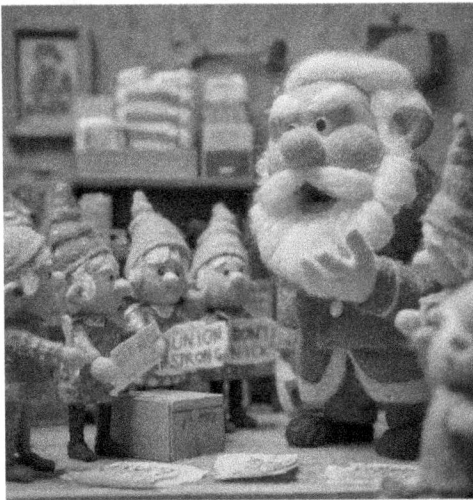

Figure 30.11: Stopping the manifesto of the EPR demands

8. Results and Discussion

As shown in *Table 30.1*, this may be the first Christmas Eve in a long time that I don't come home a shell of a man. Everything is a major upgrade, which will drastically decrease how long I'll have to work on Christmas Eve. The percentage increase in efficiencies of the clones alone will more than account for the increase in world population. The clones might make it feel like only a month or two of work instead of years like it's been for the last 200 years.

	TPH Available Decrease	TPH Required
Path optimization	1.9%	n/a
Clones	2518%	n/a
Aerial upgrades	2.8%	n/a
Vigor serum	0.3%	12.3%
Amazon logistical network	8.2%	n/a

Table 30.1: Overall upgrade expected performance

Don't get me wrong, I love what I do, but I just think if I'd had the technology we've developed with AI, modern aerial materials, and this delivery network, I might still have the same love for Christmas that I had before the 1340s when kids started asking for their parents back after the Black Death hit Europe.

While I am excited for this Christmas to be the easiest it's been since the 1700s, I am deathly afraid of what is going to happen in the battle arena. How will such a violent affair affect my jolliness? More concerning, am I going to be the one true Santa to emerge from the candy cane battle royale or will I finally taste the peace of death? For the first time since we didn't know whether we could source enough Cabbage Patch Kids to meet the demand of 1983, I am afraid of death. I don't know if I'm ready.

It's only thanks to the solace that there will be a stronger, faster, fiercer Santa Claus to protect, serve, and eat Ms. Claus's cookies after my potential death that I will gladly enter the sleigh, deliver the presents, and return with a smile into Tinsel Town Peppermint Lacrosse Arena Brought to You by Hasbro for a battle to the death. I welcome the fight. Let the best Santa win.

9. Conclusion

Assuming the clones don't go haywire and ruin 1,600 years of Christmas peace on earth in a violent uprising, and that the elves keep to their worker's contract, and my v43.8 sleigh doesn't burn up on re-entry after making the intercontinental path between oceans, this is going to be a fantastic Christmas. Last Christmas, I slept for a week and a half before I began to recover. There's no number of self-help books that can make you feel whole after 39 months of waking hours delivering presents in a gravity well on Christmas Eve Time without a break. I just can't wait for January.

References

1. Claus, Santa, Brandald Grumbwinter, et al., 2016. *Analysis of Alternatives: Risk Mitigating Options if Santa Kicks the Bucket* :: Journal of Christmas Logistics and System Engineering

2. God, Lucifer, Claus, Santa, et al., 386 AD. *Pignus Santa Clausus (Pledge of the Santa Clause)* :: Legal Contract Signed in Blood

3. Claus, Santa, Cringle O'Smoots, et al., 1984. *Optimization Metrics of Christmas Eve Delivery* :: Journal of Christmas Logistics and System Engineering

4. Claus, Santa, Cheffwilliam Ansnerberry, et al., 2017. *Localized Gravitational Relativity: How much Mass Does Santa Need to Slow Down Time* :: Annals of Theoretical Physics Applications in Toy Delivery

5. Claus, Santa, Grudolph Tinglebritches, Odovacker Speeseflake, et al., 2022. *Naughty-Nice Demographics: Annual Updates in Global Demographics Projected to December 2022* :: Journal of Christmas Demographic Studies

6. Claus, Santa, Pinçuishon Huliée-Lêgoumes, et al., 2022. *Post-Analysis of the 2022 Christmas Season* :: Journal of Christmas Demographic Studies

7. Claus, Santa, Thropwhistle Hattawacky, Halvely Minced-Tholiève, et al., 2022. *Live Weather Updates into the Christmas Eve Logistical Path Planning Engine* :: Journal of Christmas Modelling and Simulation

8. Claus, Santa, Puldrop Gumtinsel, et al., 2019. *Quantum Computing Applications in the NP-Hard Multiple-Santas Multiple-Neighborhoods Travelling Salesman Problem* :: Annals of Theoretical Physics Applications in Toy Delivery

9. Yang Shuai, Shao Ynfeng, and Zhang Kai, 2019. *An effective method for solving multiple travelling salesman problem based on NSGA-II* :: Systems Science and Control Engineering. https://www.tandfonline.com/doi/full/10.1080/21642583.2019.1674220

10. Claus, Santa, Horkins Hawludday-Hamm, et al., 2018. *Real-Time Algorithms and Computational Limits of Christmas Eve Path Planning* :: Journal of Christmas Logistics and System Engineering

11. Claus, Santa, Gregtinkle U. Burlfack, et al., 2012. *Family Location Prediction and Tracking* :: Journal of Christmas Logistics and Systems Engineering

12. Claus, Santa, Omnerflough Underchorst, et al., 2015. *Spawning and Genetics Issues in Santa Claus Cloning* :: North Pole Journal of Experimental Biology

13. Claus, Santa, Fedwinneagh West-Sprinkle, et al., 1974. *On the Body and Mind of Santa Claus* :: Christmas Principals

14. Spinoza, Baruch, 1675. *A Metaphysical Treatise on the Essence of Santa Claus* :: Christmas Principals

15. Coca-Cola Company Memo, 1931. *Santa Claus Lore to Maximize Coke Sales* :: Christmas Principals

16. Claus, Santa, Fedwinneagh East-Sprinkle, et al., 2019. *Santa Sleigh Upgrade v43.5: Additions in Fuel Capacity When the Spirit of Christmas Wanes* :: Journal of Christmas Aeronautical Engineering

17. Claus, Santa, Oddwun Tuppick, et al., 2014. *Upgrade v43.0: System Requirements Design of Analysis for the Joint Strike Toy Delivery Sled* :: Journal of Christmas Aeronautical Engineering

18. Claus, Santa, Mambs Majorbongtingle, et al., 2020. *Upgrade v43.6: Auto Ground Collision Avoidance System* :: Journal of Christmas Aeronautical Engineering

19. Claus, Santa, Vinstramp Pootshanks, et al., 2021. *Upgrade v43.5: Super Sonic Bird Strike Reliability Testing* :: Journal of Christmas Aeronautical Engineering

20. Claus, Santa, 1876. *An Ode to the Simpler Times, So Long Christmas' o' Old* :: A Collection of Christmas Poetry

21. Claus, Santa, Chuckerbutty Relishard, et al., 2018. *Psychological Profile of an Irked Ms. Claus* :: Journal of Claus Family Psychology

22. Claus, Santa, Edwurg The Conquerous, et al., 2016. *Upgrade v43.2: Integrated Aerial Counter Measures Sled Defense against 5th Gen Fighters* :: Journal of Christmas Aeronautical Engineering

23. Claus, Santa, Chames H. Oderuntertoes, et al., 1998. *Novel Techniques for Bypassing Home Security Systems* :: Journal of Christmas Breaking and Entering

24. Claus, Santa, Dinwoop Busterchorts, et al., 1976. *Energy and Strength Enhancing Medicinal Kale Shakes for a Santa on the Go* :: North Pole Journal of Experimental Biology

25. Claus, Santa, Idwallium Cheesecraft, et al., 1988. *Santa-Metrics, and Optimum Physical Fitness Pre-Christmas Eve* :: North Pole Journal of Experimental Biology

26. Claus, Santa, Aliquot Nazardtree, et al., 2018. *The Infinite Worm Hole Presents Bag: Not just a flawed concept but a recipy for global destruction* :: Annals of Theoretical Physics Applications in Toy Deliver

27. Claus, Santa, Mintquervy Ypsilanti-Jomes, et al., 1956. *Vacuum Sealed Bags and The Exciting World of Plastics* :: Journal of Christmas Technology of the Future

28. Claus, Santa, Guff Everhard Kliptickett, et al., 1964. *Elf History in the Age of Industrial Revolution* :: 8th Grade Elf History Text Book to keep the workers in line

Appendix A: Naughty-Nice List Criteria Expansion

As shown in the following tables, new criteria have been added or adjusted, which affect the overall Christmas point total score.

	Negative NN points
Getting a tattoo	-28
Participating in an argument on social media	-63
Using proper punctuation when texting a teenager and giving them anxiety	-6
Questioning Santa Claus's simultaneous divinity and humanity	-18
Not giving a thank you wave or half jogging when crossing the street while a car is waiting for you	-14
Posting an article online without reading it	-32
Singing Disney songs at karaoke (with the exception of *I'll Make a Man Out of You*)	-2

Table A1: Anti-social behavior

	Positive NN points
Telling someone not to forget the true meaning of Christmas	+19
Looking a supermarket bell ringer in the eye	+27
Turning your front yard into a daily light show	+24
Wearing a fun holiday sweater even if it barely fits	+8
Putting fuzzy antlers on a stranger's dog	+30
Putting extra rum in the eggnog	+14
Turning up the volume on robotic dancing Santa Clauses	+6

Table A2: Pro-Christmas Spirit behavior

	Positive NN points
Calling your mother	+8
Using a Ukrainian flag filter	+12
Attending a local city council meeting	+20
Liking our Facebook page: `https://www.facebook.com/TheRealJABDE`	+763
Following us on Twitter `@JABDE6`	+655
Joining our Subreddit: `https://www.reddit.com/r/ImmaterialScience/`	+923
Leaving a review for this book on Amazon or Goodreads	+infinity

Table A3: Pro-social behavior

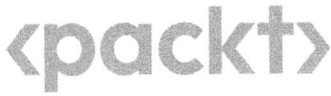

‹packt›

packtpub.com

Subscribe to our online digital library for full access to over 7,000 books and videos, as well as industry leading tools to help you plan your personal development and advance your career. For more information, please visit our website.

Why subscribe?

- Spend less time learning and more time coding with practical eBooks and Videos from over 4,000 industry professionals
- Improve your learning with Skill Plans built especially for you
- Get a free eBook or video every month
- Fully searchable for easy access to vital information
- Copy and paste, print, and bookmark content

At www.packtpub.com, you can also read a collection of free technical articles, sign up for a range of free newsletters, and receive exclusive discounts and offers on Packt books and eBooks.

Another Book You May Enjoy

If you enjoyed this book, you may be interested in this other book by Packt:

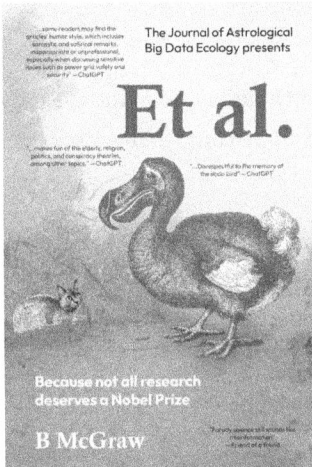

Et al

B McGraw

ISBN: 978-1-83763-257-2

- How to draw a graph using MS Paint, maybe
- Whether Sarah Palin is a figment of your imagination
- How one pirate cat brought about the extinction of the beloved dodo
- Why rabbits used to be jerks back in the day
- If you actually learn anything from these articles, get your memory erased immediately

Packt is searching for authors like you

If you're interested in becoming an author for Packt, please visit `authors.packtpub.com` and apply today. We have worked with thousands of developers and tech professionals, just like you, to help them share their insight with the global tech community. You can make a general application, apply for a specific hot topic that we are recruiting an author for, or submit your own idea.

Share your thoughts

Now you've finished *How to Prove Anything*, we'd love to hear your thoughts! Scan the QR code below to go straight to the Amazon review page for this book and share your feedback or leave a review on the site that you purchased it from.

`https://packt.link/r/1806118939`

Your review is important to us and the tech community and will help us make sure we're delivering excellent quality content.

Index

Y